Play Therapy Supervision

Play therapy is one of the fastest-growing specialty areas in mental health. Understanding the skills, knowledge, and strategies that make play therapy supervision effective is essential in supporting the integrity and needs of a thriving field.

Play Therapy Supervision: A Practical Guide to Models and Best Practices is an all-encompassing play therapy supervision compendium. In these pages, current and prospective play therapy professionals and supervisors will find effective strategies for engaging in supervision, with literature that is firmly rooted in empirical research, and practical examples. Useful for novice and experienced supervisors, this book describes best practices in supervision and contemporary topics for building an effective play therapy supervision practice. This text also emphasizes the critical importance of cultural humility in play therapy supervision. Other important features include:

- Ethical and legal issues in play therapy supervision
- Building a play therapy supervision relationship
- Evaluation in play therapy supervision
- Technology in play therapy supervision, including extended reality
- School-based play therapy supervision
- Techniques in play therapy supervision: mindfulness, sand tray, self-compassion, art and movement, and more!

Staci L. Born, EdD, LMFT, RPT-S, is an associate professor of counseling in the School of Education, Counseling, and Human Development at South Dakota State University.

Casey E. Baker, EdD, LMHC, RPT-S, is core faculty in the School of Social and Behavioral Sciences at Capella University.

Play Therapy Supervision

A Practical Guide to Models and Best Practices

Edited by Staci L. Born and Casey E. Baker

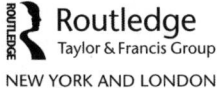

Routledge
Taylor & Francis Group

NEW YORK AND LONDON

Cover image: Getty Images

First published 2023
by Routledge
605 Third Avenue, New York, NY 10158

and by Routledge
4 Park Square, Milton Park, Abingdon, Oxon, OX14 4RN

Routledge is an imprint of the Taylor & Francis Group, an informa business

Library of Congress Cataloging-in-Publication Data
Names: Born, Staci L., editor. | Baker, Casey E., editor.
Title: Play therapy supervision: a practical guide to models and best practices/edited by Staci Born and Casey Baker.
Description: First Edition. | New York, NY: Routledge, 2023. | Includes bibliographical references and index.
Identifiers: LCCN 2022025875 (print) | LCCN 2022025876 (ebook) |
ISBN 9781032050478 (Hardback) | ISBN 9781032050461 (Paperback) |
ISBN 9781003196075 (eBook)
Subjects: LCSH: Play therapy–Methodology. | Psychotherapists–Supervision of.
Classification: LCC RJ505.P6 P5465 2023 (print) | LCC RJ505.P6 (ebook) |
DDC 618.92/891653–dc23/eng/20220716
LC record available at https://lccn.loc.gov/2022025875
LC ebook record available at https://lccn.loc.gov/2022025876

ISBN: 9781032050478 (hbk)
ISBN: 9781032050461 (pbk)
ISBN: 9781003196075 (ebk)

DOI: 10.4324/9781003196075

Typeset in Baskerville
by Deanta Global Publishing Services, Chennai, India

Contents

Contributing Authors and Affiliations

Casey E. Baker, EdD, LMHC, RPT-S
Capella University

Kenya G. Bledsoe, PhD, LPC-S, NCC, NCSC
The University of Mississippi

Staci L. Born, EdD, LMFT, RPT-S
South Dakota State University, Brookings, South Dakota

Crystal A. Brashear, PhD, LPC
Colorado Christian University, Lakewood, Colorado

Rebekah Byrd, PhD, LPC, LCMHC, NCC, RPT-S
Sacred Heart University

Janet A. Courtney, PhD, LCSW, RPT-S
Developmental Play & Attachment Therapies, Palm Beach Gardens, Florida

LaTrice L. Dowtin, PhD, LCPC, NCSP, RPT
PlayfulLeigh Psyched, LLC
Gallaudet University
School of Human Services & Sciences
Deaf and Hard of hearing Infants, Toddlers, and their Families Graduate Program

Emily Gislason, LhD, LPC-MH, RPT-S, QMHP, NCC
South Dakota State University, Brookings, South Dakota
Sprout Play Therapy and Counseling Services, Sioux Falls, South Dakota

Kenisha W. Gordon, PhD, NCC, LPC-S, ACS, RPT-S
Mississippi College, Department of Counseling

Charlotte Heckmann
South Dakota State University, Brookings, South Dakota

Donna Hickman, PhD, LPC, CSC
Texas A&M University-Commerce, Commerce, Texas

Edward (Franc) Hudspeth, PhD, LPC-S, NCC, ACS, RPT-S, RPh
Sacred Heart University

Carrie Longest, PhD, LMHC, NCC, ACS, RPT-S
Healing with Play

Rebecca Mathews, PhD, LPC-S, LCHMC
University of North Carolina Greensboro, Greensboro, North Carolina

Lynn O'Brien, EdD, LPC, NCC
Capella University

Yumiko Ogawa, PhD, LPC, ACS, RPT-S
New Jersey City University

Michelle M. Pliske, DSW, LCSW, RPT-S
Pacific University Oregon

Corie Schoeneberg, PhD, LPC, RPT-S, NCC
Play Therapy Training Institute, University of Central Missouri

Sarah D. Stauffer, PhD, LPC, NCC, NCSC, RPT-S
Association ESPAS (Espace de Soutien et de Prévention - Abus Sexuels)
Private Practice

Jessica Stone, PhD, RPT-S
CEO Virtual Sandtray, LLC
East Carolina University, College of Education Neurocognition Science
Laboratory Affiliate

Nancy Thomas, PhD, LPC
Colorado Christian University, Lakewood, Colorado

Naomi Timm-Davis, PhD, LMFT
South Dakota State University, Brookings, SD

Renee Turner, PhD, LPC-S, RPT-S
Expressive Therapies Institute, San Antonio, Texas

Amanda Winburn, PhD, LPC, RPT, NCC, NCSC
The University of Mississippi

Section 1
The Foundation

1 History and Overview of Play Therapy Supervision

Casey Baker

History and Overview of Play Therapy Supervision

At some point in a mental health professional's career, an opportunity to supervise will likely be available. It may involve overseeing an internship student, newly graduated, or even a fully licensed clinician who wants to further their expertise in play therapy. As supervisors, we can influence the future of our field by providing quality guidance to our more junior colleagues (Bernard & Goodyear, 2019). Guidance is vital in building the quality of play therapists and supervisors in the field.

The concept of using play therapeutically has been around since the inception of psychotherapy, with the founders identifying using play therapeutically in the 1921 article describing the benefits of play by Hermione von Hug-Hellmuth. She has been identified as the first practicing child psychoanalyst and advocated for continued research on the use of play in treatment (D'Angelo & Koocher, 2011; Plastow, 2011). The need to distinguish the professional identity of play therapy brought together the leaders in the field to develop a strong foundation for the field (Seymour, 2015).

In 1982, the Association for Play Therapy (APT) made its appearance as a professional organization and built momentum to make play therapy a creditable and visible approach to the treatment of children. Next, the *International Journal of Play Therapy* provides clinicians with current research and education (Seymour, 2015). This step further pushed play therapy's acceptance as a viable treatment approach.

The next step in distinguishing the profession from others was the development of the Registered Play Therapist™ (RPT™) and Registered Play Therapist-Supervisor™ (RPT-S™) in 1993. Establishing a required credential pushed the field to recognize play therapy as a specialized treatment approach for children and families (Turner et al., 2020). The initial development of both the RPT™ and RPT-S™ credentials demonstrated the value placed on clinical supervision. APT has consistently demonstrated its continuous improvement efforts regarding education and supervisory requirements.

DOI: 10.4324/9781003196075-2

Continuous Improvement: Education

Clinical supervision is a fundamental aspect of the helping field requiring many years of practice and educational training. A supervisor's development begins during their clinical training and is enhanced through continued education, experience, and engagement in professional activities (Bernard & Goodyear, 2019; Donald et al., 2015; Gardner, 2002). Early on in developing the RPT™ and RPT-S™ credentialing, Phillips and Landreth (1995, 1998) found that professionals practicing play therapy identified minimal graduate-level educational training, with little training on child development. This led to recommendations for more graduate-level clinical training to increase the need for play therapy–specific supervision (Seymour, 2015). Although there was this recommendation, APT members continued to identify a lack of graduate-level training and better supervision practices as an area of increased need (Ryan et al., 2002).

Efforts to improve members' academic knowledge were not futile. In 2004 an online professional development opportunity, the Leadership Academy, provided members with the experience to develop the high-quality skill to continue the development of APT (APT, 2022b). Additionally, written work, including a quarterly magazine, *Play Therapy*, and *The International Journal of Play Therapy*, created a vehicle to give clinicians widespread access to research, current trends, and best practices in play therapy (APT, n.d).

Further, APT has set standards for universities, organizations, and individuals providing graduate-level education. As of March 2022, 156 universities are offering graduate-level play therapy courses. To gain a higher standard of programming, a university can apply to become an Approved Center of Play Therapy Education. There are currently 30 Approved Centers of Play Therapy Education (APT, n.d). For those gaining play therapy instruction through continuing education (CE), APT developed the Approved Provider Program. This program provides the field with the peace of mind that clinicians gain quality training. There are 285 approved CE providers documented on the APT's website (APT, n.d.).

APT has continued to improve their educational requirements and have made recent changes relating to diversity, equity, and inclusion (DE&I) with the development of the APT's Inclusion, Diversity, and Equity Awareness Team (IDEA Team) (APT, n.d). In similar historical patterns, members of the IDEA team have surveyed members to get a sense of the DE&I needs for APT members, with results being put into action. Effective January 1, 2023, applicants must complete a graduate-level course in cultural and social diversity, at least six hours of play therapy specific cultural and social diversity topics, and required cultural and social diversity continuing education (APT, 2022a). This level of program evaluation and commitment to improving the education process continues to push the association forward.

Continuous Improvement: Supervision

Although many efforts were made to improve the quality of graduate and continuing education, supervisory standards continued to be lacking. Supervisors are the gatekeepers to the field, ensuring mental health professionals are qualified, ethical, and competent in their expertise. (Bernard & Goodyear, 2019). Prior to 2020, those training to become play therapists were not required to have a clinical supervisor with expertise or training in play therapy supervision to sign off on their clinical experience. This led to many concerns related to the credibility and rigor of the play therapy profession (APT, 2021; Turner et al., 2020). A significant change in credentialing came in 2020, where the requirement for those pursuing their registered play therapy credential is to have clinical supervision from a registered play therapist supervisor (APT, 2021). This move has been essential in building quality and consistency in the training and supervision of RPTs™.

Although there is a requirement for RPT-S™ status, there is still a lack of uniformity across the various disciplines' foundational clinical training, licensure, and supervision education (Falender, 2018). The lack of uniformity or consistent standards across mental health disciplines makes it difficult to identify a baseline knowledge that a mental health professional may gain from their education and professional training. Being an effective supervisor takes a significant amount of time and commitment. The role of clinical supervisor can grow out of desire or as a necessity to assist others in gaining their full licensure. Thus, not everyone has the passion, time, or desire to engage in ongoing personal or professional development. Simply relying on someone's internal drive to practice adequate supervision is insufficient. Hence, the importance of guidelines, licensure requirements, and national standards to ensure the quality of providers in the field.

Becoming an RPT-S™ begins with completing the three-phased RPT™ credentialing standards, once the RPT™ has practiced for a minimum of three consecutive years where they continue to practice play therapy, obtain a state supervisory status, and continue education. Since every state and licensure will vary in their educational and training expectation to gain supervisory status, play therapists must continue to review the requirements of their state and professional board standards.

The Foundational Guide

Having the foundational knowledge all in one book will allow supervisors to ensure they provide the best-quality supervision to their supervisees. This book pulls together the main components of supervision in a simple, hands-on, and effective way. We want this book to be something that you can go back and reflect upon throughout your career. We offer a balance of both educational and practical tools to scaffold concepts for easier digestion and application. This book is broken down into four sections: the foundation, the process, special topics, and playful strategies.

Although you may have the urge to skip right to the play-based strategies, I advise you to start at the beginning. Section 1 will assist you in gaining the foundational information regarding play therapy supervision. First, you will gain the awareness and understanding of social justice and cultural humility in supervision (Chapter 2). Supervisors inherently hold more power in the supervisory relationship (Bernard & Goodyear, 2019; Hair & O'Donoghue, 2009). While being aware and leaning into discomfort, the supervisory environment can allow supervisors and supervisees to explore their privilege, race, culture, and identities (Gardner, 2002; Mosher et al., 2017). Demonstrating humility by intentionally broaching this in supervision can promote an intellectually engaging supervisory environment where both the supervisor and supervisee continue to work on their self-reflective skills (Watkins et al., 2019). This will be your lens through which to see this entire book, and, admittedly, we hope this will be a continued lens you use in your work with supervisees and beyond.

Further, you will gain an experientially based overview of the supervisory models and best practices in play therapy supervision. Models of supervision assist clinical supervisors with theory to facilitate effective supervision (Borders & Brown, 2005). Historically, the literature on theory integration in play therapy supervision lacks models of play therapy supervision derived out of traditional clinical supervision models with elements of play therapy filtered throughout (Donald et al., 2015; Hudspeth, 2015). With the recent changes in RPT™ credentialing requirements, it is the hope that research will begin to blossom in this area as many identify that traditional supervision models are lacking in the supervision of play therapists (Donald et al., 2015; Hudspeth, 2015; Thomas, 2015). This book offers engaging case studies to gain a more hands-on experience of applying models and best practices. The cultural humility lens, models of supervision, and best practices set the stage for the next layer of supervision – the process. Play therapy supervision begins by understanding the supervisory relationship, the function of the supervisor, and the most effective ways to provide this specialized supervision (Chapters 5 to 7).

Play therapy is a widely accepted form of treatment for children. There is guidance for the education, training, and even competencies related to becoming a play therapist (O'Connor et al., 2016). However, it is likely unclear *how* a supervisor goes about evaluating, remediation, and working through issues in the supervision. Chapters 8 to 9 guide you through these essential areas that can be difficult to navigate.

As play therapists, we enjoy learning more and being creative. The last two sections of the book cover a wide variety of special topics and techniques used in play therapy supervision. It is an exciting time in the play therapy supervision field as there are endless opportunities for continued growth and research. Section 3 touches on some crucial developments in play therapy supervision, including technology (Chapter 9), school-based play therapy supervision (Chapter 10), and the use of touch (Chapter 11).

Play therapy techniques used in supervision make up the majority of the literature (Donald et al., 2015). Some of the ways supervisors are utilizing strategies in their work with supervisees include the use of the sand tray (Chapter 12), self-compassion skills (Chapter 13), mindfulness-based techniques (Chapter 14), art and movement (Chapter 15), and extended reality (Chapter 16). We hope you take what you need from this book, give yourself some grace, and know that you are doing good work with your supervisees – happy reading and playing.

References

Association for Play Therapy. (n.d.). *Education and training, association for play therapy*. https://www.a4pt.org/page/CredentialsInfo

Association for Play Therapy. (2021). Credentialing guide: Registered play therapist (RPT) and supervisor (RPT-S). https://cdn.ymaws.com/www.a4pt.org/resource/resmgr/credentials/2021_credentials/rpt_standards_2021_version.pdf

Association for Play Therapy. (2022a). Credentialing standards-summary of program changes. https://cdn.ymaws.com/www.a4pt.org/resource/resmgr/credentials/summary_of_program_changes.pdf

Association for Play Therapy. (2022b). Fact sheet-2022 class leadership academy. https://cdn.ymaws.com/www.a4pt.org/resource/resmgr/leadership_academy/APT_Leadership_Academy_Fact_.pdfq

Bernard, J. M., & Goodyear, R. K. (2019). *Fundamentals of clinical supervision* (6th ed.). Pearson.

Borders, L. D., & Brown, L. L. (2005). *The new handbook of counseling supervision*. Lahaska Press.

D'Angelo, E. J., & Koocher, G. P. (2011). Children. In J. C. Norcross, G. R. VandenBos, & D. K. Freedheim (Eds.), *History of psychotherapy: Continuity and change* (pp. 439–448). American Psychological Association. https://doi.org/10.1037/12353-024

Donald, E. J., Culbreth, J. R., & Carter, A. W. (2015). Play therapy supervision: A review of the literature. *International Journal of Play Therapy*, *24*(2), 59–77. https://doi.org/10.1037/a0039104

Falender, C. A. (2018). Clinical supervision—The missing ingredient. *American Psychologist*, *73*(9), 1240–1250.

Gardner, R. M. D. (2002). Cross-cultural perspectives in supervision. *Western Journal of Black Studies*, *26*(2), 98–106.

Hair, H. J., & O'Donoghue, K. (2009). Culturally relevant, socially just social work supervision: Becoming visible through a social constructionist lens. *Journal of Ethnic and Cultural Diversity in Social Work*, *18*(1–2), 70–88. https://doi.org/10.1080/15313200902874979

Hudspeth, E. F. (2015). Clinical supervision in play therapy: Research, practice, and application. *International Journal of Play Therapy*, *24*(2), 55–58. https://doi.org/10.1037/pla0000011

Mosher, D. K., Hook, J. N., Farrell, J. E., Watkins, C. E., Jr., & Davis, D. E. (2017). Cultural humility. In E. L. Worthington Jr., D. E. Davis, & J. N. Hook (Eds.), *Handbook of humility: Theory, research, and application* (pp. 91–104). Routledge/Taylor & Francis Group.

O'Connor, K. J., Schaefer, C. E., & Braverman, L. D. (2016). *Handbook of play therapy* (2nd ed.). Wiley.

Phillips, R. D., & Landreth, G. L. (1995). Play therapists on play therapy: I. A report of methods, demographics, and professional practices. *International Journal of Play Therapy*, *4*(1), 1–26.

Phillips, R. D., & Landreth, G. L. (1998). Play therapists on play therapy: II. Clinical issues in play therapy. *International Journal of Play Therapy*, *6*(1), 1–24.

Plastow, M. (2011). Hermine Hug-Hellmuth, the first child psychoanalyst: Legacy and dilemmas. *Australasian Psychiatry*, *19*(3), 206–210.

Ryan, S. D., Gomory, T., & Lacasse, J. R. (2002). Who are we? Examining the results of the association for play therapy membership survey. *International Journal of Play Therapy*, *11*(2), 11.

Seymour, J. (2015). An introduction to the field of play therapy. In K. J. O'Conner, C. E. Schaefer, & L. D. Braverman (Eds.), *Handbook of play therapy* (2nd ed., pp. 3–15). https://doi.org/10.1002/9871119140467.ch1

Turner, R., Schoeneberg, C., Ray, D., & Lin, Y. (2020). Establishing play therapy competencies: A Delphi study. *International Journal of Play Therapy*, *29*(4), 177–190. https://doi.org/10.1037/pla0000138

Watkins, C. E., Hook, J. N., Mosher, D. K., & Callahan, J. L. (2019). Humility in clinical supervision: Fundamental, foundational, and transformational. *Clinical Supervisor*, *38*(1), 58–78. https://doi.org/10.1080/07325223.2018.1487355

2 Cultural Humility and Social Justice in Play Therapy Supervision

LaTrice L. Dowtin

Cultural Humility and Social Justice in Play Therapy Supervision

Supervision is considered a vital part of mental health training, so much so that all mental health fields and specialties, including play therapy, require hundreds of hours of clinical supervision (Donald et al., 2015; Gardner, 2002). In that light, play therapy supervisors are responsible for providing a conducive environment for supervisees to gain and practice play therapy skills designed to help clients without harming them. Environments that are conducive for learning are what we call *safe*. Play therapy supervisors want to help supervisees feel safe to explore the challenges of learning new techniques, safe to make mistakes, admit those mistakes, and ask for help, safe to enjoy the successes that the supervisee and their clients experience as a result of attunement in play therapy, and safe to grow as a clinician. Similar to the therapist–client relationship, that sense of safety is not automatic and cannot be assumed to exist at the outset of supervision. In fact, much like the ongoing fluidity of rapport within relationships, safety in supervision needs continual attention and nurturing care throughout the supervisory relationship. Safety needs humility.

The play therapy supervisor must consider their humility and try to maintain it while in a supervisory role because the dynamic between supervisor and supervisee has intersecting layers of hierarchy and privilege. Systems of power are inherent in hierarchy, which directly impact the interactions between supervisor and supervisee (Bernard & Goodyear, 2014). Often in play therapy, supervisors are much more knowledgeable than the supervisee, and they hold seniority and responsibility under licensing and certification standards. When the supervisee is a graduate student, the supervisor may also serve as a thesis advisor or clinical faculty who determines whether or not the student will complete the program, earn a degree, and eventually have a career in this field. The reality of this power tends to leave the student dependent on the supervisor's clinical and ethical awareness. When the student or supervisee is also from a marginalized background, such as race or any areas of sociodemographic culture or identity (e.g., gender, sexual orientation, religion, ability, etc.), the student may experience an added layer or layers at the intersection (Crenshaw, 1989) of their identities. To facilitate the growth

DOI: 10.4324/9781003196075-3

and development of play therapy skills, supervisors must understand their own race, identities, and cultures, which is a necessary component of cultural humility in clinical practice (Mosher et al., 2017). A goal of supervision is to provide supervisees with the space to discuss topics that may come up for themselves and their clients in the learning process. For this to be authentically facilitated, supervisees and students need to feel emotionally safe to explore relevant topics and feel comfortable asking their supervisor whether a topic would be relevant to discuss.

From a social justice in mental health supervision framework, supervision has the potential to explore power dynamics in the supervisory relationship, allow for increased self-reflection for both supervisor and supervisee, and nurture supervisees' clinical advocacy skills that support the needs of clients. In previous literature, this area was called *cross-cultural supervision*. As researchers begin to expand the collective understanding of this concept, the language is shifting toward creating supervisory relationships that explore humility, equity, justice, and deconstruction of mental health supervision to move forward in safer ways for supervisees and their clients. This chapter has three main goals: (1) to provide the foundation for play therapy supervisors to discover and then evaluate their implicit and explicit values and beliefs, (2) to challenge current play therapy supervisors and play therapy supervisors-in-training to think about how their beliefs can influence their interactions with supervisees, and (3) to assist play therapy supervisors in gaining critical skills related to culture and justice to be used in their ongoing and future supervisory relationships.

History and Literature

Play therapy is for children and adults from a wide variety of backgrounds, which has helped people around the globe. However, all of the noted founding play therapy researchers and field experts are White cisgender people. Play therapists who notice the backgrounds of cited authors or who read researcher biographies may more easily recognize the racial disparities within play therapy teachings even though it is not readily discussed in play therapy training, workshops, or graduate courses. Moreover, it is rarely mentioned that underpinnings of the most current and popular play therapy theories did not originate from researchers or theorists from racially marginalized groups. While this omission of fact may be unintentional in the field or a result of *colorblind thinking* (Burkard et al., 2016; Neville et al., 2013), the fact that the most frequently cited and discussed play therapists over the past century are White gives the illusion that White people's theories and findings in this field are the most reputable. As a result, supervisees are encouraged to defer to them. It also ignores the systemic reasons why minoritized peoples did not have the opportunities to develop theories or how their theories were suppressed when they did create them. Creating this deference to White cisgender people is likely one of several contributing factors to why play therapy predominantly consists of White play therapists and supervisors. This deference also permeates the play therapy supervisory relationship and adds an implicit layer of discomfort when it comes to discussing race or culture in play therapy supervision. When supervisors and supervisees are from different racial or cultural backgrounds, they may clumsily navigate topics of race and culture or perhaps more commonly, fail to mention it at all.

Historically, cross-cultural supervision has been used to describe supervision that occurs when the supervisee and supervisor do not share the same primary culture. For example, in cases where the supervisee's primary cultural identity aligns with their race, such as someone who identifies as both a culturally and racially Black person and the supervisor does not share that cultural identity, those individuals would be in a cross-cultural supervisory relationship. This term has been found in literature discussing *cultural competence*, which is becoming an outdated term and way of thinking about ongoing learning in culture (Hair & O'Donoghue, 2009). Cross-cultural supervision is also often used in proximity with the word *multicultural*. According to Dollarhide et al. (2021), multicultural counseling is the "awareness of the impact of culture and context on clients" (p. 104). While these terms have helped clinicians and supervisors think about the races and cultures of clients in their work, they all fall short in fully infiltrating the play therapy supervision space. As the field grows and breathes new waves of understanding into learning and supervision, the language used in the field must naturally evolve.

Play therapy supervision needs to include more than discussions of race and culture across cultures. Currently, some practitioners maintain false beliefs of competence when working with other cultures. Contrary to the practice of focusing on cultural awareness, simply being aware of society's impact on individuals and groups due to their perceived or identified cultural membership is not enough to support clients' or supervisees' needs (Asakura & Maurer, 2018; Dollarhide et al., 2021). Therefore, instead of landing on cross-cultural supervision as the structural point, it is proposed that all of these things may be accomplished by framing play therapy supervision in the practice of cultural humility, understanding of equity, and actions of social justice.

Culture in Play Therapy Supervision

One of the most difficult types of conversations in play therapy training is conversations around race and culture (Burkhard et al., 2016; Schen & Greenlee, 2018). Research suggests that many supervisors feel uncomfortable talking about their feelings and beliefs about race when supervising others, which can cause harm to supervisees from culturally and racially marginalized backgrounds (Tummala-Narra, 2004). Some supervisors do not think that conversations about race are necessary to provide ethical supervision, and many supervisees struggle to broach this subject with their supervisors and sometimes with their clients (Burkard et al., 2016; Neville et al., 2013). While this phenomenon is not exclusive to race and often includes many sociodemographic and cultural identities, race is occasionally used here as a framework for understanding humility.

Humility in Play Therapy Supervision

While the concept of cultural humility does not have one unified definition in the literature, there are common threads that exist (Upshaw et al., 2019). In this chapter, cultural humility is defined using an amalgamation of definitions to create a fluid or expansive understanding. There are three main components defining cultural humility, starting with one's ability to self-reflect on and critically analyze one's own culture and cultural beliefs (Mosher et al., 2017; Upshaw et al., 2019). Cultural humility is also being open to the ongoing learning of other cultures, as well as holding the conscious understanding that there will always be areas one does not and cannot know about a culture that differs from their own. The final part of cultural humility is having high regard for the feelings, experiences, and beliefs of other people, while addressing imbalances of power that exist within interpersonal relationships (e.g., supervision; Mosher et al., 2017; Upshaw et al., 2019). In other words, cultural humility in play therapy supervision removes the unconscious and automatic deference to the supervisor to allow the supervisee to be the expert in their own experience.

Building Cultural Humility

The supervisor's ability to engage in metacognitive deconstruction of their ideas is at the forefront of building cultural humility. As mentioned previously, self-reflection and analysis are required at the early stages of play therapy supervisor development. Therefore, it is recommended that a play therapy supervisor or supervisor-in-training begin by asking themselves a series of questions designed to identify some of their professional and personal values related to play therapy supervision, explore their explicit beliefs, and go on an internal journey to illuminate implicit beliefs. Veach et al. (2012) identified seven areas of supervisor values that can arise as conflicts in the supervisor–supervisee relationship: (1) worldview differences, (2) power differentials, (3) managing disputes, (4) clinical versus administrative roles, (5) individual differences, (6) threatened professional standards, and (7) reconciling supervisee and client welfare. These seven areas of values conflicts can be applied to any specialty mental health field or intervention, such as play therapy, and thus are used here as a guide to inform the development of self-reflective questions. Table 2.1 contains recommended self-reflective questions and statements for play therapy supervisors and supervisors-in-training using the seven categories of supervisor values. Journaling is helpful for those looking to identify and unpack their beliefs and values (Dollarhide et al., 2019). Supervisors may want to use these questions as journaling prompts. These reflective questions and statements may also be helpful to discuss with others during supervisor training, ongoing supervision of supervisors groups, or in peer supervision/consultation encounters.

Working to discuss and prioritize one's values makes way for the exploration of *explicit beliefs*. In this context, the phrase explicit beliefs identifies the beliefs that a play therapy supervisor or supervisor-in-training holds in their conscious awareness. The supervisor can easily report that they believe a specific thing to be true. For example, when exploring beliefs of gender, a supervisor may know that they believe that there are only two genders. It is important to note that there is no inherent qualitative value placed on explicit beliefs; having an explicit belief is neither good

Table 2.1 Unpacking Play Therapy Supervisor Values

Values Conflict Category	Self-Reflective Questions and Statements
Worldview differences	To me (insert sociocultural identity or topic) is _____. Race Culture Sex (e.g., Intersex, Female, Male, etc.) Disability Sexual Orientation Gender Religion Nationality Citizenship Language (e.g., English, American Sign Language, etc.) Low income Abortion Love styles (e.g., monogamy, polyamory, etc.)
Power differentials	Which of my identities are the most salient to me? Of my identities, what factors determine whether I am in a position of power? If I use self-disclosure in play therapy or supervision, what is my barometer for determining if it is the right timing to do so or a comfortable thing for me to disclose? In the past, how have I responded to my own regrets in my work? What does authority mean to me? What does authority look like to me?
Managing disputes	When I encounter clinical dilemmas in play therapy, what tends to be the first thing that I do to work through them? How am I with situations that are neither right nor wrong, but rather in a gray area? In what ways does my work as an RPT-S™ conflict with one or more of my identities? What am I doing to help myself reconcile those felt conflicts?
Clinical versus administrative roles	When I think about being a play therapy supervisor, which role (clinical vs. administrative) comes to mind first? In the past, how have I responded to my own regrets in my clinical and administrative roles?
Individual differences	In what ways has my own experience as a supervisee in play therapy supervision shaped my beliefs and behaviors regarding supervising other supervisees? What seemed to be the values of my favorite supervisor(s)? What seemed to be the values of my least favorite supervisor(s)? What are the values that I would like to live by in my life compared to what values I am following in my life? What personal values do I have that could directly impact my beliefs and actions as an RPT-S™? In what ways do my personal values intersect or interact with my professional values?

(Continued)

Table 2.1 Continued

Values Conflict Category	Self-Reflective Questions and Statements
Threatened professional standards	What values does the field(s) of my professional identity have? Which of their values seem to be the most important as evidenced by field discussions, literature, course trainings, etc.? How does the field's prioritized values align with my own?
Reconciling supervisee and client welfare	In the triadic relationship of client–therapist–supervisor, do I have a hierarchy of needs, and if so, how do I tend to rank them? What feelings come up for me when I think about shifting that framework?

nor bad. Therefore, the supervisor is not saying whether believing that gender is binary is a good belief to have; that part can come later. Next, the supervisor can then outline some of their explicit beliefs and see how they map onto their previously identified values from Table 2.1. For example, if during the values activity the supervisor identified a worldview perspective that states gender is important for clients and supervisees, and they expressed that they believe gender is binary, they have formulated that they value gender conceptualization for those who identify as a girl, boy, woman, or man. At this stage, the supervisor would leave space to process feelings around supporting the needs of play therapy supervisees who have a different belief regarding gender (e.g., gender fluidity beliefs versus binary gender beliefs), even if they hold the same value that states gender is important in play therapy. Allowing space to process feelings is an active part of cultural humility because it means that there is an openness for multiplicity in lived experiences and beliefs.

Further, allowing space holds the supervisee's values and beliefs in high regard to say, "I can believe something to be true, and acknowledge that someone else's belief can be true simultaneously." When play therapy supervisors are working to build cultural humility into their supervisory practice, they may struggle with cognitive dissonance, particularly if they have spent time under the impression that opposite beliefs cannot co-exist or a misconception that there are right and wrong beliefs in all cases. However, this discomfort is likely to be recurrent rather than continuous, as the supervisor works through values and beliefs.

The final piece towards building cultural humility for the play therapy supervisor is the continual process of searching for *implicit beliefs*. Here, the author defines implicit beliefs to be automatic and unconscious psychological assumptions that are held by an individual and typically formed due to past experiences (e.g., how one was parented or theoretical orientation of graduate school program), incidental learning (e.g., seeing the reactions of others in certain situations), and repetitive exposure to the beliefs of others (e.g., overhearing respected members of a group share their explicit beliefs). The clincher here is that it is extremely difficult, if not impossible, for one to search for their own implicit beliefs without any outside resources or assistance because implicit beliefs are unconscious. A popular way to identify at least some explicit beliefs is to take an Implicit Association Test (IAT; http://implicit.harvard.edu/; Kurdi et al., 2021), which attempts to objectively measure if an implicit bias exists in a given area and, if so, the direction of the bias, for or against, and the degree of that direction.

However, there are other ways for supervisors to search for implicit beliefs besides the IAT. For example, external resources for this process can be engaging in community and discussion with people who have different explicit beliefs than the play therapy supervisor. Supervisors may also become more critical of the information that is readily available (e.g., examining whether things like social media content is only exposing the supervisor to content that confirms their explicit beliefs and thus may reinforce their implicit beliefs), and increase their exposure to sources of knowledge that marginalized peoples created (e.g., reading books by scholars who are neurodivergent or gender-expansive). Another key step in revealing one's own biases is decreasing impulsivity by pausing before responding. Moreover, Edgoose et al. (2019) devised an eight-piece mnemonic device to help remember these tips, IMPLICIT, which stands for: Introspection, mindfulness, perspective-taking, learn to slow down, individuation, check your messages (i.e., examine the power of your word choices and phrasing), institutionalize fairness (i.e., explore equity), and take two (i.e., acknowledge that this is a lifelong process without an endpoint). [Reproduced with permission from "How to Identify, Understand, and Unlearn Implicit Bias in Patient Care," July/August 2019, Vol 26, No 4, issue of *Family Practice Management* Copyright © 2019 American Academy of Family Physicians. All Rights Reserved.]

Destigmatizing Discussions in Play Therapy Supervision

As the supervisor or supervisor-in-training has started the journey of building cultural humility and understands what that can look like for them in their practice, they can use those underpinnings to destigmatize difficult conversations, such as topics of race and culture during play therapy supervision. There have been cases where the supervisee was the first to broach a stigmatized subject with their supervisor with success (Schen & Greenlee, 2018). However, most of the literature shows that when supervisors are comfortable gently exploring race and other sociocultural factors, such as sexual orientation, supervisees tend to feel more willing to process their feelings in supervision around those topics (Hagler, 2020; Soheilian et al., 2014; Upshaw et al., 2019). There is a consensus in the literature that it is best when supervisors have this discussion for the first time during individual supervision rather than during group supervision (Schen & Greenlee, 2018; Upshaw et al., 2019), especially in cases where the supervisee is from a minoritized identity.

Play therapy supervisors can invite conversations for race and other historically stigmatized topics in several ways. Supervisors may be able to effectively use self-disclosure as the conversation starter at the outset of supervision. Utilizing an activity or framework, such as Hay's (2007) ADDRESSING (a mnemonic device to help recall various aspects of culture), is a helpful tool in destigmatizing factors of race, sexual orientation, ability, etc. (Hagler, 2020; Watkins & Hook, 2016).

Supervisors may also invite the supervisee to engage in a dynamic interaction where the two take turns discussing aspects of the framework related to each person's identities (Hagler, 2020). It is recommended that play therapy supervisors and supervisors-in-training align this discussion with the parallel process that clients may feel in the play therapy room.

Budding play therapists may welcome opportunities to experience play therapy techniques from a first-person perspective. Doing so allows them to provide space for clients to incorporate their own cultural identities into their play. A play genogram, suggested by Gil (2003), invites the supervisee to select miniatures to represent what may be happening in a client's world. This activity has been adapted (Dowtin, 2019; Mullen et al., 2007) and could be further expanded to focus on a minoritized client's world during miniature selection by asking the supervisee to consider the client's known cultural identities and how society may view them.

Equity: Acknowledging Power in Play Therapy Supervision

Equity in play therapy supervision is first an acknowledgment that there is inherent power in the supervisor–supervisee relationship. Examining this power and being honest with oneself about such power is vital in creating space for social justice work in play therapy supervision. Like the ongoing process of building cultural humility discussed earlier in this chapter, exploring power in supervision starts with self-reflection for the Registered Play Therapist-Supervisor™ (RPT-S™)-in-training. Play therapy supervisors must ask themselves questions to better understand what power looks like and means for them as a supervisor. Furthermore, supervisors need to revisit, unlearn, and learn supervision components that commonly impact minoritized supervisees. For example, DuBois (1903) discussed the concept of double consciousness for Black people, and that concept has been carried forth and remains present in current times (Jones et al., 2018). In short, double consciousness is the heightened internal tension that Black people experience due to their exposure to historical trauma and current systemic trauma while also having obtained some privilege. While this was originally discussed solely in the context of Black people, it can be applied to other minoritized and marginalized peoples, especially those with intersecting identities. In the context of power in play therapy supervision, this would mean that a supervisee could place more emphasis on the role of power in their supervisory relationship due to their culture's history of oppression by people in power.

An additional layer of consideration for a play therapy supervisor would be the potential for marginalized supervisees to feel unsafe or afraid to address certain concerns with their supervisor due to fear of persecution, retaliation, or other negative repercussions. For example, Constantine & Sue (2007), identified the double-bind where Black supervisees opt not to discuss concerns of a supervisor's limited cultural responsiveness causing the supervisee to feel resentful or hopeless. Alternatively, if the Black supervisee decides to express their perspective regarding their supervisors' areas for growth when it comes to culture or any area, the supervisee may experience negative consequences (Constantine & Sue, 2007; Stauffer & Buckley, 2005) that can ultimately lead to more detrimental outcomes than if they were from an overprivileged community. Furthermore, Smith et al. (2012) identified self-disclosure in group supervision as an ethical dilemma for supervisees, though not specifically for those culturally marginalized, because those disclosures are often used in an evaluative manner. That means that supervisees in group supervision may struggle with worries about consequences of disclosing an identity, belief, or experience in group supervision even when it may appropriately illustrate their point, help a client or colleague, or provide needed movement in the supervision session. As a result, play therapy supervisees may be reluctant to participate in group supervision and then fear or experience negative evaluations (Stauffer & Buckley, 2005) for their lack of participation. Therefore, play therapy supervisors must realize that supervisees may not feel that supervision is safe to process cases simply because the supervisory relationship is safe. Supervisors have to work to make supervision a safe space for all parties. For many supervisees, especially those who are marginalized, supervision can be one of the scariest parts of learning to practice play therapy.

Given the understanding of power in play therapy supervision, double consciousness, and double-bind, and disclosure dilemmas, the following questions are suggested as a springboard for this needed self-reflection for play therapy supervisors to create more equitable interactions in supervision:

- As a person in a position of power, how might my implicit and explicit beliefs impact those I supervise?
- What are some of the implications of the power that I hold as an RPT-S™ or RPT-S™-in-training?
- How might the impact of my power vary depending on the identities or sociodemographics of my supervisee?
- Since play therapy trainees can already be licensed mental health practitioners, how might their professional identity influence how I use the power I have?
- What is the role of power when I engage in group play therapy supervision?
- What value do I place on power in play therapy supervisory relationships?
- What ethical dilemmas can arise for my play therapy supervisees that I may impact?

After doing some introspective work on the role of power in supervision, supervisors may need to discuss power with their supervisee openly. This discussion would facilitate modeling of this difficult task and invite supervisees to begin engaging in reflective practice for themselves.

Social Justice: Nurturing Clinical Advocacy

The phrase social justice has been used several times in this chapter to discuss play therapy supervisors building cultural humility, exploring power, and working toward equitable practices. Still, a clear definition has not been provided. Asakura and Maurer's (2018) definition of social justice in supervision is used here. Social justice is directing attention to relationship's power dynamics while encouraging the supervisee's development of reflective practice and fine-tuning their advocacy skills. This definition demonstrates that the earlier developmental activities of the play therapy supervisor support the creation of social justice, with the final part being helping supervisees find their own voice in advocacy. The play therapy supervisor helps the supervisee unpack their biases to create a more in-depth understanding of self in relation to their clients (Chang et al., 2009; Dollarhide et al., 2021). As that deeper self-awareness unfolds, the play supervisor provides the foundation for the supervisee to empower their clients to use their internal resources to identify external opportunities for healing. This approach nicely aligns with non-directive play therapy approaches that allow the client to lead. Supervisors can also provide space and support for the supervisee to begin challenging community and larger systems that engage in client marginalization (Chang et al., 2009). Play therapy supervisees learn how to use social justice to monitor client outcomes through the use of narrative supervision (Dollarhide et al., 2021) as they are shown how to ask questions of themselves rather than make definitive statements, invite curiosity and openness, create multiplicity in their own beliefs systems, and identify sources of problems all through their supervisor's modeling and engagement in such events.

Conclusion

Play therapy supervisors have a unique responsibility to help facilitate the learning and practice of play therapy skills with the next generation of play therapists in a climate that is still learning how to navigate topics of therapist identity. For that to happen, supervisees need to feel safe, but so many factors make safety difficult to achieve. Play therapy supervisors who practice building cultural humility are on their way toward creating safer spaces, perhaps compared to some of the supervision environments and interactions that existed in the past. Being in positions of authority automatically gives supervisors a firm hold on power over their supervisees regardless and inclusive of the supervisor's values and beliefs. Power is not necessarily a negative reality when wielded by someone who understands its gravity and is willing to share its privileges. To be better holders of power, play therapy supervisors are encouraged to practice introspection to allow themselves the discomfort of reflecting on who they are, what they value, why they believe what they believe, and inviting in space for the realities of their supervisees. While not easy, it is highly impactful on the lives of play therapy supervisees and their clients, and ultimately for the supervisor themself.

The role of social justice has been an emerging practice in supervision over the most recent decades. Including social justice in play therapy supervision teaches play therapy supervisees how to support clients' needs and engage with the field in a manner that begins to dismantle systemic barriers. Social justice from the lens of a play therapist means that future play therapists will better understand how to be change agents for and with clients who are marginalized, rather than primarily being part of the perpetuation of oppression.

References

Asakura, K., & Maurer, K. (2018). Attending to social justice in clinical social work: Supervision as a pedagogical space. *Clinical Social Work Journal*, *46*(4), 289–297. https://doi.org/10.1007/s10615-018-0667-4

Bernard, J. M., & Goodyear, R. K. (2014). *Fundamentals of clinical supervision* (5th ed.). Pearson.

Burkard, A. W., Edwards, L. M., & Adams, H. A. (2016). Racial color blindness in counseling, therapy, and supervision. In H. A. Neville, M. E. Gallardo, & D. W. Sue (Eds.), *The myth of racial color blindness: Manifestations, dynamics, and impact* (pp. 295–311). American Psychological Association. https://doi.org/10.1037/14754-018

Chang, C. Y., Hays, D. G., & Milliken, T. (2009). Addressing social justice issues in supervision: A call for client and professional advocacy. *Clinical Supervisor*, *28*(1), 20–35. https://doi.org/10.1080/07325220902855144

Constantine, M. G., & Sue, D. W. (2007). Perceptions of racial microaggressions among Black supervisees in cross-racial dyads. *Journal of Counseling Psychology*, *54*(2), 142–153. http://doi.org/10.1037/0022-0167.54.2.142

Crenshaw, Kimberlé (1989). Demarginalizing the intersection of race and sex: A Black feminist critique of antidiscrimination doctrine. *University of Chicago Legal Forum*, 1989: 139–168.

Dollarhide, C. T., Hale, S. C., & Stone-Sabali, S. (2021). A new model for social justice supervision. *Journal of Counseling and Development*, *99*(1), 104–113. https://doi.org/10.1002/jcad.12358

Donald, E. J., Culbreth, J. R., & Carter, A. W. (2015). Play therapy supervision: A review of the literature. *International Journal of Play Therapy*, *24*(2), 59–77. https://doi.org/10.1037/a0039104

Dowtin, L. L. (2019). Alter egos and hidden strengths: The powers of superheroes in child-centered play therapy. In L. Rubin (Ed), *Using Superheroes and Villains in Counseling and Play Therapy: A Guide for Mental Health Professionals*. London: Routledge.

Du Bois, W. E. B. (1903). *The souls of Black folk*. A. C. McClurg.

Edgoose, J. Y., Quiogue, M., & Sidhar, K. (2019). How to identify, understand, and unlearn implicit bias in patient care. *Family Practice Management*, *26*(4), 29–33. https://www.aafp.org/fpm/2019/0700/p29.html

Gardner, R. M. D. (2002). Cross-cultural perspectives in supervision. *Western Journal of Black Studies*, *26*(2), 98–106.

Gil, E. (2003). Family play therapy: "The bear with short nails". In C. E. Schaefer (Ed.), *Foundations of play therapy* (pp. 192–218). Jossey-Bass.

Hagler, M. A. (2020). LGBQ-affirming and-nonaffirming supervision: Perspectives from a queer trainee. *Journal of Psychotherapy Integration*, *30*(1), 76. https://doi.org/10.1037/int0000165

Hair, H. J., & O'Donoghue, K. (2009). Culturally relevant, socially just social work supervision: Becoming visible through a social constructionist lens. *Journal of Ethnic and Cultural Diversity in Social Work*, *18*(1–2), 70–88. https://doi.org/10.1080/15313200902874979

Hays, P. A. (2007). *Addressing cultural complexities in practice: Assessment, diagnosis, and therapy* (2nd ed.). American Psychological Association.

Jones, H. A., Perrin, P. B., Heller, M. B., Hailu, S., & Barnett, C. (2018). Black psychology graduate students' lives matter: Using informal mentoring to create an inclusive climate amidst national race-related events. *Professional Psychology: Research and Practice*, *49*(1), 75–82. http://doi.org/10.1037/pro0000169

Kurdi, B., Ratliff, K. A., & Cunningham, W. A. (2021). Can the implicit association test serve as a valid measure of automatic cognition? A response to Schimmack (2021). *Perspectives on Psychological Science, 16*(2), 422–434. https://doi.org/10.1177/1745691620904080

McCarthy Veach, P., Yoon, E., Miranda, C., MacFarlane, I. M., Ergun, D., & Tuicomepee, A. (2012). Clinical supervisor value conflicts: Low-frequency, but high-impact events. *Clinical Supervisor, 31*(2), 203–227. https://doi.org/10.1080/07325223.2013.730478

Mosher, D. K., Hook, J. N., Farrell, J. E., Watkins, C. E., Jr., & Davis, D. E. (2017). Cultural humility. In E. L. Worthington Jr., D. E. Davis, & J. N. Hook (Eds.), *Handbook of humility: Theory, research, and application* (pp. 91–104). Routledge/Taylor & Francis Group.

Mullen, J. A., Luke, M., & Drewes, A. A. (2007). Supervision can be playful, too: Play therapy techniques that enhance supervision. *International Journal of Play Therapy, 16*(1), 69. http://doi.org.proxyga.wrlc.org/10.1037/1555-6824.16.1.69

Neville, H. A., Awad, G. H., Brooks, J. E., Flores, M. P., & Bluemel, J. (2013). Color-blind racial ideology: Theory, training, and measurement implications in psychology. *American Psychologist, 68*(6), 455. https://doi.org/10.1037/a0033282

Schen, C. R., & Greenlee, A. (2018). Race in supervision: Let's talk about it. *Psychodynamic Psychiatry, 46*(1), 1–21. https://doi.org/10.1521/pdps.2018.46.1.1

Smith, R. D., Riva, M. T., & Erickson Cornish, J. A. (2012). The ethical practice of group supervision: A national survey. *Training and Education in Professional Psychology, 6*(4), 238–248. http://doi.org/10.1037/a0030806

Stauffer, J. M., & Buckley, M. R. (2005). The existence and nature of racial bias in supervisory ratings. *Journal of Applied Psychology, 90*(3), 586. https://doi.org/10.1037/0021-9010.90.3.586

Soheilian, S. S., Inman, A. G., Klinger, R. S., Isenberg, D. S., & Kulp, L. E. (2014). Multicultural supervision: Supervisees' reflections on culturally competent supervision. *Counselling Psychology Quarterly, 27*(4), 379–392. http://doi.org/10.1080/09515070.2014.961408

Tummala-Narra, P. (2004). Dynamics of race and culture in the supervisory encounter. *Psychoanalytic Psychology, 21*(2), 300–311. https://doi.org/10.1037/0736-9735.21.2.300

Upshaw, N. C., Lewis Jr., D. E., & Nelson, A. L. (2019). Cultural humility in action: Reflective and process-oriented supervision with Black trainees. *Training and Education in Professional Psychology, 14*(4), 277. http://doi.org/10.1037/tep0000284

Watkins Jr., C. E., & Hook, J. N. (2016). On a culturally humble psychoanalytic supervision perspective: Creating the cultural third. *Psychoanalytic Psychology, 33*(3), 487. http://doi.org/10.1037/pap0000044

Definition of Terms

Cross-cultural supervision – supervision where the supervisor is from a different primary cultural background than the supervisee(s).

Culture – a group of people who share a common set of values, beliefs, experiences, and language or language-use. Types of cultures include many identities not limited to, gender, socioeconomic level, race, ability, disability, religion, profession, sex, sexual orientation.

Implicit – automatic and unconscious psychological assumptions that are held by an individual and typically formed due to past experiences (e.g., how one was parented or theoretical orientation of graduate school program), incidental learning (e.g., seeing the reactions of others in certain situations), and repetitive exposure to the beliefs of others (e.g., overhearing respected members of a group share their explicit beliefs).

Humility – self-reflecting on and critically analyzing one's own culture and cultural beliefs, being open to the ongoing learning of other cultures, as well as holding the conscious understanding that there will always be areas one does not and cannot know regarding a culture that differs from their own, and having high regard for the feelings, experiences, and beliefs of other people, while addressing imbalances of power that exist within interpersonal relationships

Social Justice – direct attention to relationship power dynamics, while encouraging the supervisee's development of reflective practice and fine tuning the supervisee's advocacy skills.

3 Models of Clinical Supervision in Play Therapy Supervision

Staci Born, Naomi Timm-Davis, and Emily Gislason

Models of Clinical Supervision in Play Therapy Supervision

Supervision serves a critical role in the development of play therapists. As standards for professional education, experience, and supervision in play therapy continue to increase in specificity, play therapy supervision must become viewed as a specialized area of play therapy practice. Effective play therapy supervision is derived from clinical supervision models and incorporates elements of play therapy (Hudspeth, 2015). Therefore, the utility of clinical models of supervision for play therapists is clear. Models of supervision provide a conceptual framework for supervisors which aid in conducting cohesive supervision that addresses supervisees' needs. Prior to the introduction of revised play therapy standards by the Association for Play Therapy (APT) in 2020 (see Chapter 1 for an account of history), research suggested that 25% to 50% of play therapists received supervision related to play therapy (Phillips & Landreth, 1995; Ryan et al., 2002; VanderGast et al., 2010) and only 40% of those supervisors had significant play therapy experience (Donald et al., 2015; Phillips & Landreth, 1995; Ryan et al., 2002). Additionally, play therapy supervisees are unlikely to take a university course in play therapy and therefore receive less formal training (Donald et al., 2015; Kranz et al., 1998; Lambert et al., 2007; Ryan et al., 2002). For supervisors, this means that understanding the development of the supervisee is essential to tailor appropriate educational and clinical interventions (Donald et al., 2015).

The APT Best Practices (2020) document provides some guidance on the provision of supervision in play therapy. Supervision is defined as:

> A formal professional clinical role which is recognized and defined by the relevant state law and professional guidelines of the supervisee's professional organization and/or APT. The intent is that the supervision time will be documented and reported to a third party so that it can be applied toward professional licensure, registration and/or certification. As such, the supervisor maintains liability for the supervisee's clinical work.
>
> (APT Best Practices, 2020, p. 15)

DOI: 10.4324/9781003196075-4

Additionally, Section H.1 (APT Best Practices, 2020) recommends that supervisors establish clinical supervision contracts with supervisees, be trained in supervision methods and skills, and monitor clinical quality of play therapy supervisees. In addition, section H.3 (APT Best Practices, 2020) notes that supervisors should be aware of supervisee development, supervisor's gatekeeping responsibilities, and the necessary play therapy standards for credentialing as professional play therapists. Supervision of supervision is also an important activity supervisors engage in. In this setting, a new supervisor can meet with a more experienced supervisor for guidance and support in the development of supervision competence (Ray, 2011).

Supervision practice, just as the theories of play therapy, have evolved from a singular-model focus to an integrative approach (Seymour & Crenshaw, 2015). This chapter offers an overview of the key characteristics of models of clinical supervision. Developmental models, psychotherapy theory-based models, and process models of supervision are reviewed. While we present the models as separate categories, it is recommended that supervisors not practice within categories but across categories, to provide effective supervision to diverse supervisees (Bernard & Goodyear, 2014). Then, we briefly apply each model to an example case to illustrate some of the concepts in action and related to the specific provision of play therapy supervision.

Example Case

The following is a case example that is applied to each model of clinical supervision in this chapter. In this case, the supervisor has watched a videorecorded session of Bailey, a 26-year-old White-passing multiracial woman who is in Phase 2 of earning her RPT™ credential and is employed by a Midwestern suburban community mental health center. Her supervisor, Meredith, is a 48-year-old White woman who is a licensed counselor in her state and an RPT-S™. Meredith currently has her own private practice, has been a counselor for 15 years, and has been providing counseling and play therapy supervision for 11 years. Bailey and Meredith have been in a supervisory relationship for 9 months. Bailey sought supervision from Meredith when she decided to pursue her credential as a Registered Play Therapist. Bailey selected Meredith because she had a child-centered style of play therapy and they instantly connected over their shared interests in pop music and believing strongly in the healing powers of play.

Bailey is providing play therapy to Carlos, a 7-year-old boy who has been referred to play therapy because he is displaying defiant and aggressive behaviors at school and in his foster home. Known history of Carlos includes he and his family immigrated to the United States from Guatemala four years ago, seeking safety from escalating violence in their country. Recently, Carlos and his two sisters witnessed domestic violence between his mother and father and were removed from their care after his father threw a large plastic tote at Carlos, striking him in the head and leaving a large bruise on his forehead. Carlos and his siblings have been living with a foster family for the past 3 months. The foster family sought therapy with Bailey when searching for area play therapists and decided to work with Bailey when they noted she "had a Latinx last name."

After Bailey describes Carlos' history, she tells Meredith about pressure she has felt about how the foster family selected her as a play therapist. Bailey stated, "I'm really worried about this case and being the right fit for him. His foster mom said she scheduled with me because of my last name and the truth is, only parts of my Latino culture are known to me and I feel culturally disconnected from that part of my identity." Meredith can sense that there is a level of discomfort with Carlos and his situation. Meredith notes this and the two begin watching the recording.

In their third session together, Carlos can be seen exploring the sand tray, sifting the sand through his fingers quietly as Bailey tracks his actions. Carlos' eyes scan the playroom while he sifts the sand, and after several minutes he quietly approaches the bop bag. He smiles at first and begins pushing the bag, seeming to explore how it moves. Carlos gradually begins to kick and punch the bag. His physical intensity increases as evidenced by a grimace on his face, clenched teeth, and his hands tightly squeezing the top of the bag. Carlos can be heard grunting and yelling at the bop bag to "*cállate, idiota!*" At this time, Bailey's tracking and reflecting has nearly ceased and she appears frozen in the playroom, quietly watching Carlos' play unfold. Carlos' anger intensifies to shouting and lifting the bop bag over his head before throwing it against the wall repeatedly. After Carlos tosses the bag against the wall for a third time, a framed poster falls off the wall. Carlos pauses and stares at Bailey, first in awe and then in anger as he says, "Look what you made me do!"

Developmental Models of Supervision

Developmental models of supervision are centered on the learning processes of the supervisee (Bernard & Goodyear, 2014). It is worth noting that the process of becoming a play therapist is nonlinear by design reflecting much of what we know about the cyclical process of development overall. The APT's phase model requires play therapists in training to receive education, clinical experience, and play therapy supervision across three phases. It is also important to consider that much of the existing research related to play therapy supervisees is focused on *novice* play therapists (Donald et al., 2015). Overattention to the early career stage is critical for therapist development, however it is only a partial illustration of the developmental processes and needs of play therapists.

Loganbill, Hardy and Delworth Model

Influenced by theories of human development, Loganbill et al. (1982) applied the developmental stage theories of human growth to the supervision process. As an influential model describing counselor development, it is reviewed here. The model is composed of three stages of development while simultaneously acknowledging the complexity and uniqueness of the individual supervisee. A critical element of this model is the continuous development that is inherent to the counselor development process. Counselor development is not viewed as linear and finite but as cycling and recycling through the developmental stages at deeper levels (Loganbill et al., 1982).

Stage One is characterized by stagnation and unawareness. In this stage, supervisees are unaware of a deficiency or blind spot in their functioning. The novice supervisee in stagnation has constricted or narrow thinking that is often linear in nature. Often, supervisees believe there is only one way to define a problem and only one way to resolve the problem. At this stage, the supervisee may have a low self-concept that is characterized by high dependence on the supervisor and that new learning must come from an external source rather than from within. Additionally, because of the lack of self-awareness, a supervisee may falsely believe they are functioning well. At Stage One, the supervisor is perceived in one of two ways. The supervisor may be viewed as wise and all-knowing, which fosters greater supervisee dependence. Other times, the supervisor is viewed as irrelevant, especially if the supervisor does not align with the supervisee's narrow problem-solving approach characteristic of this stage. This irrelevance is not hostile but unaware or neutral in nature. It is worth noting that this stage serves a purpose to the supervisee's growth as it provides a space for latency and rest (Loganbill et al., 1982).

Stage Two is characterized by confusion and turbulence. Its onset may be gradual or sudden. Within Stage Two, the supervisee becomes aware of a deficit and is unsure how to resolve it. In this stage, the supervisee realizes that their supervisor does not hold all the answers or may perceive the supervisor as withholding the answer. This can result in increased frustration toward the supervisor. Anticipating this stage of development can be helpful for the supervisor and the supervisee as value in this stage comes from the replacement of unhelpful information with a fresher perspective. The supervisor viewing this stage as a sign of growth is critical as the supervisee is creating space for new learning (Loganbill et al., 1982).

Stage Three is often welcomed as it provides a reprieve from the chaos of Stage Two. Transition to Stage Three can occur gradually or abruptly and this stage is characterized by integration, calm, and new understanding. In this stage, flexible understanding is applied as supervisees gain awareness in creative problem-solving. In this stage, supervisees accept that there will be challenges and successes in their development. This stage is also characterized by growth in self-acceptance and self-confidence. The supervisor is no longer viewed as unhelpful and more realistic expectations emerge as the supervisee takes active responsibility for supervision. Stage Three provides important stability that is flexible and continuously growing (Loganbill et al., 1982).

Adapted from Chickering's (1969) seven developmental themes, Loganbill et al. (1982) identified eight key issues of supervision; a supervisee is in one of the three stages of development for each of the eight issues. The eight issues are 1) Issues of Competence, 2) Issues of Emotional Awareness, 3) Issues of Autonomy, 4) Issues of Theoretical Identity, 5) Issues of Respect for Individual Differences, 6) Issues of Purpose and Direction, 7) Issues of Personal Motivation, and 8) Issues of Professional Ethics. The complexity of the model can be felt based on the potential challenge of monitoring supervisee progress at three levels across eight domains (Bernard & Goodyear; 2014). For the field of supervision, the descriptive nature of Loganbill et al.'s (1982) work facilitated the development of additional clinical supervision models, including the Integrative Developmental Model and the Discrimination Model (Bernard & Goodyear, 2014; Stoltenberg & McNeill, 2011).

Example Case

As Meredith considers Bailey's development, she decides to briefly assess Bailey's stage of functioning across each of the eight key issues. Meredith discerns that Bailey is at Stage One for issues of:

- Autonomy: Bailey has completed much of her formal education and is in the first year of post-graduate practice. Meredith gets the sense that Bailey strives to feel confident and independent and feels she lacks knowledge for treating complex cases. In recent sessions, Bailey has shared that she lacks confidence in providing therapy – a revelation that took 9 months to be stated by Bailey but could be sensed within the supervisory relationship. Meredith needs to consider how her identity as a White, older, senior therapist may be impacting Bailey and her development.
- Professional Motivation: Meredith reflects on her 9 months with Bailey and decides that she and Bailey have not discussed Bailey's motivation for becoming a play therapist. Meredith makes note of this and considers if or how this might be impacting Bailey's present experience of Carlos. Meredith and Bailey will also benefit from discussing how Bailey's cultural identities impact her as a therapist and her clients.
- Professional Ethics: Considering the presentation of Carlos' case, Meredith concludes that Bailey does not recognize potential ethical issues in Carlos' case. This "blind spot" will need to be considered so Bailey can draw a coherent understanding of the ethical ramifications of providing play therapy.

Stage Two for issues of:

- Competence: Carlos is a more challenging case for Bailey, given his historical experiences and present experience of being in foster care and away from his family. Bailey seems frustrated by the complexity of Carlos' circumstances and doubts her professional knowledge has prepared her to help him.
- Emotional Awareness: While Bailey was aware that she became flooded in session with Carlos, she was unable to regulate herself to be emotionally present to respond to him. Meredith will need to help Bailey become presently aware of her emotions in session so she can appropriately regulate and respond to her child clients and not leave them in emotional abandonment at

that moment. Additionally, Meredith will need to support Bailey in identifying any feelings she has toward Carlos or his family.

- Theoretical Identity: Bailey is a natural child-centered play therapist. However, in the case of Carlos, Bailey seemed unable to consider alternate responses – even from different theoretical perspectives – to stay therapeutically present. Meredith decides to encourage Bailey to consider how she would respond to Carlos from multiple perspectives, and to invite Bailey to consider responding from different perspectives too; not to discredit her CCPT style, but to help Bailey integrate her skills and approach.
- Respect for Individual Differences: As a White-passing multiracial woman, Bailey presented minimal affect when she shared that Carlos' foster family had selected her based on her last name. Additionally, Meredith realizes that she has not had an explicit discussion with Bailey about the identity differences within the supervision relationship, nor within Bailey's therapeutic relationships. Meredith feels shameful and relieved that she will be able to have an important conversation with Bailey about identities and differences.
- Purpose and Direction: Bailey uses theory as a guide in her work with Carlos. However, as Carlos' play gets bigger, Bailey begins to doubt that her approach will help Carlos improve. Meredith will support Bailey by helping her reconsider how therapeutic change occurs in play therapy, especially from a child-centered approach.

Meredith will share her assessment of Bailey's functioning with her so that the two can prioritize which Stage Two issues are of utmost importance in assisting Carlos.

Integrative Developmental Model

Expanding on the model developed by Loganbill et al. (1982), the Integrative Developmental Model (IDM) continues to organize supervisee development in Levels 1 to 3 (and an additional level, 3i). However, it emphasizes that supervisee development is not global and instead is specific to important tasks related to the practice of professional helping. For example, a play therapist supervisee may be adept and confident in their ability to provide play therapy services to children in the playroom but may seriously lack skills and confidence in conducting parent consultation. In addition, the IDM supervision environment adapts in response to supervisee's developmental needs and challenges. Therefore, the supervisor needs to be diligent in evaluating supervisee functioning, making necessary supervisory shifts, and providing supervision interventions intended to facilitate increased development (Stoltenberg & McNeill, 2011).

Using IDM, supervisee development is monitored by attending to three important structures across eight domains of clinical skills. The three structures include 1) Self- and Other-Awareness: Cognitive and Affective, 2) Motivation, and 3) Autonomy. The Self- and Other-Awareness structure includes the affective awareness of self and client, and the cognitive awareness. The Motivation structure is the supervisee's invested interest in developing their clinical skills. Last, the Autonomy structure is the varying independence the supervisee demonstrates. These three structures differ across supervisee level (Stoltenberg & McNeill, 2011) and can be assessed by having the supervisee complete the Supervisee Levels Questionnaire – Revised (McNeill et al., 1992). Each of the three structures guides the understanding of a supervisee's play therapy practice skills. These eight domains are 1) Intervention Skills Competence, 2) Assessment Techniques, 3) Interpersonal Assessment, 4) Client Conceptualization, 5) Individual Differences, 6) Theoretical Orientation, 7) Treatment Plans and Goals, and 8) Professional Ethics (Stoltenberg & McNeill, 2011). The complexity of evaluation of eight skills across three structures and four levels of supervisee development add to the complexity of this developmental model.

Level 1: Level 1 supervisees may be new to the field of play therapy or new to a particular play therapy activity or approach. At Level 1, supervisees need help applying knowledge into practice and this leads to a lack of self- and other-awareness. Supervisee's preoccupation with delivery of interventions prevents them from attending to important client affective and cognitive data, as well as their own. Over-focus on implementing techniques, professional effectiveness, and competence generates increasing anxiety, too. Attention to techniques as well as the awareness of evaluation leads to elevated levels of anxiety and sometimes low levels of confidence for Level 1 play therapists. Absence of anxiety and over-confidence in novice play therapists may be problematic and supervisors should explore supervisee motivation and their ability to self-assess their skills (Stoltenberg & McNeill, 2011). Level 1 supervisees tend to be very motivated to learn and to grow beyond their uncomfortable thoughts and feelings that accompany this stage. They often seek out the "best" or "correct" techniques for their clients and are highly focused on external evaluation of their performance, therefore dependence on supervisors can be high at this level (Stoltenberg & McNeill, 2011).

Level 1 supervisees lack the knowledge and skills to perform as an autonomous play therapist. Supervisors of Level 1 play therapists serve as primary sources of knowledge and support, role models, and trainers. Supervisors of Level 1 trainees need to provide structure. Prescriptive and facilitative supervision experiences support learning and reduce anxiety. Deducing play therapy techniques into discrete and observable actions reduces fear and enhances learning. Supervisors can begin to encourage autonomy by asking supervisees to engage in self-assessment and problem-solving about their clinical work. Accurate feedback on performance is paramount as the supervisee develops a foundation for future practice and a stronger internal confidence and competence. Live supervision and reviewing session recordings are critical supervision activities (Stoltenberg & McNeill, 2011).

Level 2: An indication that a supervisee has reached Level 2 is when their primary focus is not on themselves and their performance and is instead focused on their client's thoughts and feelings. This new awareness can bring about confusion, too. At this level, with increased attention, supervisees increase their awareness of client responses to play therapy interventions – both positive and negative. This increased awareness also results in greater empathy as the supervisee can track verbal and nonverbal client responses. The vacillation between increased awareness and confusion can mimic the "dependency-autonomy conflict, not unlike what is experienced in adolescence" (Stoltenberg & McNeill, 2011). One day, the supervisee may experience themselves as confident and an internal locus of causality for their development, while on other days, the supervisee may feel incompetent, dependent, and sometimes evasive — to a supervisor it may seem like a developmental regression. These swinging feelings of motivation can lead to feelings of self-efficacy that can quickly be accompanied by self-doubt and confusion (Stoltenberg & McNeill, 2011).

Supervisors can assist Level 2 supervisees by challenging them with more complex cases, or cases that vary greatly from the supervisee's experience. Level 2 supervisees benefit from recognizing their personal influence on the therapeutic process and practice. Additionally, with greater access to empathy for clients, supervisees at this level may need support in managing feelings of enmeshment or countertransference for clients, too. Supervisors will need to pay close attention to the supervisee's vacillation in autonomy and, at times, provide Level 1 interventions to expand the supervisee's skills and understanding. To increase buy-in for these directive or didactic interventions with Level 2 supervisees, describing the purpose and rationale to supervisees will increase buy-in. As increased challenges arise in clinical and supervisory context, facilitative supervisory interventions should be frequent. Prescriptive interventions still hold importance, but are used with less frequency for Level 2 trainees. Live supervision and reviewing session recordings remain an important component of supervision of Level 2 supervisees (Stoltenberg & McNeill, 2011).

Level 3: When a supervisor observes a decreased vacillation in supervisee autonomy and reduced feelings of incompetence, Level 3 is on the horizon. At this level, the supervisee is reflective and able to provide play therapy using a more personalized approach and increased use of their self-as-therapist. Level 3 supervisees are self-aware and understand their professional strengths and challenges. Empathy continues to be well-practiced, however the danger of enmeshment or countertransference is diminished. Intrinsic motivation is high, and supervisees are motivated toward professional development. The therapist is evolving into a well-defined professional identity. At this Level, supervisees are independent and confidence in professional judgment can be observed, however consultation is still utilized as a tool when uncertainty arises (Stoltenberg & McNeill, 2011).

Supervision for Level 3 supervisees tends to be led and structured by the supervisee. Supervisors should carefully evaluate the domains that the supervisee is not yet functioning at a Level 3 so continued attention can be direct to those domains. At this stage, the supervisory relationship may begin to evolve into a mentorship relationship. Facilitative responses are still useful, yet less crucial because the therapist's self-efficacy has developed. Live supervision and reviewing session recordings remain an important part of supervision, however it is used with decreased frequency (Stoltenberg & McNeill, 2011).

Level 3i: As a supervisee develops Level 3 skills in several domains, a goal of supervision becomes integrating competence and fluidity across most of the eight domains. Additionally, the play therapist has an increased self-awareness of how their personal functioning impacts their professional functioning. Motivation continues to be mostly high across domains, and where motivation is lacking, the play therapist tends to be aware of the lowered motivation and underlying reason, too. Professional goals may shift at this stage and new training endeavors may result in revisiting Level 1 and 2 issues as integration and skill development builds (Stoltenberg & McNeill, 2011).

Example Case

From an IDM perspective, Meredith decided to draw attention to Bailey's Self- and Other-Awareness Structure with the goal of drawing attention to Bailey's affective experience with Carlos, and Carlos' affective experience with Bailey. As a result, she begins by focusing her supervisory interventions on facilitating reflections for Bailey. When Carlos throws the bop bag over his head at the wall, Meredith asks Bailey, "What is Carlos feeling at this point in the session?" Bailey thoughtfully pauses and states, "He's angry." "Yeah, we can see and hear that in the recording," replies Meredith, "What do you suppose those feelings are in response to?" Bailey thoughtfully pauses again, contemplating, and then, "Well he's probably angry about his current situation, being apart from his parents. He's probably mad at his parents too, that their actions brought him to this place." Meredith validates Bailey's insights and encourages Bailey to wonder if Carlos is also angry at himself, though it may be too therapeutically early to tell. The two also consider whether Carlos may have some anger toward Bailey and whom she may represent in his world.

Meredith later pivots to Bailey's experience in the session and asks, "What are you feeling at this point in the session?" Bailey quickly responds, "Scared and out of control, I was freaking out on the inside and had no idea what to say or do. And then when he yelled Spanish at me, I just felt completely worthless to him, I don't know what he was saying." Meredith again validates Bailey's awareness and the experience of freezing in session. The two explore Bailey's experiences with anger in personal and professional environments, and how Bailey typically responds and how she wishes to respond. Additionally, they identify skills Bailey has to draw from to stay grounded and present in session. Meredith also encourages Bailey to consider how Carlos' actions are impacting her, and that this may be the purpose of Carlos' play – to develop resolutions to the scared and overwhelmed he experiences when he witnesses his parents' conflict.

The supervision session then turns to the here and now as Bailey and Meredith process what Bailey is feeling right now. Bailey explains that she was, "terrified to share the recording but knew she had to do it if she wanted grow as a play therapist." Meredith and Bailey spend time noting where she felt the fear in her body, what she tells herself about making professional errors, and how the supervisory relationship is multifaceted and not solely evaluative in nature. Meredith and Bailey discuss how the supervisory relationship is focused on her development as a play therapist, and that together, through open and curious dialogue, they can explore challenges and successes in Bailey's professional development.

Systemic Cognitive-Developmental Supervision

The Systemic Cognitive-Developmental Supervision (SCDS) model extends the cognitive- developmental model of Piaget to assist supervisors with understanding supervisee's needs based on their cognitive style (Bernard & Goodyear, 2014; Rigazio-DiGilio & Anderson, 1994). Through this lens, supervisors can "access and assess each supervisee's unique cognitive-developmental style in the immediacy of the supervisory process, and to then co-construct supervisory environments aimed at enhancing and expanding this style toward increased conceptual and therapeutic competence" (Rigazio-DiGilio & Anderson, 1994, p. 95). The goal of utilizing a cognitive-developmental framework is to develop richer conceptualizations of their clients and have access to increased therapeutic perspectives and approaches. This is facilitated by first assessing the supervisee's primary cognitive orientation(s), building a foundation in their primary cognitive orientation(s), and then providing questions and environments that invite the supervisee to consider other orientations (Rigazio-DiGilio & Anderson, 1994).

The SCDS model presents four primary cognitive orientations. While supervisees may operate from all four orientations, they tend to have a dominant cognitive style or method of conceptualizing. Supervisors can discern supervisee orientation by attending to the language they use and structure of their thoughts, paying close attention to specific requests for help, and asking questions that explore the boundaries of the supervisee's case conceptualization (Rigazio-DiGilio & Anderson, 1994). The following summaries of each orientation are provided, including the orientation's strengths, challenges, and requests the supervisee might have of the supervisor that indicates they are operating from this orientation.

Sensorimotor

From the sensorimotor orientation, supervisees make sense of their clinical work through their immediate sensory experiences, including emotional and visceral reactions to their working with their clients. They are aware of their own personal reactions which ease access to issues of transference and countertransference. These supervisees can track client emotions well without becoming overwhelmed, yet emotional availability may interfere with their ability to be cognitively involved and execute behavioral interventions. Supervisee's clinical interventions may be widely based on what feels right at the time, which can lack structure and promote haphazard treatment planning. Supervisees may request supervisor assistance with developing behaviorally oriented treatment plans and processing strong emotional reactions. Supervisors can utilize directive techniques including recording review, co-therapy, role play, group supervision, and experiential supervision activities, with the goal of directing attention to sensory experiences (Rigazio-DiGilio & Anderson, 1994).

Concrete

Concrete supervisees see the world through a linear, cause–effect lens which offers them a sense of predictability. They are excellent at describing the events that take place and tend to be accurate and logical. However, this can also reveal rigidity and difficulty with abstract or alternative perspectives for conceptualizing client difficulty. In supervision, these supervisees may ask for specific steps to intervention and treatment planning. Supervisors can use coaching with concrete supervisees to help them articulate if/then conceptualizations, enhance their decision-making processes, and expand their therapeutic strategies. Live supervision and co-therapy, recording review focused on skill mastery, and supervision exercises focused on intervention skills are example activities to support concrete cognitive development (Rigazio-DiGilio & Anderson, 1994).

Formal

Supervisees operating from a formal orientation can analyze situations from multiple perspectives, are naturally reflective, and can integrate multiple models of therapy into cohesive treatment plans. Issues may arise when it is time to transfer knowledge into skill in session as the therapist may intellectualize content and interventions. Additionally, supervisees may have difficulty utilizing emotional and physical reactions in counseling as data. These supervisees may request supervisor assistance with identifying and deciphering therapeutic themes among clinical cases and countertransference. Supervisors can support the development of formal cognitive skills through facilitating reflection on the patterns that emerge in therapy, and supporting reflection and integration of self-as-therapist and clinical data. Supervision may include discussing patterns across cases, and analyzing preferred and other theories of therapy (Rigazio-DiGilio & Anderson, 1994).

Dialectic/Systemic

These supervisees can challenge their own assumptions that brought them to their conceptualization of clients. Additionally, they are aware of contextual implications and aim treatment at resolving issues related to the client and their environment. These supervisees can think about their thinking which can serve as a facilitator and barrier to therapeutic progress as they may be overwhelmed by multiple options and avenues in therapy and have difficulty committing. As a result, this supervisee may ask for assistance with organizing a treatment plan. Supervisors can collaborate with supervisees to enhance their awareness of assumptions that underly therapist and client behavior, thoughts, and emotions, treatment, and supervision and to enhance their awareness of the limits of our personal experiences. Supervision strategies may include reviewing recordings, conducting co-therapy, peer consultation, and supporting vulnerable dialogue of guiding beliefs and experiences (Rigazio-DiGilio & Anderson, 1994).

Supervisors using SCDS can assess and explore supervisee's use of each cognitive orientation by examining the language they use to frame and process information. Table 3.1 has been adapted from Rigazio-DiGilio and Anderson (1994) to reflect the work of play therapists. The questions are a sampling of the potential inquiries that can glean information about cognitive style and can be adapted and expanded upon. The matrix of potential questions is designed to target supervisee's cognitive orientation and understanding at four distinct levels: client, self, therapeutic process, and supervisory process.

Example Case

At the time Bailey appears frozen in response to Carlos' play, Meredith presses pause on the recording to debrief with Bailey and check in on what cognitive data Bailey has easy access to. Meredith begins by inquiring about what has stood out to Bailey while she has watched the recording. Bailey takes a deep breath and shares that she "didn't know what to do," nothing she had read in a textbook had prepared her for the intensity of play Carlos displayed and that Bailey felt like her mind was "blank." Meredith validated Bailey's experience and reflected that Bailey seemed to be searching for the *concrete self-as-play-therapist* response to Carlos' play and could not access a response in the moment. Using Bailey's strength as a concrete cognitive processor now, Meredith explored other levels (client, play therapy process, supervision process) of entry within the concrete domain. At the client level, the dyad mapped the sequence of Carlos' play that unfolded, writing them on paper in a timeline format. The timeline was meant to enhance the opportunity to visualize what unfolded. Then, they mapped the play therapy responses that Bailey was accessing during the session. Through the addition of the play therapy processes and responses to the timeline, Bailey could see a distinct time when access to her play therapy knowledge and skills seemed to cease. Critical to Bailey's growth, they had identified the point of flooding and dysregulation in this session.

Next, Meredith helped Bailey identify her sensorimotor experiences of the session. Since flooding seemed to be a critical supervision issue, exploring the sensory data Bailey encountered will assist her in identifying future moments of flooding, and rehearsing coping strategies to support her presence in play therapy. Meredith and Bailey closely explored Bailey's sensory experiences before, during, and after the encounter with Carlos, and added the emotions and physical sensations Bailey experienced to the timeline. Then, they expanded to explore the sensorimotor experiences of Carlos as well as the interplay of senses present in the play therapy relationship. By this point, the timeline had rich data to process across two cognitive domains.

In the remaining 20 minutes of supervision, Meredith makes an important supervisory shift from the relationship with Carlos to the relationship between her and Bailey. Next, the two discuss the sensorimotor experiences that Bailey has in her supervisory relationship with Meredith. They explore how Bailey is experiencing supervision in the present moment, including her affective, cognitive,

Table 3.1 Questions Associated with Each Orientation

Supervisee Cognitive orientation	Client	Self-as-Play-Therapist	Play Therapy Process	Supervision Process
Sensori-motor	How does this child express emotion? What verbal and nonverbal behaviors are helpful in understanding this child?	What did you feel during this session? Where in your body did you feel this? What did you choose to do to make sense of this feeling?	How are your feelings about this child impacting how you respond? How is this child feeling toward you?	How are your feelings about supervision affecting you now? How do you feel before you come to supervision? After?
Concrete	What did the child say? What did the child do next?	What did you do? What could you do to improve that intervention or technique?	What verbal and nonverbal data prompted your response? What did you think would happen? What happened? What did you do next?	What do we do in supervision that is helpful for you? Unhelpful? How would you describe what we have been doing in supervision?
Formal	How do you conceptualize the way this child understands and responds to the problem? Does the child always respond this way? When do they respond differently?	Does your personal reaction to this client or situation seem familiar to you? Have you behaved or responded in similar ways in relationships with other people?	What types of interventions might fit best with this child? What repeating patterns of interaction have you observed with this client?	How is our relationship like others in your life? What patterns seem to be occurring in our relationship?
Dialectic/Systemic	What rules or beliefs is this child operating from? Can these rules or beliefs be challenged? Where, when, and how were these beliefs or rules established? How is the child's culture impacting them?	What rules or beliefs are you operating from? What flaws are in these rules or beliefs? How can these rules or beliefs be changed? What would happen as a result?	What assumptions are you making about Carlos? His family? His foster family? How are these assumptions impacting your therapeutic work? What patterns of behavior or interaction are involved in your work with this child? How could you see these patterns differently?	What are our expectations of each other in supervision? How are these expectations benefiting us? Challenging us? How do our cultural differences come into play in this relationship?

and physical responses. Bailey sketches a timeline in her supervision notebook for today's meeting (there is her concrete strength again). On the timeline for today's meeting, she notes the excitement she feels before supervision because she enjoys her time with Meredith. She also notes some feelings of suspicion that she has. She wonders how Meredith perceives her time with Bailey and if she values their relationship in the same ways Bailey does. This important disclosure opens the dialogue about the nature of their supervision relationship. The two discuss how their supervision relationship is similar and dissimilar to other present and historic relationships in their professional lives. In this process, Bailey and Meredith share their affective, cognitive, and physical reactions to their present relationship. They discuss their racial and cultural differences and similarities, which continued to a discussion of the important racial and cultural differences and similarities of Bailey and Carlos, too.

Rønnestad & Skovholt Lifespan Developmental Model

Seeking to understand how therapists develop as they gain experience, Rønnestad and Skovholt (1991) explored therapist development across the lifespan. Initially, an eight-stage model of counselor development emerged from multiple interviews with 100 therapists who had diverse years of experience in the field (Rønnestad & Skovholt, 1991). Through ongoing interviews and analyses of data, authors developed a phase model of therapist development and formulated themes to describe therapist development (Rønnestad & Skovholt, 2003). It is worth noting that this model is descriptive rather than prescriptive in the work of the clinical supervisor and supervisee (Bernard & Goodyear, 2014). There are six phases of therapist development as described by Rønnestad and Skovholt (2003):

1. Lay Helper Phase includes the non-professional helping roles of parent, child, friend, and colleague. In this Lay Helper Phase, individuals help solve problems, offer emotional support, and may provide advice, all of which stem from their personal experiences. Within this phase, issues of over-involvement and boundaries are a concern.
2. Beginning Student Phase describes the exciting start of professional training. This phase is characterized by an emphasis on external feedback, dependence, vulnerability, anxiety, and self-doubt as the student encounters their first client experiences. Faculty and supervisors play a critical role in offering support and encouragement for continued therapist development. Supervisees' openness to learning and willingness to recognize the complexity of professional work is critical for growth.
3. Advanced Student Phase is characterized by the student who has begun their field placement. While there is still much to learn, the advanced student tends to rigidly apply knowledge and skills. Supervisors play a major role in this phase as they model professional behaviors, support student therapist growth, and evaluate the supervisee. This phase is also oriented toward external feedback as the supervisee is continuously evaluated by others.

4. Novice Professional Phase is typically contained in the first five years after graduation. In this phase, supervisees are experiencing independence. Supervisees seek to test the knowledge they gained from training and confirm or discredit its utility. Disillusionment can accompany this independence and assume personal responsibility for client healing. This stage typically begins the process of internal focus as increased attention is placed on integration of the personal self with professional training. At this phase, therapeutic relationships and boundary management are a major focus.

5. Experienced Professional Phase describes the therapist who has been practicing for years with a wide variety of clients. A task at this stage is to develop a congruent working style. The therapeutic relationship is understood as crucial for client success. Use of techniques and methods are fluid and personalized. Supervisees experience increased confidence in professional judgment, clinical skills, and comfort with ambiguity. While theory remains important in clinical work, greater learning is garnered from interpersonal experiences in professional and personal relationships.

6. Senior Professional Phase describes an established professional who has more than 20 years of experience in the field. The senior professional has an established authentic therapeutic style. While there may be feelings of intellectual apathy or boredom, most at this phase describe a commitment to continued professional growth. Professionals have a deep sense of self-acceptance and work satisfaction as they mentor and usher in the next generation of professional helpers.

Upon establishing the phases of development, Rønnestad and Skovholt (2003) expanded their research to examine developmental themes of therapists across the career lifespan. These themes are descriptive and describe the activities that often occur within the phases. Next is a summary of the themes. A complete review of the themes can be found in Rønnestad and Skovholt (2003).

Theme 1: Professional Development Involves an Increasing Higher Order Integration of the Professional Self and the Personal Self. Across phases of development, play therapists increase the congruence between their personality and their theory of preference. Additionally, therapists can naturally apply therapeutic techniques in their work. As a result of continued personalization of therapeutic approach, the therapist defines their role in the therapeutic relationship more effectively and more effectively connects with the client.

Theme 2: The Focus of Functioning Shifts Dramatically Over Time: From Internal to External to Internal. At the beginning phase, helping behavior is conventional as opposed to practical. Helping behaviors are internally selected by personal opinions and preferences. As formal training begins, supervisees suppress personal approaches and rigidly apply externally derived professional theories and methods. After training and with experience, supervisees renew their internal focus as increased self-awareness integrates with professional practice.

Theme 3: Continuous Reflection Is a Prerequisite for Optimal Learning and Professional Development at All Levels of Experience. The ability to reflect on professional experiences and challenges is necessary to foster learning and development. Supervision can facilitate supervisee's reflective capacities.

Theme 4: An Intense Commitment to Learn Propels the Developmental Process. A drive to learn and appropriate risk-taking increases professional functioning across phases. Of note, learning and expanding use of skills is not solely for the novice therapist but also contributes to a sense of professional growth for therapists with decades of experience.

Theme 5: The Cognitive Map Changes: Beginning Practitioners Rely on External Expertise, Seasoned Practitioners Rely on Internal Expertise. Consistent with Themes 1 and 2, early phases of development rely on supervisor instruction and didactic experiences. As phases progress, supervisee self-direction of learning emerges and experienced clinicians seek information from professional literature, peers, and professional training opportunities.

Theme 6: Professional Development Is a Long, Slow, Continuous Process That Can Also Be Erratic. Professional development is a continuous process of mastery. While it is happening, it may seem slow and unnoticeable. However, in retrospect, development can seem substantial. Additionally, critical incidents or profound personal events can intensify the development process. Regardless, development is not viewed as linear, and is instead perceived as recycling loops of uncertainty, challenges, and mastery.

Theme 7: Professional Development Is a Life-Long Process. In line with Theme 4, professional learning exists across the phases of career development. Needs, interests, and motivations may shift, however commitment to grow must remain intact.

Theme 8: Many Beginning Practitioners Experience Much Anxiety in Their Professional Work. Over Time, Anxiety is Mastered by Most. The anxiety of the beginning therapist is well documented in the literature. High performance anxiety and presence of evaluation contribute to pervasive fear for early phase clinicians. As experience increases, feelings of competence increase as anxiety decreases.

Theme 9: Clients Serve as a Major Source of Influence and Serve as Primary Teachers. Across theoretical orientation and geographic borders, therapists concur that their clients are the primary source of professional development.

Theme 10: Personal Life Influences Professional Functioning and Development Throughout the Professional Life Span. Challenges in early life and adult life exert influence on professional development – both positively and negatively.

Theme 11: Interpersonal Sources of Influence Propel Professional Development More than "Impersonal" Sources of Influence. Not meant to discount professional academic training for helpers, post-training relationships with clients, supervisors, and peers provided meaningful learning and growth opportunities.

Theme 12: New Members of the Field View Professional Elders and Graduate Training With Strong Affective Reactions. Power differentials in early phase evaluative relationships in academic and supervisory settings set up trainees to either scrutinize or admire the senior member's behaviors and actions. As the clinician develops and experiences their own professional development, they begin to recognize their professional elders humanness.

Theme 13: Extensive Experience with Suffering Contributes to Heightened Recognition, Acceptance, and Appreciation of Human Variability. Wisdom is developed by insight, introspection and reflection on personal and professional experiences, and their combined exertion of influence.

Theme 14: For the Practitioner There Is a Realignment from Self as Hero to Client as Hero. As phases of development advance, a shift in understanding of power of the therapist to power of the client is realized.

Across the career lifespan, optimal professional development at all phases is enhanced by the ability and willingness to engage in continued reflection, an attitude of openness to new learning, and acknowledgment and respect for the complexity of therapeutic work. Critical to therapist development is the process and reflection of professional difficulties and challenges. On the contrary, lack of reflection, and defensive or distorted processing of therapeutic difficulties and challenges will result in professional stagnation (Rønnestad & Skovholt, 2003).

Example Case

In the case of Bailey, who is in the Novice Professional Phase of development, Meredith recognizes that Bailey has important clinical, personal, and supervisory experiences that have shaped her professional development to date. Bailey is enjoying some confidence and independence as she gains clinical and play therapy experience. Typical of this phase, Meredith will want to pay attention to Bailey's feelings around the meaning and value of Carlos' session behavior. Bailey may internalize that something she did in session caused the play behavior, and while this may have some influence, there is more than Bailey influencing Carlos' play. Meredith may choose to explore how Bailey feels about Carlos after observing this play as well as potential indications for need for limit setting in play therapy to assist Carlos in healing. In addition, learning more about Bailey's experience of her own culture and disconnection, and how this impacts her clinical work will be critical to her professional development. Meredith and Bailey will also benefit from exploring how important supervisory themes may be influencing Bailey's responses to Carlos, and Meredith's responses to Bailey. Reviewing the list of themes together, the supervisory dyad can explore client–play therapist influences and discuss how the interplay of Bailey's development, Carlos' circumstances and development, and the supervisory relationship all influence Bailey's professional development.

Psychotherapy-Based Models of Supervision

As independent mental health practitioners, all play therapists are trained in psychotherapy theories. Early approaches to clinical supervision were commonly influenced by theoretical approaches to counseling and the same can be observed by reviewing the supervision in play therapy literature, too. In terms of play therapy theory driving supervision practice, most writing reflects on the child-centered theory that the field of play therapy was founded upon. While this seems appropriate, it also invites the opportunity to expand writing and research to reflect other play therapy theories. Psychotherapy-theory–based supervision serves an important role in teaching, refining, and evaluating the theories that drive play therapy practice.

Psychodynamic Supervision

Because of the longevity, diversity, and richness of their conceptualizations, psychodynamic approaches have been infused throughout models of supervision (Bernard & Goodyear, 2014). Psychodynamic supervision is a teaching and learning process that emphasizes the relationships between and among the client, therapist, and supervisor (Bernard & Goodyear, 2014; Ekstein & Wallerstein, 1972). As psychodynamic therapy has evolved, the focus of psychodynamic supervision has, too. Early psychodynamic supervision was patient-centered, where supervisors employed direct support for the supervisees to explore patient behaviors and select treatment accordingly (Frawley-O'Dea & Sarnat, 2001; Smith, 2009). Later psychodynamic supervision evolved to being supervisee-focused, where greater attention was placed on the process and experience of the supervisee. This approach facilitated increased supervisee self-awareness into their own thoughts, feelings, apprehensions, and learning challenges (Ekstein & Wallerstein, 1972; Frawley-O'Dea & Sarnat, 2001; Smith, 2009). Both approaches placed emphasis on the supervisor as an expert of psychodynamic theory and technique (Bernard & Goodyear, 2014).

More recently, Frawley-O'Dea and Sarnat (2001) proposed a relational model of psychodynamic supervision where supervisors focus on the therapeutic and supervisory relationship to enhance essential relationship competence in psychodynamic therapy. The relational model includes three key dimensions: (1) the supervisor's authority, (2) the supervisor's focus, and (3) the supervisor's mode of participation. First, the supervisor's authority is understood by the supervisor's power in their field through the acquisition of knowledge and experience that equips them to train and mentor supervisees. However, this power does not extend to knowing more about the knowledge and experiences of the supervisee. The supervisor and supervisee develop shared power and authority in supervisory relationship which may include the supervisor utilizing appropriate self-disclosures and open discussion of countertransference (Frawley-O'Dea & Sarnat, 2001; Sarnat, 2010).

The second dimension orients the direction of the supervisor's focus. The supervisor may focus attention on the client, the supervisee, or the relationship between the supervisor and supervisee. The third dimension is the supervisor's primary mode of participation (Frawley-O'Dea & Sarnat, 2001). Rather than approaching supervision from a didactic position, a modern and relational psychodynamic approach emphasizes the dynamics and processes of the supervisory relationship and how those may play out in the client–therapist relationship. Through the stimulation of cognitive, linguistic, affective, somatic, and relational responses within supervision, and of the supervisee and supervisors to the patient, supervisee growth is illuminated (Frawley-O'Dea & Sarnat, 2001).

Example Case

While both Bailey and Meredith resonate with a child-centered approach to play therapy, considering the utility of psychodynamic play therapy supervision strategies support the examination of the supervisory relationship between Bailey and Meredith, so that it can influence Bailey's therapeutic work with clients. Bailey and Meredith review the three key dimensions of their work together, in the context of Carlos' session they had viewed. Meredith decided to guide the conversation in exploring the impact of power in supervision. The two explore the systemic and historical influences of power among them, and then focus into the interplay of power in the supervisory relationship. Bailey notes to Meredith that she had some reservations about working with a White supervisor, as she was not confident that Meredith would understand her experiences of race and culture and a multiracial play therapist. This important dialogue illuminated the implicit expectations that can be created and maintained in supervision if not made explicit. Further, the supervisory dyad was able to clarify cognitions and emotions that had surfaced. This important dialogue enhanced Bailey's understanding of power in her play therapy relationships, too. Bailey noted that her physical presence, and what sometimes appeared to be physical similarities and differences with her clients, were creating implicit assumptions in her therapeutic work. The supervisory dyad discussed the implications of this new insight and methods for navigating important conversations in Bailey's play therapy work.

Humanistic/Child-Centered Supervision

A humanistic or child-centered approach in supervision has received more attention in play therapy literature, mainly because of their critical influence in the development of the field of play therapy. Like child-centered play therapy, humanistic supervision emphasizes the facilitative conditions provided by the supervisor that guides supervisees toward increased self-awareness and growth (Farber, 2010). The inherent attitudinal qualities of humanistic supervisors include congruence, unconditional positive regard, and empathic understanding supervisors. In supervision, congruence is a combination of self-awareness and an ability to authentically express the self. Unconditional positive regard is essential in humanistic supervision. This is an important action to make known that regardless of skill level, the supervisor is still accepting of the supervisee as a person. This is meant to reduce the sense that a supervisee is worthy only based on their skills or performance as a play therapist. Unconditional positive regard can come into conflict with the evaluative nature of supervision, though it is not impossible to navigate. Conveying empathic understanding from the supervisor to the supervisee facilitates safety and reduced anxiety (Ray, 2011).

The relationship facilitated by the humanistic approach is essential to client and supervisee growth. Humanistic supervisors' authentic display of acceptance and presence provides the felt sense of safety in a relationship that supports growth (Farber, 2010). This felt sense of safety enhances supervisee's ability to use their self as a change agent in therapy. Additionally, supervision strategies focus on in-session relationship dynamics of the supervisee and client, and empathic responding. Landreth (2012) emphasizes the critical necessity of reviewing recorded sessions and engaging in ongoing supervision, consultation, and self-supervision as necessary to continued learning about self.

The goal of humanistic supervision is to facilitate increased self-confidence and self-awareness, and to utilize the supervisory relationship to promote change (Farber, 2010; Rogers, 1961). This non-directive supervisory approach requires the supervisor to have a deep trust in the supervisee's self-growth process, the power of the supervisory relationship, and the inherent belief that humans are motivated to grow (Rogers, 1961). Rogers (1961) emphasized that supervision was about helping the therapist to gain self-confidence and self-awareness, while also increasing their understanding of the therapeutic process (Hackney & Goodyear, 1984). A humanistic approach to supervision is not solely didactic. Instead, it relies on a combination of teaching and therapeutic techniques provided by the supervisor. Humanistic supervisors support supervisees by understanding the unique developmental needs of the supervisee, increasing supervisees' knowledge of theory and technique, the person-of-the-therapist, and the use of self to facilitate change (Farber, 2010).

Landreth (2012) highlights important person-of-the-therapist qualities that are necessary for facilitating child-centered play therapy, including: (1) creating differences, (2) being with, (3) personality characteristics, (4) play therapist self-understanding, and (5) play therapist self-acceptance. First, *creating differences* in play therapy includes the felt sense of the play therapy relationship between the child and the therapist. These differences are sensed by the conditions facilitated through the play therapist's unconditional acceptance of the child, respect for the child's pace and present functioning, and attuned sensitivity to the expressions of the child. *Being with* is facilitated by the play therapist's present attention to the child including their active observation and listening, as well as the verbalizations that convey empathy, encouragement, and understanding (Landreth, 2012).

Essential *personality characteristics* of child-centered play therapists include objectivity and flexibility – this includes the ability for the therapist to appreciate and attempt to understand the child's world, and that the child's experience of their world is dynamic. Personality characteristics also include refraining from judgment and evaluation of the child because it is the therapist's responsibility to accept the child's current verbal and nonverbal behaviors and meet the child where they presently are. Further, child-centered play therapists should be open-minded, patient, and have a high tolerance for ambiguity which emphasizes the necessity for therapists to respect and trust the child's process. Additional personality characteristics include having courage and personal security to be vulnerable, take risks, and act on intuitive feelings that emerge from therapeutic encounters. Belief that children are capable of growth and not imposing restrictions on the child's desires based on historical activities or verbalizations to grow are necessary. Last, and perhaps most importantly, play therapists personality characteristics should also include warmth, sensitivity, and a sense of humor. Children are the most apt at detecting phony behaviors. Child-centered play therapists must convey these sentiments through the felt sense of the relationship, their therapeutic actions, and verbal responses (Landreth, 2012).

Play therapist self-understanding is critical for all play therapists. From a child-centered supervision perspective it includes the necessity to discuss and explore therapists' motivation and needs. Landreth (2012) suggests important points of reflection for supervisees including:

- What needs of mine are being met in play therapy?
- How strong is my need to be needed?
- Do I like this child?
- Do I want to be with this child?
- What impact do my attitudes and feelings have on this child?
- How does this child perceive me? (p. 105)

Child-centered play therapy is a function of the play therapist's beliefs about themselves and children. Exploring these items is necessary to explore the consequences of the therapist's expectations of the therapeutic relationship. As child-centered play therapists convey acceptance of the child in the present moment, they must also convey *play therapist self-acceptance*. Therapist self-acceptance allows the therapist to attend to personal reactions that may have historical and personal implications and those that may be presently associated with the child. This self-acceptance is an ongoing process of exploration and discovery, and an openness to continuously learn and grow (Landreth, 2012).

Strategies to develop the person-of-the-therapist include helping supervisees reflect on their experiences of being with clients in the present moment. Early career supervisees may benefit from supervision that is focused on increasing supervisees' self-confidence. As confidence grows, the supervisor can expand the focus of supervision to include person-of-the-therapist and use of self to facilitate change. To increase knowledge and techniques, humanistic supervisors will assist supervisees in developing clinical impressions that integrate both verbal and nonverbal aspects of sessions. With person-of-the-therapist in the primary focus of humanistic supervision, skill development is secondary (Landreth, 2012). The Play Therapy Skills Checklist (PTSC, available in Landreth, 2012) helps play therapists focus on child-centered play therapy verbal and nonverbal skills.

Example Case

After viewing the recording where Meredith and Bailey each completed the PTSC while viewing, Meredith requested that she and Bailey set the PTSC aside and focus supervision time reflecting on Bailey's experience of her self-as-therapist with Carlos. Of important supervisory focus for Meredith and Bailey will be paying close attention to Bailey's experiences of being with Carlos. Discussing the present experiences of Carlos will lead to important revelations of Bailey's self-understanding and self-acceptance – not only within her therapeutic relationship with Carlos, but also with her supervisory relationship with Meredith. It will be critical for Meredith to facilitate the felt sense of safety conveyed in her unconditional positive regard and empathy for Bailey. Meredith and Bailey discuss in detail some of Bailey's feelings about Carlos, including some resonant frustration with Carlos' foster family regarding their disclosure of picking Bailey based on the "sound" of her last name. Bringing to the surface these important feelings will help Bailey differentiate the emotions as her own and separate from her feelings about Carlos. It turns out these feelings were impacting Bailey's willingness and ability to be vulnerable, attuned, and emotionally available to Carlos as his emotions grew in play.

Cognitive-Behavioral Supervision

Cognitive-behavioral supervision is another psychotherapy-based supervision model. This approach tends to place emphasis on the foundational components of the cognitive-behavioral approach, linking cognitions and behaviors to the supervisee's therapeutic work. The supervision session therefore tends to be structured, with an agenda set and tasks assigned to bridge concepts between supervision sessions (Smith, 2009).

Cognitive behavioral therapy (CBT) was initially recognized in 1979 (Beck et al., 1979). CBT practitioners understand the scientific foundations of the theory while considering limitations related to empirical findings, cognitive styles, selective attention and recall, and schemas (Newman, 2010). The therapeutic relationship holds great importance within this model while emphasis is also placed on empirical-thinking practices and decision-making. It is within these practice principals and substantial evidence (Roth & Pilling, 2008) that CBT has gained acceptance in insurance, governmental, and managed care entities (Reiser & Milne, 2012).

CBT, from a play therapy perspective is better known as cognitive behavioral play therapy (CBPT). Susan Knell is credited for this creation, considering the theory and techniques of cognitive therapy and behavior therapy, to establish a developmentally appropriate cognitive behavioral model for work with children (Knell, 1993, 2003). Adapted interventions therefore include recording of dysfunctional thoughts, countering irrational beliefs, and using coping self-statements (O'Connor et al., 2016). Interventions are made possible by use of modeling, role-playing, and behavioral contingencies (toys, stuffed animals, puppets) (Knell, 1993). Further research pertaining to CBPT has promoted the model's effectiveness in treating trauma, depression, and post-traumatic stress disorder from a developmentally sensitive approach (Shelby, 2000; Shelby & Felix, 2005). The model has seen effectiveness treating encopresis, phobias, selective mutism, and separation anxiety (O'Connor et al., 2016).

Supervision within the cognitive behavioral therapy (CBT) model has continuously evolved over the past decade (Reiser & Milne, 2012). While research trends are limited, continued advancement efforts are taking shape. CBT supervision competencies have been further defined in the Improving Access to Psychological

Therapies (IAPT) program, which places emphasis on defining competency frameworks within each therapeutic model. CBT specific supervision therefore includes direct observation and the use of standardized outcome monitoring tools meant to track client progress (Reiser & Milne, 2012). These tools coincide with the structure implemented by a CBT session. These include a check-in, return-to-previous-session, agenda-setting, completion of agenda items, summary, homework considerations, and feedback (Reiser & Milne, 2012). However, continued research fails to conclusively detail a method for assessing competencies within the model (Roth & Pilling, 1992).

Example Case

An agenda guides Meredith and Bailey in CBT supervision. This process is similar to that of a CBT session, incorporating a check-in, discussion of the previous session, agenda, summarizing, assigning homework, and answering questions (Reiser & Milne, 2012). After observing the session between Bailey and Carlos, Meredith outlines a possible agenda to include exploration of Bailey's cognitions prior to meeting with Carlos on this specific day, along with cognitions that arose at various stages of the play therapy session. She may also wish to explore personal interpretations of the behaviors presented and how those have further developed from Session Two to Session Three. This may help Meredith to understand why Bailey stopped tracking Carlos when his behaviors became more aggressive, and subsequently froze.

Within the structure of the supervision session, Meredith would also place emphasis on understanding Bailey's problem-solving abilities, therapeutic techniques, and overall rapport with Carlos (Reiser & Milne, 2012). Bailey may be tasked with identifying goals for the supervision meeting, which could include exploration of her own hesitancies or even ideas for therapeutic interventions. Meredith would likely consider how Bailey responded to Carlos at various phases of the play therapy session and therefore explore how decisions were made. Bailey would consider the techniques implemented, which included tracking, and consider the verbal responses she offered to Carlos during his play. Meredith would also assess Bailey's rapport with Carlos and how this impacted Bailey's comfort level when Carlos began to shift his play. At the end of the supervision session, Meredith would assign a homework assignment to Bailey to support further growth in her work with Carlos. To honor Bailey's words of feeling "culturally disconnected," Meredith and Bailey co-create professional and cultural identity goals to incorporate into their supervision time. The two agree that exploring Bailey's cultural identity outside of her professional identity will be an important starting point in crystalizing her professional identity.

Systemic Models

Whereas the previously discussed psychotherapy supervision models focus on the intrapersonal and interpersonal dynamics of clients and supervisees, systemic clinical supervision expands the context to the multiple systems at play within each case. The systemic supervisor attends to the interlocking system dynamics including within the family, between the family and the supervisee (therapist), as well as the dynamics at play between the supervisor and the supervisee (Bernard & Goodyear, 2014). The following discussion will weave an overarching systems approach to clinical supervision and the specific ties to play therapy rather than review any specific family systems theory.

A systemic supervisor helps supervisees develop a systems lens of case conceptualization by inviting all relevant perspectives and exploring the family process (Celano et al., 2010; Storm & Todd, 2014). Supervisees are encouraged to reframe the family problems and dynamics to help families see more productive ways to approach them and more effectively navigate the negative interactions that unfold during therapy. Systemic supervisors also help the supervisee build a therapeutic relationship with all family members, not just the child or parental subsystems. They acknowledge the complexity of the supervision process by proactively responding to the web of intersecting relationships and isomorphic dynamics (Storm & Todd, 2014).

There are two seminal concepts within systemic clinical supervision that supervisors are keen to attend to which include the presences of isomorphism (i.e., parallel processing or the replication of dynamics that occur between therapy and supervision) and the supervisee's family of origin (i.e., the family they were born into and/or raised within). Within systems theory it is understood that a therapist inherently joins the family system during the helping process. Consequently, developing a supervisee's awareness to their potential blind-spots and/or unconscious biases and increasing their level of differentiation is integral to the supervision process. For example, a play therapist supervisee who grew up in a family where they served a role as the parentified child, may have the tendency to align with and/or unintentionally resent the parental subsystem of the family. Moreover, the isomorphic dynamic could be replicated in group supervision where the supervisee may try and overly caretake clinical cases of their peers.

Example Case

When applying the system supervision models to the case of Bailey, the Meredith may first explore elements of Bailey's personal family of origin. Meredith may ask questions such as, "In what ways was your childhood similar to Carlos's? In what ways was your childhood different from Carlos's? How are you similar to Carlos now?" These questions provide opportunity for the supervisor to help Bailey grow in her awareness of the dynamics and characteristics she is bringing into the playroom as well as foster insight into her decreased tracking of Carlos's play. Moreover, questions such as, "Who does Carlos, or this case, remind you of?" support supervision inquiry to explore isomorphic patterns. By encouraging Bailey to identify similar structures and dynamics experienced in her own life, she will expand her awareness of potential patterns in which her interactions may unintentionally be replicating or reinforcing Carlos's problematic experiences. Of course, it is important to emphasize here that supervision is not counseling, and exploration of a supervisee's family-of-origin dynamics should be carefully balanced so as to not become counseling.

In addition to family-of-origin dynamics, a systemic supervisor would help Bailey explore multiple ways of reframing Carlos's aggression and defiance both in and out of the playroom. Systemic approaches posit that problem behaviors are attempted solutions to other problems so Meredith may ask Bailey to hypothesize, "What problems does Carlos's aggression and defiance attempt to solve? What feelings, experiences, or dynamics does Carlos change when he uses his aggression and defiance?" These questions expand the perspective of the problem and facilitate a discussion that helps Bailey better understand Carlos's motivation and experience. At this point it could also be helpful to practice with Bailey ways she might test her hypotheses using reflections of meaning during Carlos's aggressive play in the playroom.

Constructivist Models

Constructivist models of supervision embrace the core philosophies of constructivist and postmodern psychotherapy models. These models are joined together by an appreciation of multiple perspectives, viewpoints, realities, and a belief that truth and knowledge are shared and created by social interactions (Bernard & Goodyear, 2014; Whiting, 2007). There is also an emphasis on meaning-making and the assumption that meaning is transitory and subject to change and evolves over time (Bobele et al., 2014). Supervision, like therapy, then becomes about co-creation and development of new meanings rather than finding the "right" way to work with a client (Philp et al., 2007). The constructivist supervisor will constantly adjust their role (i.e., teacher, consultant, supervisor, coach, etc.) to meet the needs of the supervision dynamics (Bobele et al., 2014). In doing so, they encourage and provide space to help supervisees develop new meaning to their supervision experience. Instead of viewing themselves as a trainee looking for advice from their supervisor, developing play therapists embrace their own approach to explore multiple ideas to use during therapy. Two common approaches, Narrative and Solution-Focused, are discussed to illustrate how they may be applied to the case of Bailey.

Narrative

Much like in narrative therapy, where the therapist serves as an editor to help the client consider and/or change their story to a narrative that serves them better, the supervisor helps the supervisee edit their stories as developing professionals. Supervisors help the supervisee externalize the problems they may be experiencing during therapy and identify internalized socially constructed messages that may be present during the therapeutic work (Zeligman, 2017). They walk with the supervisee to explore "the subjunctive ('as if') rather than the indicative ('this is the way it is')" (Bernard and Goodyear, 2014, p. 31) and use storying, active dialogue, to explore dynamics of power, oppression, and meaning (Zeligman, 2017).

During narrative supervision, a collaborative supervisory relationship is essential to create a safe environment to elicit and explore these stories and experiences; however, the supervisor is careful to not wade into the waters of therapy (Bobele et al., 2014). Group supervision and the use of reflecting teams can limit the blurring of boundaries and deter the discussion from becoming "therapy focused". The varied use of supervision methods (e.g., live supervision, group supervision, reflecting teams) are highly encouraged during narrative supervision to promote new perspectives on cases and greater awareness and exploration of the non-dominant discourses. Furthermore, the consideration of social influence on the supervisee's experience as well as the client's experience has made narrative supervision a natural fit for culturally diverse populations (McLean & Marini, 2008).

Example Case

Over the course of the last nine months, Bailey and Meredith have formed a collaborative, safe supervisory relationship both during individual supervision as well as group supervision. In this narrative supervision example, Bailey is joined by a fellow play therapy supervisee, Sara, for a triadic supervision session. Meredith pauses the recording following Carlos's comment, "Look what you made me do!" and begins the supervisory discussion by asking Bailey, "I am wondering what you were feeling at that moment"? She continues to explore Bailey's experience by inquiring, with Bailey, what she brings to the play therapy room with Carlos. During this storying dialogue, Bailey shares that she feels unprepared to work with Carlos despite sharing a Latino culture. She reported that she has very little experience and understanding of what life is like for those in foster care. Meredith than invites Bailey and Sara to share what they know about foster care and custody concerns in their community to explore possible biases as well as strengths. Sara then offers her unique perspective by sharing some personal stories of her time in foster care. Meredith prompts Bailey to identify any surprising insights from Sara's experience that may have challenged her local narrative about the foster care system and Carlos's experience both in and out of the playroom. This storying dialogue allows Bailey the opportunity to edit not only her understanding of the client, but also the narrative she has about her skills and knowledge as a developing play therapist.

Solution-Focused

Solution-focused supervision is grounded in the core assumptions of postmodern and constructivism discussed above. However, the emphasis on supervisee strengths and the focus on their development rather than mistakes makes this model unique (Koob, 2002). A supervisor from this approach believes that competency comes from all aspects of the play therapist's life – not just professional experiences (Thomas, 1994), and utilizes presuppositional language with the supervisee. There is also acknowledgment that solutions may not be directly related to the problem at hand. Supervisors will invite supervisees to consider the *miracle question*: "Suppose a miracle has occurred and the problem you are experiencing with your client or this case has magically disappeared. What is the first think that you notice is different that will let you know, this miracle has occurred?" Utilizing this type of questioning provides supervisees the opportunity to create a blueprint to possible solutions where the problem is no longer a problem.

Example Case

In the example with Bailey, the Meredith may start the supervisory session with strength-based prompts to foster self-efficacy (e.g., "Tell me the best thing you did with Carlos this week," "Talk about the aspects of your counseling skills that have most improved since last week"). However, despite Meredith's direct efforts to encourage successes and competency, Bailey, finds herself stuck in "problem talk" and Bailey fixates her attention on the shift in her responses during Carlos' play. She comments that she should have responded better, but found herself stuck and surprised by his play, unable to think of the best most therapeutic response. Meredith may use this opportunity to explore with Bailey what *better* and *most therapeutic* looks like. She might ask Bailey, "As you grow in your skills, how will you know your responses are better and more therapeutic? What would you be doing differently?" In this discussion, opportunities to identify past successes and skills could be explored, such as, "Tell me a time when you felt surprised by a child's play and responded therapeutically." By embracing a curiosity of past success, the supervisor encourages an assumption of competency and self-efficacy for the supervisee to continue more of what is working.

Process Models

Process models of supervision describe the process of supervision itself. Process models of supervision can be utilized with any play therapy theoretical orientation and are accordant with developmental models. A benefit of process models of supervision is their structure and multidimensionality. Further, process models illuminate diverse roles and factors that influence supervision (Bernard & Goodyear, 2014). The following is a review of Bernard's Discrimination Model and the Systemic Approach to Supervision.

Bernard's Discrimination Model

The Discrimination Model focuses attention on the supervisee in action. Supervisors respond to supervisees from one of three roles to address supervisees' skills: intervention skills, conceptualization skills, and personalization skills. Intervention skills include the purposeful behaviors the supervisee uses during session and can range from causal behaviors including greeting clients to more complex behaviors of providing empathy, immediacy, and interpretation. Conceptualization skills are more subtle and include the supervisee's ability to make sense of the client content, identify themes in session, and to discriminate what content is essential to counseling and what is not. Additionally, the conceptualization skills include the supervisee's choice of responses to client content. Personalization skills encompass the supervisee's personality and culture (Bernard, 1997).

The supervisor's role is to assess potential skill deficits and aid the supervisee in addressing the deficit. To do so, the supervisor must build a relationship with the supervisee in which identifying clinical skills and improving upon them can be done in a safe and productive manner. The supervisor assumes three roles that they may adopt for the purpose of addressing skill building: teacher, counselor, and consultant. As a teacher, the supervisor takes responsibility for what the supervisee needs to learn to increase their competency and evaluates this learning. As a counselor, the supervisee is addressing the intrapersonal or interpersonal reality of the supervisee. In the counselor role, the supervisor is "likely to instigate moments for the trainee when things 'come together,' when thoughts, behavior, and personal reality merge to enhance professional development" (Bernard, 1997, p. 312). As a consultant, the supervisor and supervisee share responsibility for the supervisee's learning. The consultant role requires the supervisee to have autonomy and confidence and for the supervisor to be comfortable creating context for learning as opposed to direction for learning. The supervisor is a resource to the supervisee, but the supervisee is encouraged to trust their own reactions and insights about the work with their clients (Bernard, 1997).

The Discrimination Model supplies supervisors with a framework of supervision choices. Within each role, the supervisor may address the focus of supervision on a particular skillset. However, the initial focus is an entry point only, as different supervisor roles and supervisee skills may be addressed as the supervision session unfolds. Additionally, supervisors should be aware of their preferred role to supervise from, and actively reflect on, the needs of the supervisee to match their role; it is worth nothing that there are many potential supervisor interventions to consider, just as there are many potential therapeutic responses. Thus, the intention of the Discrimination Model is to consider multiple responses and evaluate the response that may support the most optimal supervisee development (Bernard, 1997).

Example Case

Using the case, an example of the framework of the Discrimination Model in play therapy supervision is presented in Table 3.2.

Systems Approach to Supervision

While several systemic models of supervision exist, the Systems Approach to Supervision (SAS) Model offers a seven-dimension model that was developed

Table 3.2 Discrimination Model Example Using the Case of Bailey and Carlos

Skill of Focus	Supervisor Role		
	Teacher	Counselor	Consultant
Intervention	Supervisor may verbally model potential responses to Carlos's play.	Supervisor reflects Bailey's lack of response to Carlos's play and the power of this response to blocking therapeutic progress.	Supervisor discusses with Bailey the potential responses or interventions to Carlos's play and considers how Carlos might respond.
Conceptualization	Supervisor reviews developmental impacts of witnessing domestic violence with Bailey and discusses the implications this information has on Carlos.	Supervisor reflects on Bailey's seemingly freezing response to Carlos's play. Supervisor invites Bailey to discuss the moments before her freeze and strategies for regulating during session.	In reference to Carlos's escalating bop bag play, supervisor asks Bailey to write down as many responses as possible, encouraging her to draw from diverse skills, including encouragement, limit setting, reflecting feelings, and tracking.
Personalization	Supervisor asks Bailey to read Dion (2018), *Aggression in Play Therapy*, for the purpose of increasing Bailey's awareness of child and therapist regulation in play therapy.	Supervisor works with Bailey to understand her responses to Carlos's play, including how she felt and thought during his play. Supervisor may discuss Bailey's feelings and attitudes toward boys, aggression, and domestic violence.	Supervisor asks Bailey to identify the reactions she was having to Carlos's play as they rewatch the session moment by moment. Supervisor asks Bailey to evaluate whether her reactions added or detracted from play therapy.

from concept-clustering of existing research and practice (Holloway, 2016). Situated at the center of the model is the Supervision Relationship, created and influenced by two dimensions: the Supervisor and Supervisee. Holloway (2016) emphasized that the supervisory relationship is the most important aspect of supervision (Bernard & Goodyear, 2014). The SAS model illustrates an important conceptual map of the interaction of multiple influencing factors that impact the supervision process.

Additional dimensions include the Client, Organization or Institution, Supervisor Functions, and Learning Tasks of the Supervisees. The dimensions of the model are dynamic, interrelated, and mutually influencing. The purpose of the multiple dimensions is to "guide questions that will lead to an integrated understanding of the relationship's potential to promote individual relational learning and professional expertise," (Holloway, 2016, p. 14). Importantly, the SAS Model emphasizes the systemic influences of supervisor's decision-making and actions (Holloway, 2016). Figure 3.1 represents a visual depiction of the SAS Model.

Central to the SAS Model is the Supervision Relationship, which at the core is intended to facilitate the safe space necessary for supervisees' professional reflection and growth. The safety afforded by the relationship is meant to create optimal conditions for learning and serve as a model of the relationship qualities necessary in a therapeutic relationship, too. In SAS, three elements guide the understanding and formation of the Supervisory Relationship: interpersonal structure of the relationship, developmental phase of the supervision relationship, and contract for supervision.

First, the *interpersonal structure of the relationship* is influenced by power and involvement. Involvement includes the mutual influences present in the relationship, the intimacy between the supervisor and supervisee, and the degree to which each individual uses the other. Power implies the expert role of the supervisor and their responsibility for imparting knowledge, evaluating supervisee performance, and

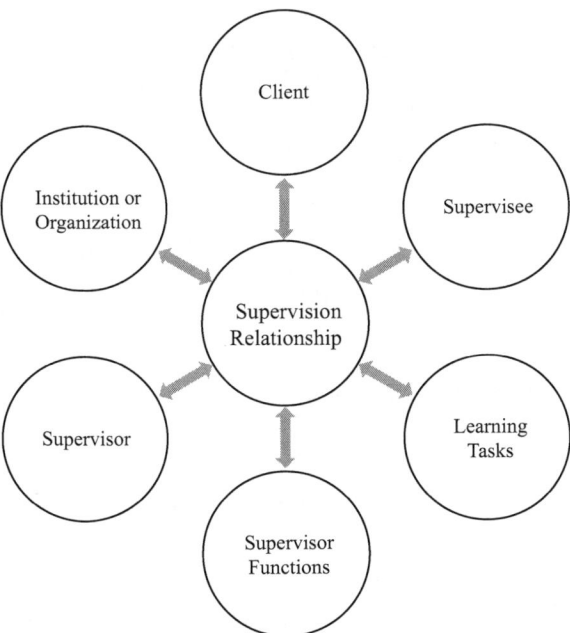

Figure 3.1 Seven dimensions of the systemic approach to supervision.

acting as gatekeeper. Supervisors must be adept at holding the relationship tension created by intimate involvement in the promotion of therapist growth as well as the need for evaluation and assessment in supervision (Holloway, 2016).

Next, the Supervision Relationship is influenced by the *developmental phase of the supervision relationship*. SAS acknowledges three phases in supervision relationship development: (1) developing phase – where the nature of the relationship is clarified, a contract is established, and initial supervisee competencies emerge; (2) maturing phase – where supervision becomes more individualized, and increases can be observed in the supervisee's skills, self-confidence, self-efficacy, and the intimacy of the supervisee-supervisor relationship; and (3) terminating phase – when distinct connections have been established between theory and practice, and there is a decrease in need for direction from the supervisor and an increase in supervisee self-reflection (Holloway, 2016).

Last, the Supervision Relationship is influenced by the *contract for supervision*. Clarifying expectations of supervision for both parties is critical. The supervisor needs to make explicit their professional responsibility and role and the supervisee needs to understand the specific tasks and parameters of the relationship. While needs may evolve as supervision develops, the explicit discussion can benefit supervisees, particularly those who are novice (Holloway, 2016).

The Supervision Relationship is influenced by the following factors:

1. Supervisor factors, including their professional experiences and role, theoretical orientation, interpersonal styles, and cultural characteristics.
2. Supervisee factors, including their experiences in counseling, theoretical orientation, interpersonal styles, cultural worldview, and learning goals.
3. Organization factors, such as the organization's mission and values, organizational structure, performance management and evaluation, culture and climate, and professional standards and ethics.
4. Client factors, including the client characteristics, client-identified problems, client history, client social and familial context, and the dynamics of the therapeutic relationship created by the supervisee and client.
5. Supervisor Functions, such as the active and dynamic roles of the supervision such as monitoring/evaluating, instructing/advising, modeling, consulting/exploring, and supporting/sharing.
6. Learning Tasks, such as counseling skills, case conceptualization, professional role, ethical practice, intrapersonal and interpersonal awareness, and self-evaluation.

The contextual factors, or Organization, Client, Supervisor Function, and Learning Task factors, are the factors that guide decisions about their engagement and active conversation in supervision. They provide multiple points of reflection for supervisors and supervisees to consider that may uncover overt and covert motivations and decision-making influences. Using the SAS Model, the Learning Tasks of supervision are influenced by the Supervisor Functions (supervision actions or strategies) (Holloway, 2016).

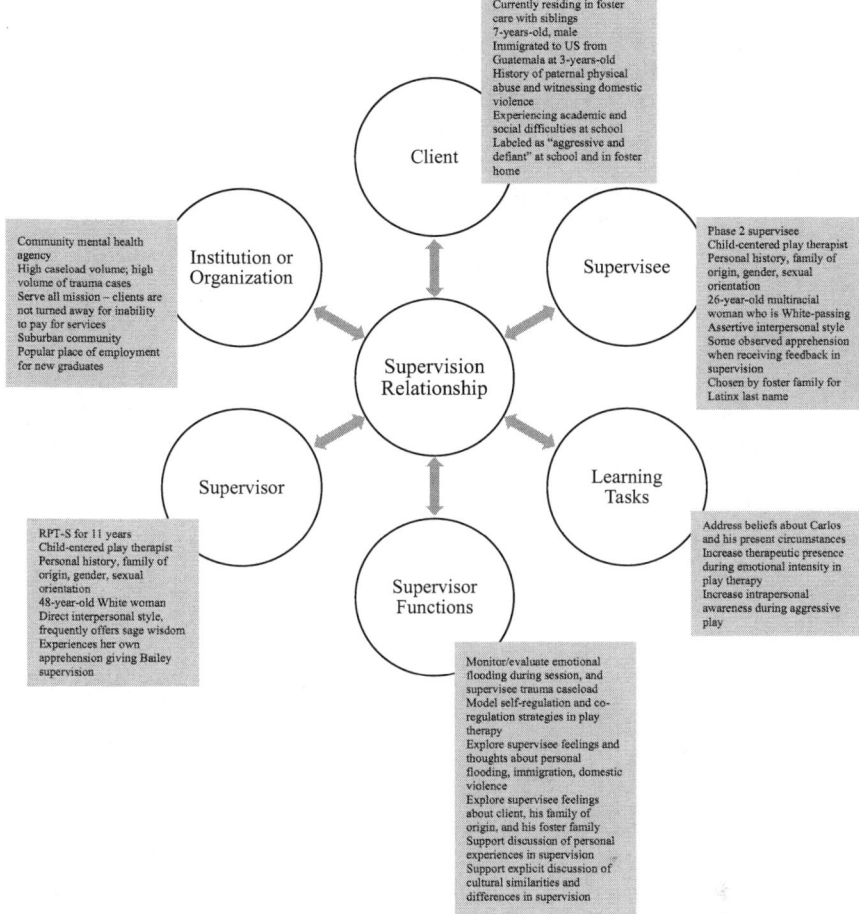

Figure 3.2 Seven dimensions of the systemic approach to supervision as applied to Bailey.

Example Case

Using her knowledge of the SAS Model, Meredith creates a map of the influencing factors of the Supervisor Relationship and the influencing factors (Figure 3.2). The process of eliciting, discussing, and influencing factors generates important insights for Bailey and Meredith. Further, Meredith has a clearer understanding of the Supervisor Functions Bailey needs from her.

Conclusion

Supporting the critical role of supervision in play therapist development is guided by the purposeful use of clinical supervision models to guide the professional development and evaluation of supervisees. Supervision models provide the framework for understanding development and developing supervisory interventions. This chapter provided an overview of key developmental, psycho-therapy-based, and process models of supervision. As standards for professional education, experience, and supervision in play therapy continue to increase in specificity, play therapy supervision must become viewed as a specialized area of play therapy practice. Effective play therapy supervision is derived from clinical supervision models which provide the essential conceptual framework for super-visors which aids in conducting cohesive supervision that addresses supervisees' needs.

References

Association for Play Therapy. (2020). Play therapy best practices: Clinical, professional, & ethical issues. https://cdn.ymaws.com/www.a4pt.org/resource/resmgr/publications/best_practices_-_sept_2019.pdf

Beck, A. T., Rush, A. J., Shaw, B. F., & Emery, G. (1979). *Cognitive therapy of depression.* Guilford Press.

Bernard, J. M. (1997). The discrimination model. In C. E. Watkins, Jr. (Ed.), *Handbook of psychotherapy supervision* (pp. 310–327). John Wiley & Sons, Inc.

Bernard, J. M., & Goodyear, R. K. (2014). *Fundamentals of clinical supervision* (5th ed.). Pearson.

Bobele, M., Biever, J. L., Solóranzo, B. H., & Bluntzer, L. H. (2014). Postmodern approaches to supervision. In T. C. Todd & C. L. Storm (Eds.), *The complete systemic supervisor: Context, philosophy, and pragmatics* (pp. 255–273). Wiley-Blackwell.

Celano, M. P., Smith, C. O., & Kaslow, N. J. (2010). A competency-based approach to couple and family therapy supervision. *Psychotherapy: Theory, Research, Practice, Training, 47*(1), 35–44. https://doi.org/10.1037/a0018845

Chickering, A. W. (1969). *Education and identity.* Jossey-Bass.

Donald, E. J., Culbreth, J. R., & Carter, A. W. (2015). Play therapy supervision: A review of the literature. *International Journal of Play Therapy, 24*(2), 59–77. https://doi.org/10.1037/a0039104

Ekstein, R., & Wallerstein, R. S. (1972). *The teaching and learning of psychotherapy* (2nd ed.). International Universities Press.

Farber, E. W. (2010). Humanistic-existential psychotherapy competencies and the supervisory process. *Psychotherapy: Theory, Research, Practice, Training, 47*(1), 28–34. https://doi.org/10.1037/a0018847

Frawley-O'Dea, M. G., & Sarnat, J. E. (2001). *The supervisory relationship: A contemporary psychodynamic approach.* Guildford Press.

Hackney, H., & Goodyear, R. K. (1984). Carl Rogers's client-centered approach to supervision. In R. F. Levant & J. M. Shlien (Eds.), *Client-centered therapy and the person-centered approach: New directions in theory, research, and practice* (pp. 278–296). Praeger Publishers/Greenwood Publishing Group.

Holloway, E. L. (2016). *Supervision essentials for a systems approach to supervision.* American Psychological Association. https://doi.org/10.1037/14942-000

Hudspeth, E. F. (2015). Clinical supervision in play therapy: Research, practice, and application. *International Journal of Play Therapy, 24*(2), 55–58. https://doi.org/10.1037/pla0000011

Knell, S. (1993). To show and not tell: Cognitive-behavioral play therapy. In T. Kottman & C. Schaefer (Eds.), *Play therapy in action: A casebook for practitioners* (pp. 169–208). Jason Aronson.

Knell, S. (2003). Cognitive-behavioral play therapy. In C. Schaefer (Ed.), *Foundations of play therapy* (pp. 175–191). John Wiley & Sons.

Koob, J. J. (2002). The effects of solution-focused supervision on the perceived self-efficacy of therapists in training. *Clinical Supervisor*, *21*(2), 161–183. https://doi.org/10.1300/j001v21n02_11

Kranz, P. L., Kottman, T., & Lund, N. L. (1998). Play therapists' opinions concerning the education, training, and practice of play therapists. *International Journal of Play Therapy*, *7*(1), 73–87. http://doi.org/10.1037/h0089419

Lambert, S. F., LeBlanc, M., Mullen, J. A., Ray, D., Baggerly, J., White, J., & Kaplan, D. (2007). Learning more about those who play in session: The national play therapy in counseling practices project (phase I). *Journal of Counseling and Development*, *85*(1), 42–46. http://doi.org/10.1002/j.1556-6678.2007.tb00442.x

Landreth, G. L. (2012). *Play therapy: The art of the relationship* (3rd ed.). Routledge.

Loganbill, C., Hardy, E., & Delworth, U. (1982). Supervision: A conceptual model. *Counseling Psychology*, *10*(1), 3–27. https://doi.org/10.1177/0011000082101002

McLean, R., & Marini, I. (2008). Working with gay men from a narrative counseling perspective: A case study. *Journal of LGBT Issues in Counseling*, *2*(3), 243–257. https://doi.org/10.1080/15538600802120085

McNeill, B. W., Stoltenberg, C. D., & Romans, J. S. (1992). The integrated developmental model of supervision: Scale development and validation procedures. *Professional Psychology*, *23*(6), 504–508. https://doi.org/10.1037/0735-7028.23.6.504

Newman, C. F. (2010). Competency in conducting cognitive-behavioral therapy: Foundational, functional, and supervisory aspects. *Psychotherapy: Theory, Research, Practice, Training*, *47*(1), 12–19. https://doi.org/10.1037/a0018849

O'Connor, K., Schaefer, C., & Braverman, L. (2016). *Handbook of play therapy*. John Wiley & Sons.

Phil, K., Guy, G., & Lowe, R. (2007). Social constructionist supervision or supervision as social construction? Some dilemmas. *Journal of Systemic Therapies*, *26*(1), 51–62.

Phillips, R. D., & Landreth, G. L. (1995). Play therapists on play therapy I.: A report of methods, demographics and professional practices. *International Journal of Play Therapy*, *4*(1), 1–26. https://doi.org/10.1037/h0089404

Ray, D. C. (2011). *Advanced play therapy: Essential conditions, knowledge, and skills for child practice*. Routledge.

Reiser, R. P., & Milne, D. (2012). Supervising cognitive-behavioral psychotherapy: Pressing needs, impressing possibilities. *Journal of Contemporary Psychotherapy*, *42*(3), 161–171. https://doi.org/10.1007/s10879-011-9200-6

Rigazio-DiGilio, S. A., & Anderson, S. A. (1994). A cognitive-developmental model for marital and family therapy supervision. *Clinical Supervisor*, *12*(2), 93–118. https://doi.org/10.1300/J001v12n02_07

Rogers, C. R. (1961). *On becoming a person*. Houghton Mifflin.

Rønnestad, M. H., & Skovholt, T. M. (1991). Professional development and stagnation of therapists and counselors. *Norwegian Psychology Journal*, *28*, 555–567.

Rønnestad, M. H., & Skovholt, T. M. (2003). The journey of the counselor and therapist: Research findings and perspectives on professional development. *Journal of Career Development*, *30*(1), 5–44. https://doi.org/10.1177/089484530303000102

Roth, A., & Pilling, S. (1992). IAPT supervision competencies framework. University College London. http://www.ucl.ac.uk/clinical-psychology/CORE/supervision_framework.htm

Roth, A., & Pilling, S. (2008). A competence framework for supervision of psychological therapies. University College London. http://www.ucl.ac.uk/clinical-psychology/CORE/supervision_framework.htm

Ryan, S. D., Gomory, T., & Lacasse, J. (2002). Who are we? Examining the results of the association for play therapy membership survey. *International Journal of Play Therapy*, *11*(2), 11–41. http://doi.org/10.1037/h0088863

Sarnat, J. (2010). Key competencies of the psychodynamic psychotherapist and how to teach them in supervision. *Psychotherapy: Theory, Research, Practice, Training*, *47*(1), 20–27. https://doi.org/10.1037/a0018846

Seymour, J. W., & Crenshaw, D. A. (2015). Reflective practice in play therapy and supervision. In D. A. Crenshaw & A. L. Stewart (Eds.), *Play therapy: A comprehensive guide to theory and practice* (pp. 483–495). The Guilford Press.

Shelby, J. S. (2000). Brief therapy with traumatized children: A developmental perspective. In H. G. Kaduson & C. E. Schaefer (Eds.), *Short-term play therapy for children* (pp. 69–104). The Guilford Press.

Shelby, J. S., & Felix, E. D. (2005). Posttraumatic play therapy: The need for an integrated model of directive and nondirective approaches. In L. A. Reddy, T. M. Files-Hall, & C. E. Schaefer (Eds.), *Empirically based play interventions for children* (pp. 79–104). American Psychological Association. https://doi.org/10.1037/11086-005

Smith, K. L. (2009). A brief summary of supervision models. https://www.gallaudet.edu/documents/Department-of-Counseling/COU_SupervisionModels_Rev.pdf

Stoltenberg, C. D., & McNeill, B. W. (2011). *IDM supervision: An integrative developmental model for supervising counselors and therapists* (3rd ed.). Routledge. https://doi.org/10.4324/9780203893388

Storm, C. L., & Todd, T. C. (2014). Core premises and a framework for systemic/relational supervision. In T. C. Todd & C. L. Storm (Eds.), *The complete systemic supervisor: Context, philosophy, and pragmatics* (2nd ed., pp. 2–16). Wiley.

Thomas, F. N. (1994). Solution-oriented supervision: The coaxing of expertise. *Family Journal*, *2*(1), 11–18. https://doi.org/10.1177/1066480794021003

VanderGast, T. S., Culbreth, J. R., & Flowers, C. (2010). An exploration of experiences and preferences in clinical supervision with play therapists. *International Journal of Play Therapy*, *19*(3), 174–185. https://doi.org/10.1037/a0018882

Whiting, J. B. (2007). Authors, artists, and social constructionism: A case study of narrative supervision. *American Journal of Family Therapy*, *35*(2), 139–150.

Zeligman, M. (2017). Supervising counselors-in-training through a developmental, narrative model. *Journal of Creativity in Mental Health*, *12*(1), 2–14. https://doi.org/10.1080/15401383.2016.1189370

4 Best Practices and Ethical Considerations in Play Therapy Supervision

Carrie Longest

Best Practices and Ethical Considerations in Play Therapy Supervision

Supervision is the cornerstone of the training and development of students and new counseling professionals. In the play therapy field, supervision is critical to ensure prospective play therapists integrate theory and practice as well as practicing ethically. Therefore, play therapy supervisors need to have established supervision practices including a solid foundation of best practices and ethical considerations before engaging in a supervisory relationship. Ethical codes and best practices are often confused with one another, but they do serve different purposes in the mental health field. Ethical standards provide the rules in professional practice (Cottone, Tarvydas, & Hartley, 2022). Best practices are guidelines created from case-based research intended to support professionals in their work and decisions (Borders et al., 2011). Best practices guidelines provide support to the ethical codes but do not replace them.

Within the literature, there is a lack of guidance on best practices in play therapy supervision. The Association for Play Therapy's (2020) document, *Play Therapy Best Practices*, serves as a staple to guide supervisors toward making the best possible decisions regarding best practices in play therapy supervision. Each discipline's (psychologist, social work, mental health counseling, and school counseling) code of ethics is tailored to the specific discipline's needs. However, each of the codes are rooted in the five moral principles identified by Kitchener (1984).

This chapter will serve to provide an overview of ethical considerations and best practices in play therapy supervision and outline the Principles, Principals, and Process (P³) model for play therapy ethics problem-solving (Seymour & Rubin, 2006).

Learning objectives for this chapter are:

- Describe the five cornerstone ethical principles – autonomy, nonmaleficence, beneficence, justice, and fidelity
- Identify best practices for play therapy supervision
- Identify common ethical dilemmas for play therapy supervisors

DOI: 10.4324/9781003196075-5

- Gain an understanding of dual roles, informed consent, competency, and liability related to play therapy supervision
- Describe the ethical decision-making model: P³ Model (Seymour & Rubin, 2006)

What are ethics?

Ethics provide professionals with standards of practice for professional behavior and accountability. Principle ethics are rooted in moral principles and represent the shared beliefs of a professional group (Remley & Herlihy, 2020). Kitchener (1984) identified five ethical moral principles – autonomy, nonmaleficence, beneficence, justice, and fidelity. These principles provide the foundation for the professional, ethical codes (AAMFT, 2015; ACA, 2014; AMHCA, 2020b; APA, 2017; ASCA, 2016; NASW, 2021). For each specific discipline, the ethical codes provide general guidance on professional behavior to protect the welfare of the client. However, very little guidance is provided in the ethical codes specific to children. Often conflict arises between legal and ethical obligations when counseling children (Remley & Herlihy, 2020). For play therapists, the Association for Play Therapy (APT) provides best practices guidance in the documents Play Therapy Best Practices (2020) and the Paper on Touch (2022a).

Ethics in play therapy is multidimensional. It is critical for play therapists to understand their ethical and legal responsibilities to the children and guardians. For the play therapy supervisor, ethical responsibility is layered and can be complex. The ethical responsibilities of play therapy supervisors include the play therapy supervisee and the supervisee's clients. Possible ethical dilemmas in play therapy supervision identified in the literature include informed consent, confidentiality, competence, and dual relationships (Ashby et al., 2017; Barnett & Molzon, 2014; Carmichael, 2006; Carnes-Holt et al., 2016). When ethical conundrums arise, play therapy supervisors should have an ethical decision-making process to guide their decisions and limit ethical errors (ACA, 2014). An ethical decision-making model provides play therapy supervisors with an approach to examine and resolve the ethical dilemma objectively (Cottone & Clause, 2000; Evans et al., 2012). There are various generic ethical decision-making models available (Cottone & Claus, 2000). However, specific play therapy ethical decision-making models are limited. Seymour and Rubin (2006) provide play therapists with the Principles, Principals, and Process (P³) ethical decision-making model (covered later in the chapter) to guide ethical decisions.

Best Practices in Play Therapy Supervision

Effective supervision is established by utilizing theoretically grounded supervision practices (Borders et al., 2011). Play therapy supervisors can establish a supervision framework by implementing a supervision model to guide their play therapy supervision practices (covered in Chapter 4). Best practices provide clinical supervisors with guidance grounded in research (ACES, 2011; Borders et al., 2014;

Falender & Shafranske, 2008). These guidelines offer support to supervisors and are intended to enhance their judgment in supervision (Borders et al., 2011). Best practices are intended to supplement rather than replace the established ethical codes.

Best Practice in Clinical Supervision (ACES, 2011) outlines 12 areas of supervision best practices: initiating supervision, goal-setting, giving feedback, conducting supervision, the supervisory relationship, diversity and advocacy considerations, ethical considerations, documentation, evaluation, supervision format, supervisor training and supervision preparation including supervision training and supervision of supervision. These best practices offer play therapy supervisors guidance in providing effective play therapy supervision to develop the supervisee while protecting the welfare of the client. In addition, these guidelines could be used to train and develop future play therapy supervisors and play therapy supervision trainings.

As described prior, the *Play Therapy Best Practices* and the "Paper on touch" guide clinical, professional, and ethical behavior for play therapists, supervisors, and consultation (APT, 2020). Best practices identified for supervisors include supervision preparation, responsibility for services to clients, and the clinical supervision contract (APT, 2020a Section H.1) and distance and online supervision are outlined in Section J.6 (APT, 2020). While there are numerous ethical issues that may arise in play therapy supervision, this chapter will focus on the issues of competence, informed consent, evaluation, dual relationships, confidentiality, and technology issues in play therapy supervision.

Competence

According to the ACA *Code of Ethics* (2014), counselors are expected to practice "within the boundaries of their competence." Competency relates to a professional's knowledge, skills, activities, and attitudes that cumulatively represent the capabilities, qualifications, understanding, and effectiveness that is required to the standard by which the treatment will produce its intended therapeutic outcomes (Turner et al., 2020). Play therapy supervisors need to demonstrate competency in counseling practices, play therapy practices, and supervision practices including assessing the play therapy supervisee's competency level (Borders & Brown, 2005).

The APT (2022b) outline the expectations for Registered Play Therapist-Supervisors™ in the Credentialing Standards for Registered Play Therapist-Supervisor document. The RPT-S™ is expected to demonstrate knowledge of supervision practices and advanced play therapy practices (APT, 2022b). In addition, the RPT-S™ is expected to facilitate play therapist development and self-awareness and insight. While competencies related to the practice of play therapy have been identified and outlined (APT, 2021; Turner et al., 2020), there are no supervision specific competencies for Registered Play Therapist-Supervisors. As a result, it is unclear how the competency of a play therapy supervisor can be determined.

Competency as a play therapist does not create a competent play therapy supervisor (Remley & Herlihy, 2020). Play therapy supervision is a separate function in the counseling field contributing to the development of new play therapy professionals and ensuring client welfare (Bernard & Goodyear, 2014). Determining competency as a play therapy supervisor should include various aspects including formal training, evaluation, and supervised experience (Ashby et al., 2017). However, the literature suggests play therapy supervisors have limited instruction on supervision practices and rely on their experiences of supervision (Longest, 2020). It is critical for play therapy supervisors to evaluate their supervision competency. Swank et al. (2021) developed the Supervision Competencies Scale (SCS) to assist in developing competent supervisors. The scale addresses four areas: supervision skills, supervision laws and ethics, supervision modalities, and supervision knowledge (Swank et al., 2021). Play therapist supervisors can use the SCS as a tool to evaluate their competency in play therapy supervision.

Another consideration around competence includes the play therapist supervisor's ability to assess the play therapy supervisee's competence and training needs (Barnett & Molzon, 2014). It is critical for play therapy supervisors to evaluate each play therapy supervisee's developmental level and training needs using the play therapy competencies (APT, 2021). The play therapy competencies include knowledge and understanding of play therapy, clinical play therapy skills, and professional engagement in play therapy (see the chapter on evaluation in play therapy supervision).

Informed Consent

Informed consent is the process of informing a play therapy supervisee and a client of the purposes, goals, limitations, and foreseeable risks and possible benefits of supervision or therapy (ACES, 2011; Bernard & Goodyear, 2014; Remley & Herlihy, 2020). Informed consent is an ongoing process and should be reviewed regularly. Each specific discipline (social work, psychology, school counseling) addresses informed consent in their respective code of ethics. In the ACA code of ethics (2014), client informed consent is addressed in Section A (A.2.a.) and supervisee informed consent is addressed in Section F (F.4.a.). The American Psychological Association (APA, 2016) addressed client informed consent in Section 3 (3.10) and the American Association for Marriage and Family Therapy (AAMFT, 2015) covers client informed consent in Section I (1.2). However, informed consent for supervision is not explicitly discussed.

In play therapy supervision, obtaining informed consent is layered. A play therapy supervisor must provide the supervisee with informed consent and determine if the supervisee informs clients about the parameters of therapy and the parameters of supervision that affects them (Bernard & Goodyear, 2014; Borders & Brown, 2005). Informed consent in the play therapy supervision process should be a formalized process. Providing the play therapy supervisee with a written supervision disclosure statement is identified as a best practice (ACES, 2011; APT, 2020). A written agreement formalizes the process of play therapy supervision and clarifies the expectations (Remley & Herlihy, 2020; Thomas, 2007). It is recommended a supervision disclosure statement includes the following topics: purpose of play therapy supervision, play therapy supervisor's background and training, supervisory methods, scheduling and emergency contact information, play therapy supervisor's responsibilities and requirements, play therapy supervisee's responsibilities, confidentiality policies, documentation and evaluation of supervision, financial policies, risks and benefits, complaint procedures and due process, and the duration and termination of the supervision contract (Barnett & Molzon, 2014; Thomas, 2007, 2010). The supervision disclosure statement addresses the possible ethical issues that could arise during the supervision process and minimizes the potential for their occurrence (Cobia & Boes, 2000).

Evaluation

Evaluation of the play therapy supervisees skills is essential to the play therapy supervision process and developing competent play therapists. As gatekeepers for the play therapy field, RPT-Ss™ are expected to evaluate the play therapy supervisee using the play therapy competencies. The methods of evaluation should be outlined in the informed consent and reviewed with the supervisee (Barnett & Molzon, 2014). Evaluation in the play therapy supervision process is ongoing. It includes formal and informal evaluations, supervision plans, and ongoing documentation. Formal evaluations should have an established schedule while informal evaluations will be provided on an ongoing basis (Barnett & Molzon, 2014). Historically, evaluating play therapy skills has been unclear. There are several checklists that allow supervisors to evaluate the application of basic play therapy skills (Ray, 2004; Demanchick, 2007). However, there is no empirical evidence in the literature to show their effectiveness (Donald et al., 2015.)

Dual relationships in Play Therapy Supervision

The supervisory relationship can be complex and layered. Play therapy supervisors often engage in several roles within the supervisory relationship. The most common roles identified in the literature are teacher, counselor, and consultant (Remley & Herlihy, 2020). Multiple relationships become problematic when there is unequal power distribution and the person with less power is at risk of harm (Bernard & Goodyear, 2014).

The ACA *Code of Ethics* (2014) addresses dual relationships in Section F.3. Supervisory Relationship. In the supervisory relationship it is important for the supervisor to define and maintain clear professional, personal, and social relationships with supervisees (ACA, 2014; F.3.a.). Research shows boundary violations in supervision occur frequently (Welfel, 2016). It is important for supervisors to enter supervisory relationships where objectivity can be maintained (Welfel, 2016).

The experiential nature of play therapy allows for play therapy supervisors to integrate creative methods in play therapy supervision to promote play therapy supervisee's professional identity development (Drewes & Mullen, 2008).

Intentional use of expressive techniques creates a parallel process and promotes self-awareness for the play therapy supervisee. Additionally, it allows for the play therapy supervisee to learn and apply the skills. However, the deeper exploration of self in the supervision process may create a complicated supervisory relationship (Purswell & Stulmaker, 2015). Play therapy supervisors are responsible for ensuring the play therapy supervisee has the space to process their experience using the creative techniques (Purswell & Stulmaker, 2015). However, play therapy supervisors need to maintain the line between supervision and therapy.

Confidentiality

Confidentiality is another common ethical issue in play therapy supervision. In play therapy supervision, confidentiality is an overarching issue and needs to be addressed by the play therapy supervisor and the play therapy supervisee. Play therapy supervisors should ensure supervisees inform their clients of the limits of confidentiality (ACA, 2014; F.1.c.). Play therapy supervisees must inform the parents/guardians they are under supervision and there will be other professionals (play therapy supervisor) involved (Ashby et al., 2017). Often this will be included in the informed consent. However, the play therapy supervisee may want to discuss this with the parents/guardians.

Due to the evaluative relationship, information about the play therapy supervisee is not considered confidential (Bernard & Goodyear, 2014). Therefore, play therapy supervisors should present clear guidelines at the onset of supervision. These limits are similar to those in the therapeutic relationship, including the supervisee granting permission and when ethically and legally required to breach confidentiality. These guidelines should be provided in the supervision disclosure statement and discussed at the start of play therapy supervision (outlined above).

Technology Issues in Play Therapy Supervision

Distance supervision is one method of providing play therapy supervision. Play therapy supervisors need to understand the use of technology in the play therapy supervision process and supervisory relationship. There are benefits and limitations with using distance supervision in play therapy supervision. It is critical that play therapy supervisors are knowledgeable in best practices regarding the use of distance supervision (see Chapter 9, Technology in Play Therapy Supervision).

Resolving Ethical Dilemmas in Supervision

When ethical dilemmas arise, it is critical an ethical decision-making model is applied to assist with the decision (ACA, 2014; I.1.b.). Cottone and Claus (2000) reviewed various general ethical decision-making models. Central to every ethical dilemma are the moral principles of autonomy, beneficence, nonmaleficence, justice, and fidelity. Play therapy supervisees should have a basic understanding of the code of ethics that guides their discipline (professional counselor, social worker, school counselor, psychologist, psychiatry, psychiatric nurse practitioners, and MFT).

Principles, Principals, and Process (P³) Model

Seymour and Rubin (2006) proposed the Principles, Principals, and Process (P3) Model as an ethical decision-making model specifically for play therapists. This integrative and collaborative model combines the ethical codes from the various professional disciplines of play therapists and provides a process to dissect ethical dilemmas with the input of those affected by the ethical dilemma (Seymour & Rubin, 2006). The P³ Model acknowledges the various backgrounds from which play therapists originate and allows for supervisors using moral reasoning and social context when approaching ethical dilemmas (Seymour & Rubin, 2006).

The P³ Model is comprised of three steps: first, the ethical principles (specific professional ethical codes, legal codes, and virtue ethics) and principals (client, counselor, collateral, and community voices) are identified by the play therapist; next, each principle is examined from the perspective of each principal identified; last, a discussion with the principals regarding the principles is facilitated to develop a shared understanding. The discussion will inform an ethical decision (Figure 4.1).

Applying the P³ Model

The following case study will illustrate application of the P³ Model.

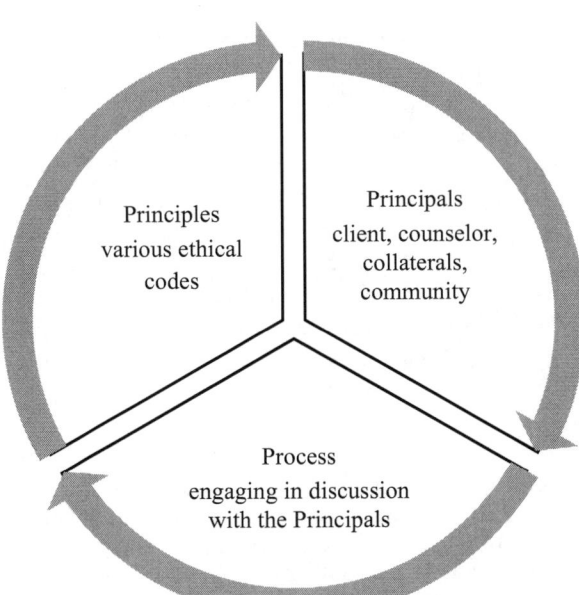

Figure 4.1 Principles, Principals, and Process (P³) Model

Maureen's Story

Hope is a play therapy supervisee working at a local mental health agency. Maureen is a Registered Play Therapist-Supervisor. Currently, Maureen is supervising ten aspiring play therapists, including Hope. Hope is struggling with obtaining the required direct client hours. In supervision, Hope has discussed ways to obtain the hours with Maureen. Maureen has an 8-year-old daughter (June) who has started to exhibit emotional regulation struggles at home and at school. Maureen has had some difficulty finding a play therapist in her area to work with her daughter. During a conversation with Hope, Maureen suggests she "practice" with June. Hope agrees but is worried about working with her play therapy supervisor's daughter.

P^1: *Identify the Principles.* In this scenario, the ethical principles to consider are beneficence, autonomy, fidelity, and non-malfeasance.

P^2: *Identify the Principals.* The primary principal in this case is the supervisee, Hope. Additional principals include June and The Association for Play Therapy.

P^3: *Identify the Process.* This situation illustrates how easy dual relationships can be established within the supervisory relationship. Maureen should consider the power differential that is present in the supervisory relationship. It is important Maureen examine how this situation may affect Hope who has less power within the supervisory relationship. Additionally, Maureen should consider consulting with another play therapy supervisor.

Conclusion

In play therapy, ethics are complicated due to the obligation to the child and to multiple stakeholders such as parents/guardians, teachers, and other professionals. Ethical obligations in play therapy supervision are layered and require the play therapy supervisor to be competent in supervision practices and play therapy practices. This chapter examined possible ethical issues relevant to play therapy supervision, including informed consent, dual roles, competency, and evaluation. The P^3 Model (Seymour & Rubin, 2006) was provided as an ethical decision-making model. Play therapy supervisors should continually assess their practices to ensure ethical professional practice. It is critical play therapist supervisors always remember the basic ethical principles – autonomy, beneficence, non-malfeasance, and fidelity when examining possible ethical dilemmas.

Key Readings and Resources

2014 ACA code of ethics. https://www.counseling.org/resources/aca-code-of-ethics.pdf
ACES best practices in clinical supervision. https://acesonline.net/wp-content/uploads /2018/11/ACES-Best-Practices-in-Clinical-Supervision-2011.pdf
American Association for Marriage and Family Therapy. (2015). Code of ethics. https:// aamft.org/Legal_Ethics/Code_of_Ethics.aspx
American Association for Marriage and Family Therapy. Approved supervision resources. https://aamft.org/AAMFT/ENHANCE_Knowledge/Approved_Supervisor_

Resources/Supervision/Supervision.aspx?hkey=f3fe9160-efbc-490e-b6f7-7a493fa
47632
Approved Clinical Supervisor (ACS) Credential. Center for credentialing & education.
https://www.cce-global.org/credentialing/acs
Association for play therapy resource page (for APT members). https://www.a4pt.org/
page/ResourceCenter
National Association of Social Workers. (2021). Code of ethics. https://www.socialworkers
.org/About/Ethics/Code-of-Ethics/Code-of-Ethics-English

References

American Association for Marriage and Family Therapy. (2015). Code of ethics. https://
www.aamft.org/Legal_Ethics/Code_of_Ethics.aspx
American Counseling Association. (2014). 2014 ACA code of ethics. https://counseling
.org/knowledge-center
American Mental Health Counselors Association. (2020a). Considerations for supervisors
related to ethical supervision. https://www.amhca.org/HigherLogic/System/Dow
nloadDocumentFile.ashx?DocumentFileKey=73ff672f-c5fc-b132-f95a-f4771c8607ff
&forceDialog=0
American Mental Health Counselors Association. (2020b). AMHCA code of ethics.
https://www.amhca.org/HigherLogic/System/DownloadDocumentFile.ashx
?DocumentFileKey=24a27502-196e-b763-ff57-490a12f7edb1&forceDialog=0
American Psychological Association. (2017). Ethical principles of psychologists and code
of conduct (2002, amended effective June 1, 2010, and January 1, 2017). https://www
.apa.org/ethics/code/index.aspx
American School Counselors Association. (2016). ASCA ethical standards for school
counselors. https://www.schoolcounselor.org/getmedia/f041cbd0-7004-47a5-ba01
-3a5d657c6743/Ethical-Standards.pdf
Ashby, J. S., Wood, L., & Kiperman, S. (2017). Ethics in play therapy consultation and
supervision. In R. L. Steen (Ed.), *Emerging research in play therapy, child counseling, and
consultation* (pp. 214–231). IGI Global. https://doi.org/10.4018/978-1-5225-2224-9
.ch012
Association for Counselor Education and Supervision. (1993). Ethical guidelines for
counseling supervisors. https://acesonline.net/wp-content/uploads/2018/11/ACES
-Best-Practices-in-Clinical-Supervision-2011.pdf
Association for Counselor Education and Supervision. (2011). Best practices in clinical
supervision. https://acesonline.net/wp-content/uploads/2018/11/ACES-Best
-Practices-in-Clinical-Supervision-2011.pdf
Association for Play Therapy. (2020). Play therapy best practices. https://cdn.ymaws.com
/www.a4pt.org/resource/resmgr/publications/apt_best_practices_-_june_20.pdf
Association for Play Therapy. (2021). Credentialing standards for the registered play
therapist. https://cdn.ymaws.com/www.a4pt.org/resource/resmgr/credentials/rpt
_standards.pdf
Association for Play Therapy. (2022a). Paper on touch. https://cdn.ymaws.com/www
.a4pt.org/resource/resmgr/resource_center/Paper_on_Touch_2022__-_Final.pdf
Association for Play Therapy. (2022b). Credentialing standards for the registered play therapist-
supervisor. https://cdn.ymaws.com/www.a4pt.org/resource/resmgr/credentials
/RPT-S_Standards__updated_.pdf

Barnett, J. E., & Molzon, C. H. (2014). Clinical supervision of psychotherapy: Essential ethics issues for supervisors and supervisees. *Journal of Clinical Psychology, 70*(11), 1051–1061. https://doi.org/10.1002/jclp.22126

Bernard, J. M., & Goodyear, R. K. (2014). *Fundamentals of clinical supervision* (5th ed.). Routledge.

Borders, L. D., & Brown, L. L. (2005). *The new handbook of counseling supervision.* Lawrence Erlbaum Associates Publishers.

Borders, L. D., DeKruyf, L., Fernando, D. M., Glosoff, H. L., Hays, D. G., Page, B., & Welfare, L. E. (2011). Best practices in clinical supervision. https://acesonline.net/wp-content/uploads/2018/11/ACES-Best-Practicesin-Clinical-Supervision-2011.pdf

Borders, L. D., Glosoff, H. L., Welfare, L. E., Hays, D. G., DeKruyf, L., Fernando, D. M., & Page, B. (2014). Best practices in clinical supervision: Evolution of a counseling specialty. *Clinical Supervisor, 33*(1), 26–44. https://doi.org/10.1080/07325223.201.905225

Carmichael, K. D. (2006). Legal and ethical issues in play therapy. *International Journal of Play Therapy, 15*(2), 83–99.

Carnes-Holt, K., Maddox, R. P. II., Warren, J., Morgan, M., & Zakaria, N. S. (2016). Using bookmarks: An approach to support ethical decision making in play therapy. *International Journal of Play Therapy, 25*(4), 176–185.

Center for Credentialing & Education. (2008). The approved clinical supervisor (ACS) code of ethics. https://www.cce-global.org/Assets/Ethics/ACScodeofethics.pdf

Cobia, D. C., & Boes, S. R. (2000). Professional disclosure statements and formal plans for supervision: Two strategies for minimizing the risk of ethical conflicts in post-master's supervision. *Journal of Counseling and Development, 78*(3), 293–296.

Cottone, R. R., & Claus, R. E. (2000). Ethical decision-making models: A review of the literature. *Journal of Counseling and Development, 78*(3), 275–283. http://doi.org/10.1002/j.1556-6676.2000.tb01908.x

Cottone, R. R., Tarvydas, V. M., & Hartley, M. T. (2022). *Ethics and decision making in counseling and psychotherapy* (5th ed.). Springer.

Demanchick, S. P. (2007). The development of an observational assessment for studying therapist behaviors in child-centered play therapy (Doctoral dissertation). Retrieved from ProQuest dissertations & theses. (UMI No. 3279137)

Donald, E. J., Culbreth, J. R., & Carter, A. W. (2015). Play therapy supervision: A review of the literature. *International Journal of Play Therapy, 24*(2), 59–77. http://doi.org/10.1037/a0039104

Drewes, A. A., & Mullen, J. A. (Eds.). (2008). *Supervision can be playful: Techniques for child and play therapist supervisors.* Jason Aronson.

Evans, A. M., Levitt, D. H., & Henning, S. (2012). The application of ethical decision-making and self-awareness in the counselor education classroom. *Journal of Counselor Preparation & Supervision, 4*(2), 41–52. https://repository.wcsu.edu/jcps/vol4/iss2/3

Falender, C. A., & Shafranske, E. P. (2008). Best practices of supervision. In C. A. Falender & E. P. Shafranske (Eds.), *Casebook for clinical supervision: A competency-based approach* (pp. 3–15). American Psychological Association.

Kitchener, K. S. (1984). Intuition, critical evaluation, and ethical principles: The foundation for ethical decisions in counseling psychology. *Counseling Psychologist, 12*(3), 43–55. https://doi.org/10.1177/0011000084123005

Longest, C. H. (2020). The integration of supervision theory in play therapy supervision: A generic qualitative study (Doctoral dissertation). Retrieved from ProQuest dissertations & theses. (UMI No. 28150471)

National Association of Social Workers. (2021). Code of ethics. https://www.socialworkers.org/About/Ethics/Code-of-Ethics/Code-of-Ethics-English

Purswell, K. E., & Stulmaker, H. L. (2015). Expressive arts in supervision: Choosing developmentally appropriate interventions. *International Journal of Play Therapy*, *24*(2), 103–117. http://doi.org/10.1037/a0039134

Ray, D. (2004). Supervision of basic and advanced skills in play therapy. *Journal of Professional Counseling: Practice, Theory, & Research*, *32*(2), 28–41.

Remley, T. P., & Herlihy, B. (2020). *Ethical, legal, and professional issues in counseling* (6th ed.). Pearson.

Seymour, J. W., & Rubin, L. (2006). Principles, principals, and process: A model for play therapy ethics problem solving. *International Journal of Play Therapy*, *15*(2), 101–123.

Swank, J. M., Liu, R., Neuer Colburn, A. A., & Williams, K. A. (2021). Development and initial validation of the supervision competencies scale (SCS). *International Journal for the Advancement of Counselling*, *43*(2), 195–206. https://doi.org/10.1007/s10447-021-09427-z

Thomas, J. T. (2007). Informed consent through contracting for supervision. *Professional Psychology: Research and Practice*, *38*(3), 221–231.

Thomas, J. T. (2010). *The ethics of supervision and consultation*. American Psychological Association.

Turner, R., Schoeneberg, C., Ray, D., & Lin, Y. (2020). Establishing play therapy competencies: A Dephi study. *International Journal of Play Therapy*, *29*(4), 177–190. https://doi.org/10.1037/pla0000138

Welfel, E. R. (2016). *Ethics in counseling and psychotherapy: Standards, research, and emerging issues* (6th ed.). Cengage.

Section 2

The Process

5 Building the Play Therapy Supervisory Relationship

Utilizing the Therapeutic Powers of Play Can Support Effective Supervision

Kenisha W. Gordon

Beginning the Supervisory Relationship

The journey to becoming a registered play therapist can be both exciting and anxiety-provoking. The therapist commits to gaining additional training and education in the form of supervision. Identifying a play therapist supervisor can be a challenging task. The Association for Play Therapy (n.d.) website outlines qualifications for supervisor credentialing. Along with identifying a supervisor with these qualifications, other areas should be assessed. Bernard and Goodyear (2019) addressed the issue of supervision style. The authors explain that supervisors are seen as attractive based on their ability to focus on task completion, handling of multicultural concerns, and professional competency. Therefore, when beginning a play therapy supervision relationship, one of the first areas to consider is understanding what supervision entails and what it requires of each person. The supervisor serves as a gatekeeper for the profession, but both the supervisor and the supervisee need to have a clear concept of what they are agreeing to do (Amaro et al., 2020). This connection is evaluative and time-sensitive. Bernard and Goodyear described supervision as a relationship to improve the professional skills of a beginning clinician who is providing services to a certain population. The quality of services delivered can be reflected in the working alliance. The working alliance is the connection between the supervisor and supervisee regarding tasks and goals (Morrison & Lent, 2018). More specifically, Bernard and Goodyear explained that the combination of the supervisor, supervisee, and the client represents a three-person system. This system becomes the groundwork for the acquisition of awareness, knowledge, and skills. The authors also encourage supervisors and supervisees to complete the supervisory working alliance survey to assess the strength of the relationship.

Trust and truthfulness are two significant elements in building a strong relationship. Trust is established from truthfulness. Supervisors are ethically bound to practice within their scope of competency. Supervisors should be truthful about their experiences, preferences, and knowledge. This truthfulness can assist the supervisee in selecting a supervisor. Supervisors should also present themselves as genuine and authentic, practicing within their scope of competency. Singh-Pillay

DOI: 10.4324/9781003196075-7

and Cartwright (2019) discussed how self-disclosure can impact the relationship in a multitude of ways (e.g., learning opportunities, strong supervisory alliance, etc.) based on the response to the disclosure. Due to the evaluative nature of the relationship, the supervisee may feel vulnerable or guarded about relinquishing control while in the relationship (Boyle & Kenny, 2020). Considering the imbalance of power, supervisors must be aware that attachment trauma can result from a lack of trust and truthfulness (Kidwell & Kerig, 2021), making it difficult for either person to fully commit. In situations of premature termination, the supervisor or supervisee may hesitantly enter a supervisory relationship or may altogether avoid engaging in another supervisor relationship (Wrape et al., 2017).

A caring personality is another important part of the supervisory relationship. It does not begin and end once the supervision contract has been signed but transitions into the care of the play therapy client. If empathy is unilateral, either person may feel they are being taken for granted. Equal sensitivity within the supervisory relationship can create a shared protection between the supervisor and supervisee when delivering feedback. Empathy can clarify intentions and encourage professional and personal growth (Aponte & Ingram, 2018).

Therapeutic Powers to Begin the Supervisory Relationship

When beginning the play therapy relationship, self-expression, attachment, positive emotions, therapeutic relationship, and social competence, are five therapeutic powers of play that can support the initial curiosity about the other person, establish trust, and convey a caring attitude. In play therapy, the therapist can gain a plethora of information about the child through observation (Parson, 2021). Self-expression, demonstrated either directly or indirectly, is a crucial component of language and understanding. The therapeutic power of self-expression in play therapy occurs when the therapist provides a safe environment in which the client has space to change. Bennett and Eberts (2014) associated self-expression with freedom and happiness in experiences and interactions with others. Conversely, when self-expression is suppressed, individuals may internalize a negative view of themselves and others. When emphasizing the power of self-expression in supervision, supervisors should be attentive to information communicated (verbally or nonverbally). Encouraging the supervisee's authenticity and validating them as a person acts as feedback about how they will be understood in the relationship (Yerushalmi, 2021).

A direct connection to self-expression is the therapeutic power of attachment. Attachment in play therapy is an affectional bond that occurs between the client and the therapist. The therapist serves as a secure base for the client. The availability of the therapist and acceptance from the therapist allow the client to explore parts of themselves, maximizing the potential for change (Whelan & Stewart, 2014). When supervisors focus on the therapeutic power of attachment, they can similarly represent security for the supervisee to fully experience both positive and negative emotions that come into the supervision process (Wrape et al., 2017). When supervisees present with insecure attachment styles, the supervisor should respond with care and honesty. In meeting the needs of the supervisee, supervisors can draw correlations from the circle of security model (Hoffman et al., 2017). Supervisors should support the need to explore, be observant of how the supervisor approaches play therapy, convey excitement about the supervisee while tailoring lessons and information about play therapy, and value moments together that may or may not be directly related to supervision. Additional supervisor characteristics are openness, protecting the supervisee both ethically and morally, and helping the supervisee regulate emotions. Lastly, the supervisor can normalize the process by appropriately disclosing their own experience of being a supervisee.

Clients can experience the therapeutic power of positive emotions when engaged in the process of play therapy with a patient play therapist in a safe environment (Kottman, 2014). This combination can provide an overall sense of emotional and cognitive well-being. Kottman summarized resources that could result from a positive emotional experience, such as excitement, delight, and contentment. When a child experiences, or rather feels, the adult sharing an emotion, their connection with both the adult and their own positive internal state is enhanced. Similar to the therapeutic power of positive emotions in play therapy, the supervisor who guides the supervision process and conveys a welcoming attitude provides feedback to the supervisee that the supervision process can be enjoyable. Creating positive energy and the use of humor and fun can strengthen the therapeutic alliance (Hutchby & Dart, 2019).

The therapeutic power of a strong relationship between the client and the therapist is important to play therapy. A strong relationship can influence the client's motivation toward change and can create an example for the development of other relationships (Stewart & Echterling, 2014). Motivation in the supervisory relationship is also an important element when focusing on how the supervisor and supervisee work together to accomplish tasks and meet goals. Bernard and Goodyear (2019) described several factors that affect the therapeutic alliance, such as social skills, openness, and clear expectations of the evaluation process. With familiarity, the supervisor and supervisee create their own shared language and should work toward attunement of each other. Often, clients add a dynamic to the therapeutic relationship that the supervisee may be unprepared to address. However, the supervisory relationship can serve as a safe space to express uncertainty. The security of the relationship contributes to the growth of the supervisee.

Social competence as a therapeutic power of play therapy assists the client with gaining skills necessary to engage with others. Social competence involves understanding and appropriately demonstrating societal standards when interacting with others (Nash, 2014). The therapist supports the client's learning and practice of new behaviors. Competency in the context of play therapy supervision reflects awareness, knowledge, and skills that support the supervisory relationship. McGarry et al. (2021) described three categories of social competency: the ability to express emotions, the ability to be sensitive when interpreting the environments, and the ability to demonstrate control in their conversations. Watkins et al. (2019) explained that cultural humility in supervision is the combination of being open, reflecting on one's own limitations and abilities, and intentionally focusing on others. Demonstration of social competence by the supervisee and the supervisor can also determine compatibility during the initial onset of the relationship.

Strategies to Begin the Supervisory Relationship

Similar to traditional play therapists' philosophy that toys should be selected, not collected (Altvater et al., 2017), strategies for beginning the supervision relationship should be tailored to fit the need. Ramos and Linstrum (2017) discussed the shift in how people express themselves. Self-expression has changed from the traditional written forms to include social media presence, music, poetry, electronic journaling, and text messaging. When utilizing any technology as a means of self-expression, supervisors and play-therapists-in-training must practice online safety and security to maintain confidentiality (Martin et al., 2017).

Implementing sandtray work is another avenue that has a place in both the play therapy sessions and supervision. Hartwig and Bennett (2017) described four diverse interventions (i.e., consultation, group supervision, supervisee awareness, and teaching) of using sandtray in supervision. The authors emphasized that the appropriate use of sandtray can assist both the supervisor and supervisee with their professional growth.

Maintaining the Supervisory Relationship

Maintaining the relationship in the play therapy supervision requires a great deal of effort and energy. Commitment to the process of supervision is a fundamental aspect of the relationship. Partial or no commitment can result in both people feeling that the relationship is a reluctant chore. A shared commitment to the work of play therapy and the profession should be shared. As supervisees continue to develop and engage with others, the supervisor must address any issues of role conflict, transference, and countertransference (Bernard & Goodyear, 2019). When supervisors broach these issues from a cultural perspective, the supervisee feels supported to explore other ideas, increasing their awareness. Both supervisor and supervisee should continuously seek to understand each other's identity, biases, and prejudices. Jones et al. (2019) discussed the benefits of having difficult conversations with one another and the disadvantages of not engaging in meaningful conversations. Supervisors who used broaching as an intervention experienced higher supervisee satisfaction and supervisees also experienced higher client satisfaction.

The supervisory relationship is asymmetrical due to its evaluative nature (Bernard & Goodyear, 2019); however, equality is still important in that each person should make an equal effort in solidifying the relationship. If, at any point, one or the other is not fulfilling their responsibilities, having low to no intention of meeting goals or simply unprepared to accomplish specific tasks, this will lead to resentment. Inequality of effort can become more complicated if one person lacks awareness and/or the other lacks the confidence to address the issue. A periodic review of the supervision contract can increase opportunities to communicate areas for improvement and support.

Humility, an intentional act, is another fundamental component of the play therapy supervisory relationship. Although a high level of competence is an ideal professional goal, demonstrating humility can promote an uplifting atmosphere. Valuing another while not taking excessive pride in oneself requires a delicate balance of each person's thoughts, emotions, and behavior (Watkins et al., 2019). More specifically, when examining humility within a cultural context, mental health professionals are ethically and morally bound to approach each engagement from a multicultural perspective (Patallo, 2019). Although these two basic skills are essential in the counseling process, in supervision these qualities are demonstrated via constructive feedback and realistic recommendations for improvement. How this information is delivered and received can impact the amount of conflict in the relationship, extend the relationship, or help bring the relationship to premature closure.

With the understanding that each person in the play therapy supervision relationship has other responsibilities, keeping the relationship a priority is important. Being present and prepared are highly sought-after qualities for any relationship. Kemer et al. (2019) examined several studies in which supervisors described desired supervisee behavior. Being accountable in their responsibilities, demonstrating a level of maturity, having an openness to feedback, and being motivated toward professional and personal growth were behaviors deemed positive by supervisors. Alternately, undesired supervisee behaviors consisted of inflexibility or resistance to the process, poor dispositional issues, an abnormal amount of anxiety, being uncooperative in supervision, defensive, and unprofessional (Kemer et al., 2019). Each person must take inventory of strengths and areas of improvement early in the relationship so that there is awareness of expectations. This awareness decreases the likelihood of misplaced assumptions.

To maintain a high-quality relationship, reflective supervision allows each person to identify how decisions should be handled based on thoughts, emotions, and behaviors (Rankine, 2017). Reflective supervision is especially important for the play therapy supervisor due to the evaluative nature of the relationship. The therapist is expected to practice introspection for personal and professional development in play therapy. This same challenge should take place within the supervisory relationship. Modeling the reflective process can create a pathway to acknowledge spaces of resolve and healing (Dollarhide et al., 2020).

Therapeutic Powers to Maintain the Supervision Relationship

I propose that a majority of the therapeutic powers of play are beneficial to the middle phase of the supervisory relationship, as this is the space where more effort is required to maintain the relationship. Several therapeutic powers of play, such as moral development and self-regulation, social competence, access to the unconscious, abreaction, catharsis, accelerated psychological development, direct and indirect teaching, creative problem-solving, and resiliency can all assist the supervisor and supervisee in maintaining the relationship.

The therapeutic power of moral development in the supervision relationship is reflected in the care each takes to understand the other's value system. From the supervisor's role, this knowledge can direct training needs and inform feedback delivery (Nejati & Shafaei, 2018). Supervisors are responsible for upholding professional ethics and modeling a high level of moral development. When moral development complements ethical values, supervisees are more autonomous and demonstrate appropriate decision-making skills.

Self-regulation involves the ability to organize thoughts and behaviors to meet a goal. In play therapy, the therapist assists the client with recognizing their own emotions through self-monitoring. The therapeutic power of self-regulation in supervision can assist the supervisee with intentionality regarding the three-person system. Additionally, as training progresses, the supervisee will face more complex situations and will need to learn to adjust their focus. Inzlicht et al. (2021) discussed how self-regulating enables individuals to resolve conflicts, efficiently manage time, and demonstrate better self-control. The supervisor can serve as a secure base for encouragement of the supervisee.

In play therapy, the therapist accesses the unconscious of the client as a therapeutic power to bring unknown emotions and cognitions to the conscious. This information provides transparency about behaviors or tendencies. Symbolic play creates a safe platform to work with the unconscious material. The goal is to restructure memories, giving control to the client so that the memories no longer trigger unwanted behaviors or emotions.

Abreaction and catharsis are often connected and have generally been associated with trauma recovery or as a reaction to traumatic experiences; both therapeutic powers of play are associated with healing and transformation. Abreaction is the mental repeating of a traumatic experience (E. Prendiville, 2014; Yasenik, 2021). Catharsis is the building up and release of a repressed or suppressed emotion (Yasenik, 2021) but is not appropriate for all clients (Drewes & Schaefer, 2014). When the therapist determines that catharsis is beneficial to the client, combining catharsis and abreaction transforms subconscious emotions into conscious material. This combination can be used to develop coping skills and insight (Drewes & Schaefer). In play therapy, when the therapist accesses the unconscious, through abreaction the client can release and manage overwhelming emotions and experiences, while catharsis provides the safe space to hold the release of emotions.

Supervisors can utilize the therapeutic powers of access to the unconscious, abreaction, and catharsis to support the supervisee who may experience challenges within the supervisory or client relationship that hinder professional or personal growth. These challenges can include traumatic experience, role conflict, transference, countertransference, or cultural biases and prejudices. Supervisors must create a safe environment, be observant, be comfortable with ambiguity and tension, and be creative when identifying interventions to assist the supervisee (O'Neill & del Mar Fariña, 2018). The authors remind supervisors to be reflective in their approach due to the imbalance of power.

Play therapists use the therapeutic power of accelerated psychological development to close the gap if there is a delay in emotional, or cognitive development. Accelerated psychological development is the idea of seeing progress from a forward-thinking perspective (S. Prendiville, 2014). When supervisors project the development of the play-therapist-in-training, they review characteristics of a master-level therapist and compare this with what the supervisor's current awareness, knowledge, and skills. Similar to the play therapist, the supervisor will discuss possible goals with the supervisee that can maximize the supervisee's potential.

As it relates to the therapeutic powers of teaching, the play therapist implements indirect and direct teaching to facilitate learning and assist the client in developing new skills that are transferable to real-life situations. While direct teaching involves modeling or practice (Fraser, 2014), indirect teaching requires the therapist to convey theme-related messages that are appropriate to the client's comprehension (de Faoite, 2014). Indirect teaching is best suited for the client who is defensive or resistant to direct teaching as it creates a mental separation from the emotion or situation. These powers of play can easily translate into supervision. Bernard and Goodyear (2019) addressed the role of the supervisor-teacher in the discrimination model for supervision. Different from other forms of supervision, the play therapy supervisor may use play media as a mode to assist the supervisee's understanding of themselves and their clients. The supervisor should tailor methods of direct teaching to complement the supervisee's learning styles and match client scenarios. Supervisors using the therapeutic power of indirect and direct teaching can further increase the supervisees' awareness, knowledge, and skills in play therapy.

Clients supported by the therapeutic power of creative problem-solving gain the advantage of learning emotional regulation, rehearsing conflict resolutions, and an opportunity to understand their fears (Russ & Wallace, 2014). Supervisees may lack the ability to use problem-solving skills appropriately. The integrated developmental model (Stoltenberg, et. al., 1998, as cited in Bernard & Goodyear, 2019) highlights anxiety as a component in determining the transition from novice to master-level supervisee. Supervisees with high levels of anxiety are more likely to not disclose information related to supervision (Tolleson et al., 2017). While anxiety can motivate some supervisees, it can hinder others. When supervisees experience stagnation with a clinical case or with their own development, the supervisory relationship can act as a supportive structure. Play therapists use the relationship to understand and motivate clients to develop alternatives to difficult situations. Likewise, the supervisor can assist the supervisee in establishing their own creative problem-solving abilities. Play-therapists-in-training who benefit from the therapeutic power of creative problem-solving may feel more confident in the supervisory relationship, which can further support the supervisor's evaluation of their progress.

Frey (2014), explained that self-esteem describes how an individual approaches life. It involves two components: competency and worthiness. When play therapists guide their work using the therapeutic power of self-esteem, they provide the client with a supportive environment to begin the work of merging their self-esteem with their self-concept, with the goal of self-growth. Frey encouraged therapists to offer both positive feedback and constructive criticism to the client. Supervisees are certainly not immune from doubt about themselves and their work. Regardless of the supervisees' internal hesitations, the supervisor must maintain integrity in their evaluation of the supervisee (Miller et al., 2019). Supervisors should evaluate dispositional issues (i.e., personal and professional functionings that influence fit for the profession) from the therapeutic power of self-esteem. The supervisor needs to encourage the supervisee to reflect on the origins of their doubt and help the supervisee understand the connection between disposition and progress toward the goal of becoming a registered play therapist. Within a safe supervisory relationship, the supervisor and supervisee can identify a plan to resolve any dispositional matters and provide support for the supervisee to implement the plan. Supervisors who include the therapeutic power of self-esteem in the supervisory relationship can elevate the supervisee's professional competency.

The play therapist who incorporates the therapeutic powers of stress management and resiliency maintains ideals that success and the ability to overcome are both learned and innate (Seymour, 2014). Bemis (2014) explained that stress is difficult to define since every individual responds to stressful events differently. Bemis described how play can provide an opportunity for the client to reduce and manage their stress levels. Therapists also understand that resiliency can be beneficial in reducing self-blame, increasing self-esteem, and creating meaning from experiences. Helping others can also improve resiliency (Russ, 2004 as cited in Seymour, 2014). Like clients in play therapy, supervisees may experience moments of uncertainty. Supervisors can use the therapeutic power of resiliency to encourage supervisees to focus on successes and to remain focused on the reasons they sought play therapy training. Hitchcock et al. (2021) emphasized that supervisees are accountable for their own professional resilience, but supervisors should be supportive in assisting supervisees in identifying ways to manage stress and find resilience.

Strategies to Maintain the Supervision Relationship

Sandtray is a flexible intervention that can be utilized throughout the developmental process of the supervision relationship. Sandtray allows the supervisee to utilize symbolism to express any thoughts or emotions about a variety of situations or interactions with others (Saltis et al., 2019).

Peer supervision is also another strategy that can be used to maintain the relationship. Somerville et al. (2019) discussed how supervisees were able to benefit from peer collaboration without the structure from the supervisor. Supervisees can receive feedback from peers without the anxiety of formal evaluation.

Tolleson et al. (2017) described experiential activities focused on mindfulness ("brief mindfulness"), opportunities to practice skills ("guess and reflect the feeling"), and creative ways to receive feedback ("find the apple"). Other strategies to consider are the use of social media (Ingram et al., 2017), bibliotherapy (Bradley et al., 2019), and game-based learning (Pietrantoni et al., 2019).

Transitioning the Supervisory Relationship to a Collegial Relationship

Much like termination of the therapist–client relationship, ending the supervision relationship can be very emotional, particularly if the termination is premature, resulting in missed learning opportunities for both the client and therapist. When successful termination occurs, it indicates that goals have been met and standards have been maintained. Understanding that there may be some self-doubt on the part of the supervisee about operating independently, the supervisor can continue to serve as a secure base in the form of consultation (Copenhaver & Crandell-Williams, 2020). Although not every supervisory relationship will continue beyond the contractual obligation, supervisors who have established a strong bond with the supervisee can seize the opportunity to form a collegial relationship with the former supervisee (Bernard & Goodyear, 2019). A relationship where both are now registered play therapists can help decrease stagnation within the profession.

Therapeutic Powers to Transition the Supervisory Relationship to a Collegial Relationship

Stress inoculation and counterconditioning fears are two therapeutic powers to assist the supervisor and supervisee in transitioning the supervision relationship to a collegial relationship. Play therapists use the therapeutic power of stress inoculation to assist clients in managing future stress or anxiety, while counterconditioning fears can reduce or eliminate fear or anxiety. Cavett (2014) provided examples of situations in which children may experience fear. These examples include a terminal illness of a family member, life or school transitions, or a child's own medical procedures. Related to the focus of fears and anxiety, van Hollander (2014) explained the goal of counterconditioning fears is to pair the fear with something enjoyable. The therapy session can act as a safe holding environment for clients to act out their fears. The supervisory relationship can also serve as a place for calming fears that might exist for the play-therapist-in-training who is nearing the end of the supervision term. Although fears of conducting a first session alone may create anxiety, there may still be anxiety regarding the ending of the relationship. The supervisor must discuss these fears with the supervisee and prepare them for full autonomy (Levendosky & Hopwood, 2017).

Strategies for Transitioning the Relationship to a Collegial Relationship

Socratic questioning is a widely used approach to encourage critical thinking and reflection (Feinstein, 2020). When supervisors pose challenging questions to the supervisee, they can process their thoughts and emotions about the supervision experience and future work. The use of photovoice is a creative method to discuss specific themes, that is, having supervisees take photos to represent what supervision termination may mean to them (Zeglin et al., 2019). Supervisors can also use guided imagery which allows supervisees to visualize new possibilities and expectations (Marshall & Farrell, 2019). Other options to transition from supervision to a collegial relationship could entail narrative work, sandtray activities, collaborative academic contributions, attending/presenting at local or state conferences together, or creating community platforms to provide play therapy information.

Conclusion

This chapter provided an overview of the intersection of play therapy supervision with the 20 therapeutic powers of play. Suggestions for transitioning the relationship from beginning to termination were also provided. Play therapist-supervisors can use this chapter as a guide to strengthening the supervisory relationship but are encouraged to tailor all therapeutic powers and strategies to the needs of the supervisee.

References

Altvater, R. A., Singer, R. R., & Gil, E. (2017). Part 1: Modern trends in the playroom—Preferences and interactions with tradition and innovation. *International Journal of Play Therapy, 26*(4), 239–249. https://doi.org/10.1037/pla0000058

Amaro, C. M., Mitchell, T. B., Cordts, K. M. P., Borner, K. B., Frazer, A. L., Garcia, A. M., & Roberts, M. C. (2020). Clarifying supervision expectations: Construction of a clinical supervision contract as a didactic exercise for advanced graduate students. *Training and Education in Professional Psychology, 14*(3), 235–241. https://doi.org/10.1037/tep0000273

Aponte, H. J., & Ingram, M. (2018). Person of the therapist supervision: Reflections of a therapist and supervisor on empathic-identification and differentiation. *Journal of Family Psychotherapy, 29*(1), 43–57. https://doi.org/10.1080/08975353.2018.1416233

Association for Play Therapy. (n.d.). Association for play therapy. Retrieved July 30, 2021, from https://www.a4pt.org/page/WhyPlayTherapy

Bemis, K. S. (2014). Stress management. In C. E. Schaefer & A. A. Drewes (Eds.), *The therapeutic powers of play: 20 core agents of change* (2nd ed., pp. 143–152). Wiley.

Bennett, M. M., & Eberts, S. (2014). Self-expression. In C. E. Schaefer & A. A. Drewes (Eds.), *The therapeutic powers of play: 20 core agents of change* (2nd ed., pp. 11–24). Wiley.

Bernard, J., & Goodyear, R. (2019). *Fundamentals of clinical supervision* (6th ed.). Pearson.

Boyle, S. L., & Kenny, T. E. (2020). To disclose or not to disclose: Examining supervisor actions related to self-disclosure in supervision. *Journal of Psychotherapy Integration, 30*(1), 36–43. https://doi.org/10.1037/int0000181

Bradley, N., Stargell, N., Craigen, L., Whisenhunt, J., Campbell, E., & Kress, V. (2019). Creative approaches for promoting vulnerability in supervision: A relational-cultural approach. *Journal of Creativity in Mental Health, 14*(3), 391–404. https://doi.org/10.1080/15401383.2018.1562395

Cavett, A. M. (2014). Stress inoculation. In C. E. Schaefer & A. A. Drewes (Eds.), *The therapeutic powers of play: 20 core agents of change* (2nd ed., pp. 131–143). Wiley.

Copenhaver, M., & Crandell-Williams, A. (2020). A safe place: Using clinical supervision groups to build interprofessional collaborative practice skills. *Advances in Social Work, 20*(2), 320–337. https://doi.org/10.18060/23318

de Faoite, A. T. (2014). Indirect teaching. In C. E. Schaefer & A. A. Drewes (Eds.), *The therapeutic powers of play: 20 core agents of change* (2nd ed., pp. 51–67). Wiley.

Dollarhide, C. T., Hale, S. C., & Stone-Sabali, S. (2020). A new model for social justice supervision. *Journal of Counseling and Development, 99*(1), 104–113. https://doi.org/10.1002/jcad.12358

Drewes, A. A., & Schaefer, C. E. (2014). Catharsis. In C. E. Schaefer & A. A. Drewes (Eds.), *The therapeutic powers of play: 20 core agents of change* (2nd ed., pp. 71–81). Wiley.

Feinstein, R. E. (2020). Descriptions and reflections on the cognitive apprenticeship model of psychotherapy training & supervision. *Journal of Contemporary Psychotherapy, 51*(2), 155–164. https://doi.org/10.1007/s10879-020-09480-6

Fraser, T. (2014). Direct teaching. In C. E. Schaefer & A. A. Drewes (Eds.), *The therapeutic powers of play: 20 core agents of change* (2nd ed., pp. 39–50). Wiley.

Frey, D. (2014). Self-esteem. In C. E. Schaefer & A. A. Drewes (Eds.), *The therapeutic powers of play: 20 core agents of change* (2nd ed., pp. 295–318). Wiley.

Hartwig, E. K., & Bennett, M. M. (2017). Four approaches to using sandtray in play therapy supervision. *International Journal of Play Therapy, 26*(4), 230–238. https://doi.org/10.1037/pla0000050

Hitchcock, C., Hughes, M., McPherson, L., & Whitaker, L. (2021). The role of education in developing students' professional resilience for social work practice: A systematic scoping review. *British Journal of Social Work, 51*(7), 2361–2380. https://doi.org/10.1093/bjsw/bcaa054

Hoffman, K., Cooper, G., Powell, B., Siegel, D. J., & Benton, C. M. (2017). *Raising a secure child: How circle of security parenting can help you nurture your child's attachment, emotional resilience, and freedom to explore* (1st ed.). The Guilford Press.

Hutchby, I., & Dart, A. (2019). The interactional workings of laughter in group supervision for psychotherapeutic counsellors. *Counselling and Psychotherapy Research, 19*(2), 167–175. https://doi.org/10.1002/capr.12206

Ingram, M. V., Speedlin, S., Cannon, Y., Prado, A., & Avera, J. (2017). A seat at the table: Using social media as a platform to resolve microaggressions against transgender persons. *Journal of Creativity in Mental Health, 12*(3), 289–304. https://doi.org/10.1080/15401383.2016.1248266

Inzlicht, M., Werner, K. M., Briskin, J. L., & Roberts, B. W. (2021). Integrating models of self-regulation. *Annual Review of Psychology, 72*(1), 319–345. https://doi.org/10.1146/annurev-psych-061020-105721

Jones, C. T., Welfare, L. E., Melchior, S., & Cash, R. M. (2019). Broaching as a strategy for intercultural understanding in clinical supervision. *Clinical Supervisor, 38*(1), 1–16. https://doi.org/10.1080/07325223.2018.1560384

Kemer, G., Sunal, Z., Li, C., & Burgess, M. (2019). Beginning and expert supervisors' descriptions of effective and less effective supervision. *Clinical Supervisor, 38*(1), 116–134. https://doi.org/10.1080/07325223.2018.1514676

Kidwell, M. C., & Kerig, P. K. (2021). To trust is to survive: Toward a developmental model of moral injury. *Journal of Child & Adolescent Trauma.* https://doi.org/10.1007/s40653-021-00399-1

Kottman, T. (2014). Positive emotion. In C. E. Schaefer & A. A. Drewes (Eds.), *The therapeutic powers of play: 20 Core agents of change* (2nd ed., pp. 103–120). Wiley.

Levendosky, A. A., & Hopwood, C. J. (2017). Terminating supervision. *Psychotherapy, 54*(1), 37–46. https://doi.org/10.1037/pst0000096

Marshall, R. C., & Farrell, I. C. (2019). Career guided imagery: A narrative approach for emerging adults. *Journal of Creativity in Mental Health, 14*(2), 193–204. https://doi.org/10.1080/15401383.2019.1586612

Martin, P., Kumar, S., & Lizarondo, L. (2017). Effective use of technology in clinical supervision. *Internet Interventions, 8,* 35–39. https://doi.org/10.1016/j.invent.2017.03.001

McGarry, K. A., West, M., & Hogan, K. F. (2021). Perspective-taking and social competence in adults. *Advances in Cognitive Psychology, 17*(2), 129–135. https://doi.org/10.5709/acp-0323-5

Miller, S. M., Larwin, K. H., Kautzman-East, M., Williams, J. L., Evans, W. J., Williams, D. D., Abramski, A. L., & Miller, K. L. (2019). A proposed definition and structure of counselor dispositions. *Measurement and Evaluation in Counseling and Development, 53*(2), 117–130. https://doi.org/10.1080/07481756.2019.1640618

Morrison, M. A., & Lent, R. W. (2018). The working alliance, beliefs about the supervisor, and counseling self-efficacy: Applying the relational efficacy model to counselor supervision. *Journal of Counseling Psychology, 65*(4), 512–522. https://doi.org/10.1037/cou0000267

Nash, J. B. (2014). Social competence. In C. E. Schaefer & A. A. Drewes (Eds.), *The therapeutic powers of play: 20 core agents of change* (2nd ed., pp. 185–212). Wiley.

Nejati, M., & Shafaei, A. (2018). Leading by example: The influence of ethical supervision on students' prosocial behavior. *Higher Education, 75*(1), 75–89. https://doi.org/10.1007/s10734-017-0130-4

O'Neill, P., & del Mar Fariña, M. (2018). Constructing critical conversations in social work supervision: Creating change. *Clinical Social Work Journal, 46*(4), 298–309. https://doi.org/10.1007/s10615-018-0681-6

Parson, J. A. (2021). Children speak play: Landscaping the therapeutic powers of play. In E. Prendiville & J. A. Parson (Eds.), *Clinical applications of the therapeutic powers of play: Case studies in child and adolescent psychotherapy* (1st ed., pp. 1–10). Routledge. https://bookshelf.vitalsource.com/books/9781000359404

Patallo, B. J. (2019). The multicultural guidelines in practice: Cultural humility in clinical training and supervision. *Training and Education in Professional Psychology, 13*(3), 227–232. https://doi.org/10.1037/tep0000253

Pietrantoni, Z., Henning, J., Totten, J., Shindelar, L., & Keene-Orton, B. (2019). Game-based learning in counselor education: Strategies for counselor training. *Journal of Counselor Preparation and Supervision, 12*(2). https://repository.wcsu.edu/jcps/vol12/iss2/3

Prendiville, E. (2014). Abreaction. In C. E. Schaefer & A. A. Drewes (Eds.), *The therapeutic powers of play: 20 Core agents of change* (2nd ed., pp. 83–102). Wiley.

Prendiville, S. (2014). Accelerated psychological development. In C. E. Schaefer & A. A. Drewes (Eds.), *The therapeutic powers of play: 20 Core agents of change* (2nd ed., pp. 255–268). Wiley.

Ramos, J., & Linstrum, K. S. (2017). Written forms of self-expression: Changes from 1985 to 2016. *College Student Journal, 51*(3), 424–428.

Rankine, M. (2017). Making the connections: A practice model for reflective supervision. *Aotearoa New Zealand Social Work, 29*(3), 66–78. https://doi.org/10.11157/anzswj-vol29iss3id377

Russ, S. W. (2004). *Play in child development and psychotherapy: Toward empirically supported practice.* Erbaum.

Russ, S. W., & Wallace, C. E. (2014). Creative problem solving. In C. E. Schaefer & A. A. Drewes (Eds.), *The therapeutic powers of play: 20 Core agents of change* (2nd ed., pp. 213–223). Wiley.

Saltis, M. N., Critchlow, C., & Smith, J. A. (2019). Teaching through sand: Creative applications of sandtray within constructivist pedagogy. *Journal of Creativity in Mental Health, 14*(3), 381–390. https://doi.org/10.1080/15401383.2019.1624995

Seymour, J. (2014). Resiliency. In C. E. Schaefer & A. A. Drewes (Eds.), *The therapeutic powers of play: 20 core agents of change* (2nd ed., pp. 225–242). Wiley.

Singh-Pillay, N., & Cartwright, D. (2019). The unsaid: In-depth accounts of non-disclosures in supervision from the trainees' perspective. *Counselling and Psychotherapy Research, 19*(1), 83–92. https://doi.org/10.1002/capr.12203

Somerville, W., Marcus, S., & Chang, D. F. (2019). Multicultural competence–focused peer supervision: A multiple case study of clinical and counseling psychology trainees. *Journal of Multicultural Counseling and Development, 47*(4), 274–294. https://doi.org/10.1002/jmcd.12158

Stewart, A. L., & Echterling, L. G. (2014). Therapeutic relationship. In C. E. Schaefer & A. A. Drewes (Eds.), *The therapeutic powers of play: 20 Core agents of change* (2nd ed., pp. 157–169). Wiley.

Stoltenberg, C. D., McNeil, B., & Delworth, U. (1998). *An integrated developmental model for supervising counselors and therapists.* San Francisco, CA: JosseyBass.

Tolleson, A. M., Grad, R., Zabek, F., & Zeligman, M. (2017). Teaching helping skills courses: Creative activities to reduce anxiety. *Journal of Creativity in Mental Health, 12*(4), 428–439. https://doi.org/10.1080/15401383.2017.1281186

van Hollander, T. (2014). Counterconditioning fears. In C. E. Schaefer & A. A. Drewes (Eds.), *The therapeutic powers of play: 20 core agents of change* (2nd ed., pp. 121–130). Wiley.

Watkins, C. E., Hook, J. N., Mosher, D. K., & Callahan, J. L. (2019). Humility in clinical supervision: Fundamental, foundational, and transformational. *Clinical Supervisor, 38*(1), 58–78. https://doi.org/10.1080/07325223.2018.1487355

Whelan, W. F., & Stewart, A. L. (2014). Attachment. In C. E. Schaefer & A. A. Drewes (Eds.), *The therapeutic powers of play: 20 core agents of change* (2nd ed., pp. 171–182). Wiley.

Wrape, E. R., Callahan, J. L., Rieck, T., & Watkins, C. E. (2017). Attachment theory within clinical supervision: Application of the conceptual to the empirical. *Psychoanalytic Psychotherapy, 31*(1), 37–54. https://doi.org/10.1080/02668734.2016.1261927

Yasenik, L. (2021). Polly meets Maddie: Fostering emotional wellness. In E. Prendiville & J. A. Parson (Eds.), *Clinical applications of the therapeutic powers of play: Case studies in child and adolescent psychotherapy* (1st ed., pp. 128–143). Routledge. https://bookshelf.vitalsource.com/books/9781000359404

Yeager, M., & Yeager, D. (2014). Self-regulation. In C. E. Schaefer & A. A. Drewes (Eds.), *The therapeutic powers of play: 20 core agents of change* (2nd ed., pp. 269–293). Wiley.

Yerushalmi, H. (2021). Authentic voices in supervision. *British Journal of Psychotherapy, 37*(1), 116–129. https://doi.org/10.1111/bjp.12609

Zeglin, R. J., Niemela, D. R. M., Rosenblatt, K., & Hernandez-Garcia, J. (2019). Using photovoice as a counselor education pedagogical tool: A pilot. *Journal of Creativity in Mental Health, 14*(2), 258–268. https://doi.org/10.1080/15401383.2019.1581116

6 Delivering Play Therapy Supervision

Function, feedback, and formats

Lynn O'Brien

The Function of Supervision

There is an ongoing and increasing need for professional supervision as the field of play therapy continues to grow (Association for Play Therapy, 2021; Donald et al., 2015), especially as supervision by a Registered Play Therapist-Supervisor™ (RPT-S™) is required to become a Registered Play Therapist™ (RPT™)(Association for Play Therapy, 2021). For many play therapists working with children, there are barriers to receiving supervision, such as a lack of access to an RPT-S™, and affordability (VanderGast et al., 2010). Additionally, play therapists report a lack of supervisors who are experienced with working with children and have knowledge related to expression through play (Thomas, 2015).

In general, supervision refers to "an intervention provided by a more senior member of a profession to a more junior colleague or colleagues who typically (but not always) are members of that same profession" (Bernard & Goodyear, 2019, p. 9). Clinical supervision is the cornerstone of professional development for therapists and a complex process for examining complex situations (Christman-Dunn, 1998; Veilleux et al., 2014). Along with gatekeeping for the profession, the purpose of supervision enhances the professional competencies of the junior supervisee through the development of an ongoing evaluative and hierarchical relationship (Bernard & Goodyear, 2019). Although clinical supervision requires managerial and organizational skills, it is not administrative in nature (Bernard & Goodyear, 2019).

The role of the supervisor is of utmost importance to the development of supervisees. Supervisors who identify as a play therapist positively impact supervisee satisfaction with supervision (VanderGast & Hinkle, 2015). To be effective, supervision must be perceived as helpful by the supervisee (Edwards, 2013). Not only does clinical supervision play a critical role in the professional field of therapy, but the supervisory process can also foster the development of play therapists, thus impacting mental health services provided to children (VanderGast et al., 2010).

Supervisors fulfill a variety of roles depending on clinical and supervisory theoretical orientation of the supervisor and supervisee, the developmental level of the supervisee, the format of the supervision, and the goals of the supervisee (Mullen, 2015; Mullen et al., 2007). Many supervisors learn how to supervise through

DOI: 10.4324/9781003196075-8

their own experience as a supervisee (Mullen, 2015). Previously, supervisors without play therapy experience felt confident in their supervision of play therapists (Bergeron, 2004), with less than 30% of RPT-Ss™ completing a course in supervision and most not receiving supervision of their supervision (Donald et al., 2015; Fall et al., 2007). Supervisors who provide supervision to play therapists, yet lack knowledge and are unfamiliar with play therapy, may be limiting supervisee's work (Allen, et al. 2007). Additionally, play therapist supervisees prefer experienced and credentialed supervisors (VanderGast et al., 2010).

Not only is supervision that is specific to play therapy required to preserve the integrity of the profession (Thomas, 2015), play therapist supervisors need to possess past and ongoing play therapy experience along with advanced knowledge, skill, and experiences (Ray, 2011). In 2016, APT updated the standards to be a RPT-S™ and now requires supervisors to have play therapy–specific supervisor training (Association for Play Therapy, 2021). During clinical supervision, the supervisee's growth and development are enhanced through processing counseling experiences, including clinical skills, ethical competency, and case conceptualization (Bernard & Goodyear, 2019; Bradley & Ladany, 2010; Thompson & Moffett, 2010). Similarly, play therapists are interested in supervision goals related to improvement of skills and techniques and case conceptualization, professional support, identifying play themes, and an increase in self-awareness (VanderGast et al., 2010). Recognizing the importance of skill as a play therapist is secondary to focusing on the personhood of the play therapist themselves (Blanco et al., 2014; Landreth, 2012).

When supervising play therapists, intentional supervision can promote supervisee growth and development through teaching and protecting the welfare of the client. Assessing the developmental level of supervisees prior to providing supervision will give play therapy supervisors a framework to begin work from (Mullen, 2015). Additionally, play therapy supervisors need to identify with a model of supervision. To assist clinical supervisors with the task of supervising competent therapists, multiple models of supervision have been developed (Borders & Brown, 2005); "most traditional supervision has paralleled conventional counseling, looking for what the supervisee was doing incorrectly or not doing enough of, mostly in the area of technique, and attempting to devise remedial solutions" (Edwards & Chen, 1999, p. 350). However, traditional supervision models do not consistently meet the needs to effectively supervise play therapists because the models do not focus on using play with child clients who communicate through the manipulation of objects, nor do they provide understanding of the power differential within the therapeutic relationship (Allen et al., 2007; Thomas, 2015). Philosophical approaches to play therapy supervision may vary by models of supervision or theoretical orientation, even though the purpose is consistent across helping professions (Thomas, 2015).

Supervisees report continuous feedback from supervisors contributes to their development as a play therapist through supervisee self-evaluation and supervisor teaching and evaluation (Aguilera, 2010). Continuous monitoring of supervisee performance is not only an important gatekeeping measure for the profession, it empowers the supervisee to self-supervise and achieve goals (Thomas, 2015). While the focus during supervision for beginning play therapists is on mistakes made, intermediate and advanced play therapists focus more on case conceptualization and unique challenges that enhances professional growth (Mullen, 2015).

Supervision by a supervisor with play therapy experience allows the supervisee to receive more targeted feedback related to play therapy knowledge and skills without needing to interpret and self-guide the learning process during supervision (Bergeron, 2004). Issues that play therapist supervisors face include setting limits, ethical issues, issues with abuse, and transference and countertransference (Metcalf, 2003). Furthermore, multicultural concerns arise more often in supervision when clinicians provide services to more children who are minoritized (Ceballos et al., 2012). Supervision impacts the effectiveness of counseling. Leadership development in multicultural counseling and social justice competencies may also present as opportunities through supervision (Kozol, 2005). Racial identity, cultural biases, and prejudicial attitudes can be explored during supervision, thus allowing play therapists time and space to engage in self-awareness (Ceballos et al., 2012). To meet the needs of all children, multicultural competence challenges personal biases of the supervisee and creates the ability to see the world through the child client's eyes while applying appropriate techniques and interventions (Strohmer & Shivy, 1994).

Social justice advocacy training for play therapists is necessary to address impacts of childhood exposure to social adversity on psychological and socioemotional well-being (Smith et al., 2009). When play therapists take societal factors that impede growth into consideration, empathy and understanding drive interventions that have long-term positive results (Ceballos et al., 2012; Kiselica & Robinson, 2001). Supervisors can provide opportunities for supervisees to increase incorporation of social justice into their play therapy work. Encouraging reflection from a holistic perspective and focusing on self-awareness shed light on comfort levels of supervisees with social justice issues and can directly impact their willingness to advocate on behalf of child clients who are marginalized (Glosoff & Durham, 2010; Cebellos et al., 2012).

Play therapist supervisors can grow professionally as they serve an important gatekeeping role for the profession by seeking supervision of their supervision (Mullen, 2015). Supervision of their role as supervisor, additional training on supervision, and receiving mentoring as a play therapist supervisor elevates the field of play therapy (Mullen, 2015). Play therapy supervisors should be aware of the experiences they bring to the supervisory relationship and be mindful of the relationship itself, thus enhancing the experience for themselves as well as the supervisee (Glazer & Stein, 2015). APT is committed to deepening credibility of RPT-Ss™ through increased preparation demonstrated through credentialing, thus affording RPT-Ss™ the ability to better serve clients and supervisees (Association for Play Therapy, 2021).

Prior to registering as a play therapist, supervisees must complete direct play therapy experiences while participating in play therapy supervision. Additionally, supervisor observations are required to assess supervisee competencies, qualifications, professionalism, and other issues pertaining to the play therapy practice (Association for Play Therapy, 2021). Supervision may be scheduled for convenience, but time also needs to be provided when the need for supervision is pressing (Disney & Stephens, 1994). However, satisfaction seems to be higher for supervisees when feedback is delivered immediately (Bernard & Goodyear, 2019). Supervision provided within 4 hours of a therapy session tends to be more consultative rather than content-oriented, with more follow-through with use of strategies by the clinician in subsequent sessions (Couchon & Bernard, 1984).

Feedback

While supervision models provide the framework for conducting clinical supervision, the use of supervision formats provides strategies for delivering feedback or providing interventions to supervisees within various settings. Within the context of clinical supervision, feedback is information that supervisors communicate to inform supervisees of their performance based on professional standards and competencies (Claiborn et al., 2001). The delivery of feedback can be either positive or corrective-focused and given hierarchically or be strengths-based, each having its usefulness or drawbacks (Edwards, 2013). Hierarchical feedback is direct and linear, as it is delivered from the supervisor to the supervisee. Also assumed is that the supervisor holds the power within the supervisory relationship (Bernard & Goodyear, 2019; Claiborne et al., 2001; Edwards, 2013). Moreover, strengths-based feedback focuses on supervisee assets which affirms the supervisee is on the right path with application of skills and knowledge (Bernard & Goodyear, 2019; Claiborne et al., 2001; Edwards, 2013).

Another approach to play therapy supervision is the use of play. Creative approaches to play therapy supervision that include play activities and techniques allow playfulness into the relationship, thus facilitating an increase in risk-taking (Crocker & Wroblewski, 1975). Toys and other expressive means enhance communication between supervisors and supervisees (Fall & Sutton, 2004). Creative play to use during supervision include use of sandtray (Perryman et al., 2016), metaphor (Guiffrida et al., 2007), art techniques (Deaver & Shiflett, 2011), psychodrama and bibliosupervision (Graham et al., 2014), mythology and fairy tales (Sommer et al., 2009), and Legos (Peabody, 2015).

Using creative interventions in play therapy supervision helps lower supervisee defenses and provides for better understanding of the child client's perspective while focusing on the supervisee's self as therapist (Blanco et al., 2014; Donald et al., 2015; Drewes & Mullen, 2008; Mullen et al., 2007). "Just as children use toys rather than words to express themselves in play therapy, so too can supervisees use play therapy techniques when words fail to express their experience or understanding of their clients" (Mullen et al., 2007, p. 69). Play therapists should be playful and play therapy feedback can be delivered in playful ways (Landreth, 2012). Furthermore, feedback can be categorized in several different ways and processed through self-report, print, recording, live, and virtual.

Self-report

Self-report is one format to use during clinical supervision for play therapists. Play therapist supervisees describe what happened during the play therapy session, providing valuable insights into the play therapist's thoughts and emotions (Noelle, 2002). However, the limitations include the risk of distortion in the withholding of information by the supervisee (Mullen, 2015). Case presentation is the most-used mode for keeping supervisors up-to-date about clinician's cases (Edwards, 2013). A case presentation format provides the opportunity for clinicians and supervisors to discuss the process and expectations of the supervisory relationship (Biggs, 1998). Issues with case presentation relate to the accuracy of describing the case by the clinician and clinicians wanting to be perceived positively (Edwards, 2013).

Supervisees can also self-report, using process notes and case notes. Process notes include initial impressions and observations by the supervisee regarding the play therapy sessions. Case notes are more formal and provide written explanation of the content and the interventions used during therapy sessions. Process notes and case notes can be used to direct the supervisory session and "should be used in conjunction with any other supervision modality" (Bernard et al., 2019, p. 165).

Print

Print forms allow supervisees to notice faulty intervention strategies and the opportunity to critique their approaches (Bernard et al., 2019). Transcripts provide written content of therapy sessions including the actual interchanges between the play therapist and client. Pauses are also noted along with the length of time between responses and client nonverbal behavior. The transcript can be studied to identify areas for improvement or highlight effective practice (Arthur & Gfroerer, 2002).

Another form of print is written feedback provided by the supervisor to supervisees. Written feedback can include supervisory thoughts and impressions regarding skills and interventions utilized during play therapy sessions. Progress toward goals and suggestions might also be included and be shared in-between supervision meetings. Written feedback can help to coordinate supervision meetings through the sharing of the supervisor's conceptualization and the supervisee's review of the comments prior to supervision (Bernard et al., 2019).

As a play therapist, a primary catalyst for growth is working through difficult or challenging experiences (Rønnestad & Skovholt, 2013). However, maintaining a reflective practice is essential to bring functional closure to difficult challenges (Seymour & Crenshaw, 2014). Supervision is not something a supervisor does; rather, it is more reflective in nature (Carroll, 1996). Reflective practices can be facilitated through any configuration of supervision and require dedication to self-examination as a supervisor (Seymour & Crenshaw, 2014). Journal writing is one way to reflect as a play therapist. Supervisors can help supervisees identify patterns and themes within the entries to stimulate reflection and evaluate their effectiveness and development. (Bernard et al., 2019). Topics for entries might include supervisees' values, strengths, skills, and thoughts and feelings regarding play therapy sessions (Seymour & Creshaw, 2014).

Recording

Interpersonal Process Recall (IPR) is one strategy to help with case recall, as identified as an issue in self-reporting. In IPR, recorded audio or video is used to process sessions and to promote recollection of thoughts and feelings of the supervisee that occur during play therapy sessions (Kagen & Kagen, 1991). When something of importance occurs, the recording is stopped and explored through questioning, not statements (Bernard et al., 2019). Socratic questions can be used with IPR and are designed to increase the insight of the supervisee to help shed light on blind spots, as clinicians are "the best authority of their own dynamics and the best interpreter of their own experience" (Kagan, 1980, pp. 279–280).

The use of audio and video recordings during supervision has a long history from which rich clinical and relational data has been gleaned (Mullen, 2015; Rogers, 1942; Protinsky, 2003). Audio can highlight stellar moments within a session or help clinicians explore more challenging issues such as feeling stuck with a client (Edwards, 2013). Video-recorded supervision has become commonplace (Protinsky, 2003). Video allows for immediate feedback by supervisors, thus enhancing learning opportunities through correction and practice (Edwards, 2013). Moving the video-recorder is not advised as that would cause disruption to the play therapy session, yet the fixed position of the camera might inhibit capturing all the important pieces (Mullen, 2015). Perhaps the biggest drawback of recordings is the intimidation factor for the supervisee to be seen or heard, leaving play therapists self-critical of their words and gestures (Mullen, 2015).

Live

Live observation allows supervisors to directly view the play therapy session through a one-way mirror or other technological means, such as phoning-in or bug-in-the-ear (Mullen, 2015). This type of observation might not involve interacting with the supervisee during the therapy session. Rather, the supervisor observes the session while safeguarding client welfare through immediate availability to intervene if needed. Live observation provides a more complete picture of the session compared to audio or video tape (Bernard et al., 2019). Supervisors can come to conclusions regarding the client child, the child's play, the supervisee's skills, and the relationship and interaction between the play therapist and child (Mullen, 2015). Space, setup, scheduling, time, and cost are all limiting factors to direct observation (Mullen, 2015).

Live supervision is similar to live observation with the inclusion of embedding a teaching component (Mullen, 2015). Supervisors can make phone calls to provide suggestions to supervisees while in session (Montalvo, 1973). Phone-ins allow for immediate feedback regarding skill development (Wright, 1986). However helpful, stopping forward momentum during a session to provide feedback needs to be considered (Edwards, 2013). Bug-in-the-ear allows clinicians to receive immediate feedback using a receiving devise like a Bluetooth device (Boylston & Tuma, 1972). Feedback is given by the supervisor who watches and listens to the session behind a one-way mirror. Directions to provide additional input or to correct a mistake in clinical procedure are given through a microphone to the clinician (Edwards, 2013). Time and cost are two noted limitations to supervisors providing live supervision (Bernard & Goodyear, 2019). Additionally, there is potential for supervisees to become dependent on the supervisor, thus compromising growth for the play therapist (Mullen, 2015).

Co-therapy provides a unique experience for play therapists to participate in a session while also watching and learning from a more-seasoned clinician (Hendrix et al., 2001; Levinger, 1994; Roller & Nelson, 1991). One form of co-therapy allows one therapist to engage in play with the child client while the supervising therapist watches the process and reflects, thus benefitting the child and the play therapist (Levinger, 1994). Although immediate feedback and multiple perspectives enhance new understanding of clients and issues, co-therapy can be costly as it involves the time of two therapists for one session and can be complicated for clinics and agencies who are short on providers (Edwards, 2013; Levinger, 1994).

Another form of feedback is through the use of a team. Taking a team-break during play therapy sessions can provide time to discuss and devise strategic interventions or help course correction from a team perspective (Boscoloe et al., 1987; Edwards, 2013). Hearing multiple voices and meanings lessens the hierarchy of supervision and reduces individual culpability (Edwards, 2013). Reflecting teams are made up of a small group of colleagues who watch the clinician and child client behind a one-way mirror. Halfway through the session, the reflecting team becomes the focus for the clinician and child client as they reflect upon their thoughts regarding what they are seeing in the session (Edwards, 2013).

Virtual

There has been an explosion in the number of technologies used in supervision and for providing feedback to supervisees (Rousmaniere, 2014). The use of the Internet provides for use of videoconferencing, emailing, and text chatting for supervision. Additionally, web-based software and routine outcome monitoring is a technology that allows clients to complete outcome assessment forms electronically that graph progress of client symptoms and risk factors (Bernard et al., 2019). Cases that are not showing improvement can be prioritized during supervision. Supervisory bias is diminished, as the outcome data provides an empirical perspective (Bernard et al., 2019).

Virtual supervision increases accessibility to RPT-Ss™ for supervision, especially for play therapists in rural or remote areas. Additionally, there is reduced cost for travel and improved flexibility of scheduling, increased access to peer consultation via teleconference, web forums, and electronic list servs, and potentially enhanced diversity of supervisees and supervisors due to accessibility (Rousmaniere, 2014). Other considerations regarding the use of technology in play therapy supervision include legal, regulatory, and ethical issues, as well security of information. This topic is discussed further in the chapter on technology.

The next section focuses on formats for delivering supervision. Configurations include individual, dyadic, and group supervision, as well as peer consultation.

Formats

Play therapists supervisees typically receive supervision in either an individual or group supervision format (Ryan et al., 2002). However, APT specifies supervisees should have no more than 10 hours of group supervision under an RPT-S™ (Association for Play Therapy, 2021). With individual, dyadic, or group supervision for play therapist supervisees, the supervisor has a level of expected expertise (Mullen, 2015). Although with peer supervision, it is likely that all group members have similar levels of expertise and provide alternate perspectives and input to each other's play therapy cases (Mullen, 2015).

Individual Supervision

Individual supervision is one-on-one supervision between the supervisor and supervisee (Edwards, 2013) and is the cornerstone of professional development for therapists (Bernard et al., 2019). The relationship between supervisor and supervisee is crucial to successful supervision (Mullen, 2015). Supervisors' general functions include assessing supervisee learning needs, enhancing supervisee professional behavior, and evaluating supervisee performance (Borders & Brown, 2005; Bernard & Goodyear, 2019). The supervisors' preference for delivering supervision often relates to the supervisors' theoretical orientation, worldview, experience, and goals for the supervisee and self as supervisor. Learning goals and developmental levels of the supervisee also influences the supervisors' choice of format. Additionally, agency policies, facility capabilities, and client difficulty are influential (Borders & Brown, 2005).

APT states individual supervision consists of one supervisor and one supervisee. The focus of the supervision meeting is to discuss case notes, reports, or session video. There is not a limit to the number of hours obtained in-person or through distance supervision. APT allows dyadic supervision to be considered "individual" when the focus of the supervision session is on individual cases (Association for Play Therapy, 2021).

Dyadic Supervision

Dyadic supervision involves one supervisor and two supervisees and is the bridge between individual supervision and group supervision (Bernard et al., 2019). Dyadic supervision can be split-focus by dividing the available time between two supervisees or single-focus by allowing one supervisee to present their work for the entire time and the other supervisee to present the next supervisory session (Nguyen, 2004).

92   *Lynn O'Brien*

When supervisees are not the main focus of supervision, it is reported that the dyadic configuration allows supervisees to be more comfortable and relaxed, contributing to feeling psychologically safer than when participating in individual supervision (Lawson et al., 2009). It also provides for functional flow of information and synergy among the supervisees and supervisor and a sense of community (Oliver et al., 2010). Diverse perspectives and vicarious learning are valuable products of triadic supervision (Borders et al., 2012; Hein & Lawson, 2009; Lawson et al., 2009).

Supervisors also find it to be a more relaxed atmosphere while increasing the possibility for diversity (Hein & Lawson, 2008, Hein & Lawson, 2009), thus, reducing the sense of hierarchy and increasing a sense of collegiality. This is especially prevalent when the non-presenting supervisee provides feedback that normalizes challenges inherent in supervisee development (Felton et al., 2015).

Limitations with dyadic supervision include lack of time, which might leave few opportunities to go deeper with each supervisee (Bernard et al., 2019). Attention should be paid to time allotted for each supervisee, possibly supplementing with individual supervision. Another limitation is the compatibility of the peers receiving supervision (Hein et al., 2011). Carefully selecting pairs and identifying the roles of each supervisee during each session can help ensure compatibility. When the triad between supervisor and supervisees is not functional, the context of supervision becomes less safe, thus restricting peer feedback and self-disclosure while limiting immediacy (Lawson et al., 2009). Although triadic supervision might be perceived as more relaxed, it could be more taxing due to the supervisor's required preparation and skills sets (Borders et al., 2012), including orienting supervisees to the process and format.

Group Supervision

Group supervision involves a group of supervisees who meet with a designated supervisor to monitor the therapeutic services being provided and to continue gaining understanding as a therapist and the clients with whom they work (Bernard & Goodyear, 2019). Goals and feedback are provided by the supervisor and through interactions with other group members. The size of the supervisee group can greatly impact the group dynamics. APT allows group supervision to include up to no more than ten supervisees (Association for Play Therapy, 2021). Membership can also affect the outcomes depending on if supervisees are constant or constantly changing (Bernard & Goodyear, 2019).

There are many benefits to group supervision. Time and cost are the most obvious (Bernard & Goodyear, 2019; Mullen, 2015). Other benefits include opportunities for observing and vicarious learning from other supervisees as supervisees conceptualize and discuss interventions utilized with clients (Proctor & Inskipp, 2001). Hearing supervisees discuss cases also provides exposure for others to learn about a variety of client issues and diagnoses. Supervisees can also provide diverse perspectives when providing feedback and normalize the supervisee experience for others. Supervisees can also learn supervisory skills during group supervision to prepare for a supervisory role (Bernard & Goodyear, 2019).

However, group supervision may not provide sufficient time for supervisees to review their cases if their load is heavier than other supervisees or if other supervisees have greater needs. Confidentiality can be a concern and group phenomena, such as between-member competition and insensitivity to cultural differences, can impede learning (Bernard & Goodyear, 2019). Additionally, supervisors may need to prepare clinicians who have negative experiences with corrective-feedback in childhood, as this can impact how feedback is received in group supervision (Alexander & Hulse-Killacky, 2005).

Other considerations for providing group supervision include the supervisor's comfort level with group work (Bernard & Goodyear, 2019). Group supervision is likely to mirror group counseling and group supervisors can hinder the process with poor facilitation skills (Bernard & Goodyear, 2019; Grigg, 2006). Just as supervision of group work is in its infancy (Riva, 2014), so is the literature regarding supervision of group work within play therapy. Nonetheless, this is an important consideration for supervisors as supervisees can learn vicariously through the experiences of group members who are leading play therapy groups (Riva, 2014). It would behoove supervisors to be familiar with the literature around Supervision of Group Work (SGW) to broaden their conceptualization of running client groups and supervision groups (Bernard & Goodyear, 2019).

Peer group consultation

Peer group consultation involves play therapist supervisees gathering together to provide support and suggestions to each other with difficult cases. Joining with peers can help supervisees counter isolation and burnout, especially when considering the availability and affordability of additional supervisory support (Bernard & Goodyear, 2019; Mullen, 2015). Another benefit is the absence of hierarchy which changes the dynamics and can decrease supervisee anxiety, increase self-efficacy and confidence, and enhance learning opportunities (Edwards, 2013). Benefits of peer group consultation include increased collegiality and motivation, strengthening connection with peers, building a sense of community, increased knowledge, and vicarious learning (Kassan, 2010; Newman et al., 2013). As with any group, attention should be paid to establishing ground rules and group norms (Bernard & Goodyear, 2019). Group dynamics can pose challenges, as there is no designated leader, and each supervisee must hold themselves and others to ethical and professional codes of conduct (Mullen, 2015).

Conclusion

There is a myriad of approaches to play therapy supervision. Supervisors must decide not only on their preferred model of supervision, but also formats, configurations, and other considerations. Play therapists prefer a combination of individual and group supervision with self-report and videotape review being of interest focusing on identifying play themes and case conceptualization (VanderGast, et al. 2010). Communication and intentionality are essential to any supervisory relationship (Bernard & Goodyear, 2019). Play therapy supervisors should consider seeking supervision of their supervision. Having support, knowing yourself, gathering additional resources, and getting feedback are building blocks for the essential work of supervision (Bernard & Goodyear, 2019).

Bernard et al. (2019) formed a list of questions supervisors might ask when selecting types of feedback and format for delivering supervision:

- How will the supervisee receive this method of supervision?
- Am I considering the functions of supervision?
- Am I considering the timing or relative structure of the supervision?
- What are the administrative constraints, if any; and can I advocate for appropriate time and/or equipment required?
- What does the supervisee need to learn? Am I using the best method for this purpose?
- Am I skilled in the use of this method?
- Have I considered the ethical safeguards?
- Is it time to try something new?
- Can I document the success of the method used?
- Am I willing to confront my own assumptions?
- Are clients getting better as a result of the supervision being provided?

The intent of the APT Credentialing Program is to increase play therapy competencies and to promote the value of play (Association for Play Therapy, 2021). Supervision is one component that strengthens the play therapist and play therapy practices. The increased need for play therapy supervision highlights the importance of understanding the function of supervision, ways to provide feedback, and format options to deliver supervision.

References

Aguilera, M. E. (2010). *An exploratory study of the developmental process of novice play therapist.* Dissertation Abstract International Section A: Humanities and Social Sciences, 70, 3500.

Alexander, A., & Hulse-Killacky, D. (2005). Childhood memories and receptivity to corrective feedback in group supervision. *Journal for Specialists in Group Work, 30*(1), 23–45.

Allen, V. B., Folger, W. A., & Pehrsson, D. E. (2007). Reflective process in play therapy: A practical model for supervising counseling students. *Education, 127*(4), 472.

Arthur, G. L., & Gfroerer, K. P. (2002). Training and supervision through the written word: A description and intern feedback. *Family Journal, 10*(2), 213–219.

Association for Play Therapy. (2021). Credentialing guide: Registered play therapist (RPT) and supervisor (RPT-S). https://cdn.ymaws.com/www.a4pt.org/resource/resmgr/credentials/2021_credentials/rpt_standards_2021_version.pdf

Bergeron, K. (2004). Supervisors' perceptions of the process of supervision with counselors who utilized play therapy. *Dissertation Abstracts International, 65,* 1259.

Bernard, J. M., & Goodyear, R. K. (2019). *Fundamentals of clinical supervision* (6th ed.). Pearson.

Bernard, J. M., Goodyear, R. K., & Rousmaniere, T. (2019). Individual supervision. In J. M. Bernard & R. K. Goodyear (Eds.), *Fundamentals of clinical supervision* (6th ed.). Pearson.

Biggs, D. A. (1998). The case presentation approach in clinical supervision. *Counselor Education and Supervision, 27*(3), 240–248.

Blanco, P. J., Muro, J. H., & Stickley, V. K. (2014). Understanding the concept of genuineness in play therapy: Implications for supervision and teaching of beginning play therapists. *International Journal of Play Therapy, 23*(1), 44–54.

Borders, L. D., & Brown, L. L. (2005). *The new handbook of counseling supervision.* Lahaska Press.

Borders, L. D., Welfare, L., Greason, P. B., Paladino, D. A., Mobley, K., Villalba, J. A., & Wester, K. L. (2012). Individual and triadic and group: Supervisee and supervisor perceptions of each modality. *Counselor Education and Supervision, 51*(4), 281–295.

Boscolo, L., Cecchin, G., Hoffman, L., & Penn, P. (1987). *Milan systemic family therapy.* Basic Books.

Boylston, W. H., & Tuma, J. M. (1972). Training of mental health professionals through the use of the "bug in the ear". *American Journal of Psychiatry, 129*(1), 92–95.

Bradley, L. J., & Ladany, N. (Eds.). (2010). *Counselor supervision: Principles, process, and practice* (4th ed.). Brunner-Routledge.

Carroll, M. (1996). *Counseling supervision: Theory, skills, and practice.* Cassell.

Ceballos, P. L., Parikh, S., & Post, P. B. (2012). Examining social justice attitudes among play therapists: Implications for multicultural supervision and training. *International Journal of Play Therapy, 21*(4), 232–243.

Christman-Dunn, R. (1998). *The necessity of providing clinical supervision for school counselors* (Report No. CG 028994). (ERIC Document Reproduction Service No. ED 426 320).

Claiborn, C. D., Goodyear, R. K., & Horner, P. A. (2001). Feedback. *Psychotherapy, 38*(4), 401–405.

Couchon, W. D., & Bernard, J. M. (1984). Effects of timing of supervision on supervisor and counselor performance. *Clinical Supervisor, 2*(3), 3–20.

Crocker, J. W., & Wroblewski, M. (1975). Using recreational games in counseling. *Personnel and Guidance Journal, 53*(6), 453–458.

Deaver, S. P., & Shiflett, C. (2011). Art-based supervision techniques. *Clinical Supervisor, 30*(2), 257–276.

Disney, M. J., & Stephens, A. M. (1994). *Legal issues in clinical supervision.* American Counseling Association.

Donald, E. J., Culbreth, J. R., & Carter, A. W. (2015). Play therapy supervision: A review of the literature. *International Journal of Play Therapy, 24*(2), 59–77.

Drewes, A. A., & Mullen, J. (2008). *Supervision can be playful: Techniques for child and play therapist supervisors.* Jason Aronson.

Edwards, J. K. (2013). *Strengths-Based supervision in clinical practice.* Sage.

Edwards, J. K., & Chen, M. W. (1999). Strength-based supervision: Frameworks, current practice, and future directions. *Family Journal, 7*(4), 349–357.

Fall, M., Drew, D., Chute, A., & More, A. (2007). The voices of registered play therapists as supervisors. *International Journal of Play Therapy, 16*(2), 133–146.

Fall, M., & Sutton, J. M., Jr. (2004). *Clinical supervision: A handbook for practitioners.* Allyn & Bacon.

Felton, A., Morgan, M., & Bruce, M. A. (2015). Lessons from triadic supervisors: Maximizing effectiveness. *Journal of Counselor Preparation and Supervision, 7*(3), 133–160.

Glazer, H. R., & Stein, D. (2015). Mindfulness and the play-therapist supervisor: A study in transformative learning. *International Journal of Play Therapy, 24*(1), 41–53.

Glosoff, H. L., & Durham, J. C. (2010). Using supervision to prepare social justice counseling advocates. *Counselor Education and Supervision, 50*(2), 116–129.

Graham, M. A., Scholl, M. B., Smith-Adcock, S., & Wittmann, E. (2014). Three creative approaches to counseling supervision. *Journal of Creativity in Mental Health, 9*(3), 415–426.

Grigg, G. (2006). Designs and discriminations for clinical group supervision in counseling psychology: An analysis. *Canadian Journal of Counseling, 40*(2), 110–122.

Guiffrida, D. A., Jordan, R., Saiz, S., & Barnes, K. L. (2007). The use of metaphor in clinical supervision. *Journal of Counseling and Development, 85*(4), 393–400.

Hein, S. F., & Lawson, G. (2009). A qualitative examination of supervisors' experiences of the process of triadic supervision. *Clinical Supervisor, 28*(1), 91–108.

Hein, S. F., Lawson, G., & Rodriquez, C. P. (2011). Supervisee incompatibility and its influence on triadic supervision: An examination of doctoral student supervisors' perspectives. *Counselor Education and Supervision, 50*(6), 422–436.

Hein, S., & Lawson, G. (2008). Triadic supervision and its impact on the role of the supervisor: A qualitative examination of supervisors' perspectives. *Counselor Education and Supervision, 48*(1), 16–31.

Hendrix, C. C., Fournier, D. G., & Briggs, K. (2001). Impact of co-therapy teams on client outcomes and therapist training in marriage and family therapy. *Contemporary Family Therapy, 23*(1), 63–82.

Kagan, N. (1980). Influencing human interaction-eighteen years with IPR. In A. K. Hess (Ed.), *Psychotherapy supervision: Theory, research, and practice* (pp. 262–286). Wiley.

Kagan, N. I., & Kagan, H. (1991). Interpersonal process recall. In P. W. Dowrick (Ed.), *Practical guide to using video in the behavioral sciences* (pp. 221–230). John Wiley & Sons.

Kassan, L. D. (2010). *Peer supervision groups: How they work and why you need one.* Jason Aronsol.

Kiselica, M. S., & Robinson, M. (2001). Bringing advocacy counseling to life: The history, issues, and human dramas of social justice work in counseling. *Journal of Counseling and Development, 79*(4), 387–397.

Kozol, J. (2005). *The shame of the nation: The restoration of apartheid schooling in America.* Three Rivers Press.

Landreth, G. L. (2012). *Play therapy: The art of the relationship* (3rd ed.). Brunner-Routledge.

Lawson, G., Hein, S. F., & Stuart, C. L. (2009). A qualitative investigation of supervisees' experiences of triadic supervision. *Journal of Counseling and Development, 87*(4), 449–457.

Levinger, A. C. (1994). Co-play therapy. *International Journal of Play Therapy, 3*(2), 53–62.

Metcalf, L. M. (2003). Countertransference among play therapists: Implications for therapist development and supervision. *International Journal of Play Therapy, 12*(2), 31–48.

Montalvo, B. (1973). Aspects of live supervision. *Family Process, 12*(4), 343–359.

Mullen, J. A. (2015). Play therapy supervision. In K. J. O'Connor, C. E. Shaefer, & L. D. Braverman (Eds.), *Handbook of play therapy.* John Wiley & Sons, Inc.

Mullen, J. A., Luke, M., & Drewes, A. (2007). Supervision can be playful too: Play therapy techniques that enhance supervision. *International Journal of Play Therapy, 16*(1), 69–85.

Newman, D. S., Nebbergall, A. J., & Salmon, D. (2013). Structured peer group supervision for novice consultants: Procedures, pitfalls, and potential. *Journal of Educational and Psychology Consultation, 23*(3), 200–216.

Nguyen, T. V. (2004). A comparison of individual supervision and triadic supervision. *Dissertation Abstracts International: Section A. Humanities and Social Sciences, 64*(9), 3204.

Noelle, M. (2002). Self-report in supervision: Positive and negative slants. *Clinical Supervisor, 21*, 125–134.

Oliver, M., Nelson, K., & Ybanez, K. (2010). Systemic processes in triadic supervision. *Clinical Supervisor, 29*(1), 51–67.

Peabody, M. A. (2015). Building with purpose: Using Lego serious play in play therapy supervision. *International Journal of Play Therapy*, *24*(1), 30–40.

Perryman, K. L., Moss, R. C., & Anderson, L. (2016). Sandtray supervision: An integrated model for play therapy supervision. *International Journal of Play Therapy*, *25*(4), 186–196.

Proctor, B., & Inskipp, F. (2001). Group supervision. In J. Scaife (Ed.), *Supervision in the mental health profession: A practitioner's guide* (pp. 99–121). Routledge.

Protinsky, H. (2003). Dismounting the tiger: Using tape in supervision. In T. C. Todd & C. L. Storm (Eds.), *The complete systemic supervisor: Context, philosophy, and pragmatics* (pp. 298–307). IUniverse.

Ray, D. (2011). *Advanced play therapy: Essential conditions, knowledge, and skills for child practice.* Routledge.

Riva, M. T. (2014). Supervision of group leaders. In J. L. DeLucia-Waack, C. R. Kalodner, & M. T. Riva (Eds.), *Handbook of group counseling & psychotherapy* (2nd ed., pp. 146–158). Sage Publications.

Rogers, C. R. (1942). The use of electrically recorded interviews in improving psychotherapeutic techniques. *American Journal of Orthopsychiatry*, *12*(3), 429–434.

Roller, B., & Nelson, V. (1991). *The art of co-therapy: How therapists work together.* Guilford Press.

Rønnestad, M. H., & Skovholt, T. M. (2013). *The developing practitioner: Growth and stagnation of therapists and counselors.* Routledge.

Rousmaniere, T. (2014). Using technology to enhance clinical supervision and training. In C. E. Watkins & D. Milne (Eds.), *International handbook of clinical supervision* (pp. 204–237). Wiley Publishers.

Ryan, S. D., Gomory, T., & Lacasse, J. R. (2002). Who are we? Examining the results of the association for play therapy membership survey. *International Journal of Play Therapy*, *11*, 11–41.

Seymour, J. W., & Crenshaw, D. A. (2014). Reflective practice in play therapy and supervision. In D. A. Crenshaw & A. L. Stewart (Eds.), *Play therapy: A comprehensive guide to theory and practice* (pp. 483–495). Guilford Publications.

Smith, L., Chambers, D., & Bratini, L. (2009). When oppression is in pathogen: The participatory development of socially just mental health practice. *American Journal of Orthopsychiatry*, *79*(2), 159–168.

Sommer, C. A., Derrick, E. C., Bourgeois, M. B., Ingene, D. H., Yang, J. W., & Justice, C. A. (2009). Multicultural connections: Using stories to transcend cultural boundaries in supervision. *Journal of Multicultural Counseling and Development*, *37*(4), 206–218.

Strohmer, D. C., & Shivy, V. A. (1994). Bias in counselor hypothesis testing: Does accountability make a difference? *Journal of Counseling and Development*, *73*(2), 191–197.

Thomas, D. A. (2015). *Intentionality in supervision: Supervising play therapy interns and practitioners.* VISTAS Online.

Thompson, J. M., & Moffett, N. L. (2010). Clinical preparation and supervision of professional school counselors. *Journal of School Counseling*, *8*(30), 1–24.

VanderGast, T. S., Culbreth, J. R., & Flowers, C. (2010). An exploration of experiences and preferences in clinical supervision with play therapists. *International Journal of Play Therapy*, *19*(3), 174–185.

VanderGast, T. S., & Hinkle, M. S. (2015). So happy together? Predictors of satisfaction with supervision for play therapist supervisees. *International Journal of Play Therapy*, *24*(2), 92–102.

Veilleux, J. C., Sandeen, E., & Levensky, E. (2014). Dialectical tensions supervisor attitudes and contextual influences in psychotherapy supervision. *Journal of Contemporary Psychotherapy*, *44*(1), 31–41.

Wright, L. M. (1986). An analysis of live supervision "phone-ins" in family therapy. *Journal of Marital and Family Therapy*, *12*(2), 187–190.

7 Evaluation in Play Therapy Supervision

Corie Schoeneberg and Renee Turner

Evaluation in Play Therapy Supervision

In her timeless book, *Dibs in Search of Self,* Virginia Axline (1964) presents a powerful theme: "Experience that never disappoints or saddens or stirs up a feeling is a bland experience with little challenge or variation in color" (p. 215). While Axline was referring to her work with children, this same principle can be applied to the supervisory process. Play therapy supervision is often experienced by supervisees as challenging, emotional, and exposing, and these elements are primarily due to the evaluative component needed for the professional growth process. Evaluation is a defining feature of clinical supervision yet many play therapist supervisors struggle to provide effective, formative, and summative feedback vital to the supervisory process.

As mentioned in previous chapters, supervisions models, approaches, and practices have evolved over time, but the most recent progressions in the supervisory field highlight the need for integration of relational (Fitch et al., 2010) and attuned supervision approaches that emphasize cultural humility (Watkins et al., 2019a; Watkins et al., 2019b). Unfortunately, the exploration and emphasis of evaluation (i.e., assessment, feedback, gatekeeping) in the context of the supervisory relationship remains underdeveloped and may feel counter to relational approaches, a cornerstone of play therapy practice. In this chapter, the authors discuss the importance of working from a developmentally sensitive and attachment-oriented supervision theory, highlight the challenges associated with feedback in play therapy supervision, and identify formal and informal evaluation measures to gauge and promote supervisee development. From this discussion, play therapy supervisors will glean practical and playful strategies to evaluate the progress of play therapy supervisees while preserving the relationship central to all play therapy theories and models.

Critical Concepts in Play Therapy Evaluation

Supervision is recognized as a distinct professional competence, separate from the obtention and application of therapeutic skills. Despite this, specialized training to strengthen supervisor competence is lacking and inconsistent (Falender, 2018).

DOI: 10.4324/9781003196075-9

Supervisor training must emphasize the essential use of evaluation measures and consistent feedback, which is imperative for fostering and cultivating a supervisee's clinical knowledge and skills in play therapy. For Registered Play Therapist-Supervisors™ (RPT-S™), effective evaluation in play therapy supervision must include a strong understanding of the credentialing standards and processes, the play therapy competencies, a theoretical framework for supervisee assessment, and a relationship-oriented perspective.

Conceptualizing Evaluation Along the Phase Model and Play Therapy Competencies

Evaluation in the context of play therapy supervision poses unique challenges. Chiefly, at the time of this writing, there is no standardized evaluation tool specific to play therapy supervision; therefore, supervisors must establish their own consistent measures and protocols for assessing play therapy competence. This is complicated by the fact that individuals pursuing the Registered Play Therapist™/School Based-Registered Play Therapist™ (RPT™/SB-RPT™) credential come from a range of mental health–related disciplines, converging into one specialized field of play therapy practice. As a result, the RPT-S™ is approved to supervise those who may fundamentally view presenting problems and clinical progress through a distinctly different disciplinary lens and professional perspective. Additionally, supervisors may supervise individuals from differing play therapy theories, models, and approaches, which requires a deep and wide knowledge of play therapy theory and application as well as subsequent evaluation. With these complications in mind, the Association for Play Therapy (APT) revised credentialing standards by outlining a three-phase model that layers play therapy education with supervised practice in a learning hierarchy. APT's intended purpose of the phase-model approach is to encourage the development of integrated and theoretically grounded play therapists across disciplines and approaches resulting in increased consistency within the field of play therapy (K. Lebby, personal communication, June 15, 2021).

The phase model gives rise to a scaffolded, integrated approach to play therapy training. Phase One is characterized by supervisees gaining foundational knowledge of theory and basic skills, Phase Two is characterized by alignment with one's primary theoretical orientation, and developing and demonstrating intermediate skills, while Phase Three is characterized by deepening knowledge of specialized populations and demonstrating advanced skills. The current standards also introduced a set of play therapy competencies (Turner et al., 2020) and can be utilized as a practical and valuable tool in evaluating supervisee development. The current play therapy competencies can be referenced in Table 7.1. The competencies are intentionally broad in order to encompass a wide range of disciplines and approaches, and the umbrella competencies are divided into three domains: Competency 1: Knowledge and Understanding of Play Therapy; Competency 2: Clinical Play Therapy Skills; and Competency 3: Professional Engagement in Play Therapy. Within each of the three umbrella competencies, a series of indicators are identified, which provides greater specificity and clarity for the multifaceted aspects of the competency. The competencies are a supportive tool for both supervisor and supervisee and promote consistency within the growing field of play therapy. In tandem with the phase model, the competencies serve as a guide for supervisors to establish clear and measurable goals to support the development and evaluation of play therapy supervisees' professional growth.

Table 7.1 Association for Play Therapy - Play Therapist Competencies

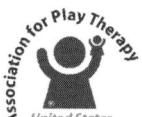

Play Therapy Competencies
APT Professional Credentialing Program

APT identifies the following areas of competencies as essential to the competent practice of play therapy, irrespective of theoretical orientation:

Competency 1: Knowledge & Understanding of Play Therapy
The play therapist will:

1a.   Demonstrate knowledge of the history of play therapy
1b.   Demonstrate understanding of the therapeutic powers of play
1c.   Demonstrate knowledge of the therapeutic relationship in play therapy
1d.   Demonstrate knowledge of seminal/historically significant play therapy theories and models
1e.   Apply theories and stages of childhood development in play therapy
1f.   Identify and apply ethical practices in play therapy
1g.   Demonstrate an understanding of the play therapy treatment process (e.g., treatment goals and plans, documentation, intake/termination, and tracking of treatment progress)
1h.   Demonstrate knowledge of family & systemic theories in play therapy
1i.   Demonstrate knowledge of childhood-related problems and mental health diagnosis/disorders
1j.   Demonstrate an understanding of the diverse impacts of childhood trauma (e.g., neurobiological, systemic, social) and the implications in play therapy
1k.   Demonstrate knowledge of assessment in play therapy

Competency 2: Clinical Play Therapy Skills
The play therapist will:

2a.   Apply and articulate the therapeutic powers of play
2b.   Demonstrate relationship and rapport building skills (e.g., empathy, safety, unconditional positive regard) by utilizing 'self' in relationships with children, caregivers, stakeholders in play therapy
2c.   Apply assessments that highlight various aspects of the child and/or system and the play therapy process (e.g. conceptualization, diagnosis, family dynamics, treatment suitability and effectiveness, termination)
2d.   Articulate and explain the play therapy process
2e.   Demonstrate basic play therapy skills (e.g., tracking, reflection of feeling, limit setting, pacing with the client)
2f.   Identify play dynamics (e.g., types of play, themes, stages) and incorporate clinical considerations in treatment
2g.   Develop play therapy treatment goals and plans congruent with theoretical orientation
2h.   Demonstrate understanding of own cultural and social identity and its influence in the play therapy process
2i.   Exhibit multicultural orientation to diversity, equity, and inclusion through a culturally and socially diverse playroom and play therapy process
2j.   Demonstrate play therapy treatment skills congruent with   theoretical orientation (e.g., conceptualization, interventions)

<u>**Competency 3: Professional Engagement in Play Therapy**</u>
The play therapist will:

3a. Maintain play therapy credentials and involvement in professional play therapy organizations
3b. Consistently evaluate and adjust play therapy practices to meet state and discipline ethical guidelines and codes
3c. Apply ongoing integration of APT's guidelines within the Best Practices and Paper on Touch
3d. Recognize and adhere to the limits of professional scope of competence in play therapy
3e. Seek and integrate play therapy-specific continued education, research, and literature
3f. Seek and integrate play therapy-specific supervision and consultation
3g. Practice self-care to maintain quality play therapy services
3h. Seek and integrate ongoing knowledge regarding cultural and social diversity in play therapy

Turner, R., Schoeneberg, C., Ray, D., & Lin, Y. (2020). Establishing play therapy competencies: A Delphi study. *International Journal of Play Therapy. 29*(4), 177–190. https://dx.org/10.1037/pla0000138

Conceptualizing Evaluation from a Developmentally Sensitive Supervision Theory

Play therapist supervisors must be knowledgeable not only in *what* needs to be evaluated, such as the play therapy competencies, but also in *how* to evaluate. The *how* of the evaluation process must be structured along a theoretical model specific to supervision. As discussed in Chapter 3, the Integrative Developmental Model (IDM) of supervision (Stoltenberg et al., 1998) may be particularly helpful for play therapist supervisors as they evaluate and assess supervisees. As a result of APT's phase model approach, supervisors must carefully consider the current developmental phase of learning and growth of the play therapy supervisee when providing evaluation and feedback, and a helpful theoretical orientation for this consideration is the IDM. The IDM conceptualizes supervisees along three stages of professional development, which lends itself fluidly to APT's three phases of play therapy education and experience for emerging RPT's™, and provides eight domains (or targets) for supervisor evaluation (Table 7.2). The IDM proposes that effective supervisors apply a developmental lens when evaluating supervisees in these eight areas. Just as adults need to manage and adjust expectations around the developmental stage of a child, supervisors must likewise tailor standards of evaluation to be congruent with a supervisee's stage of professional development as a growing play therapist. The IDM's eight domains of evaluation provide a helpful checklist for supervisor evaluation and can be easily applied in play therapy supervision. Again, these domains are constructs intended to assess from a developmentally sensitive perspective and in conjunction with the play therapy competencies.

Conceptualizing Evaluation from an Attachment Lens

As child mental health specialists, play therapists are keenly aware of the critical role of the parent–child relationship and positive attachment in the child's overall well-being and success in therapy. While attachment is most frequently discussed in relation to childhood, the role and function of attachment is have relevant in adulthood and in the context of supervision. Grounded in the attachment theory

Table 7.2 IDM's Eight Domains of Evaluation and the Play Therapy Competencies

IDM Domain	Paralleled Play Therapy Competency Indicators
Intervention skills	Theory-based play therapy skills
Assessment techniques	Play-based assessments, diagnosis
Interpersonal assessment	Play therapy relationship, parent consultation
Client conceptualization	Childhood development, family systems, impacts of childhood trauma, play dynamics
Individual differences	Social and cultural diversity
Theoretical orientation	Seminal theories and historically significant approaches in play therapy
Treatment plans and goals	Application of play therapy theory in treatment, documentation practices in play therapy, stages of play
Professional ethics	Unique ethical issues in play therapy, APT's Play Therapy Best Practices, APT's Paper on Touch, and issues of confidentiality

created by Bowlby (1969), connections between attachment and the supervisory relationship began with the work of Hill (1992) and were then later expanded by Watkins (1995), Pistole and Watkins (1995), and Bennett and Saks (2006) before Fitch et al. (2010) formalized this attachment-based conceptualization of supervision into the Attachment-Caregiving Model of Supervision (ACMS).

The ACMS parallels the parent–child relationship to the supervisor–supervisee relationship by highlighting the various shared parent/supervisor characteristics. The parallels between the parent and supervisor include the parent/supervisor's authoritative status in which evaluative conclusions are made toward a child/supervisee (the person in the relationship with limited authority). Other shared relationship dynamics include the parent/supervisor's role as a significant source for learning and a sought-after safe-haven presence during moments of anxiety and risk (Fitch et al., 2010). Because supervisees often find themselves in unfamiliar and anxiety-provoking situations as novice clinicians, effective supervisors function as an attachment figure by serving as an affective-regulatory agent, a caregiver of greater strength and knowledge, and a secure base for psychological safety and refuge for the supervisee (Fitch et al., 2010).

Viewed in conjunction with the Integrated Developmental Model, a supervisee's safe-haven seeking and need for a secure base from the supervisor varies according to professional developmental stages. For example, some supervisory attachment-activating "threats" include structure-seeking to ease feelings of anxiety during the early phases in the supervisory relationship, feelings of incompetence and the "imposter syndrome" in middle phases, and feelings of ambivalence regarding completion of supervision as the relationship nears termination. Other continuous attachment-activating "threats" include in-session stress and client crisis, undertaking new learning and tasks, and making oneself vulnerable to evaluation and subsequent feedback (Bernard & Goodyear, 2014; Fitch et al., 2010). Threats and anxiety-activating events specific to play therapy may include moments of significant countertransference with a child client, challenges when working with resistant, hostile, or abusive caregivers, and unique legal and ethical dilemmas that accompany working with children. With RPT™ credentialing status and measurement of competence on the line, the supervisor's evaluation and feedback are, arguably, some of the most anxiety-provoking yet defining aspects of supervision. Therefore, framing the supervisory process, especially during moments of evaluation, within an attachment framework is critical for the success of the supervisory relationship.

Supervisors can apply ACMS conceptualizations by asking themselves:

- How am I actively creating a secure-base and safe-haven relationship for the supervisee?
- Am I keeping the relationship the central priority above the tasks associated with supervision?
- How am I relationally attending to the supervisee during moments of great risk, vulnerability, and new learning?
- Am I modeling the characteristics of a secure caregiver, especially when I provide feedback and engage in evaluation?

Theoretical models specific to supervision provide supervisors with an operational map for how to navigate the functions of supervision, including evaluation. However, even with an attachment-focused mindset, the process of feedback and evaluation naturally stimulates incidents of relational ruptures. As suggested by Bowlby (1969), attending to ruptures that occur within a relationship is foundational to fostering healthy attachment and a secure sense of self, and these principles are equally important in supervisory relationships. Moreover, emerging literature emphasizes the need to approach relational repair from a stance of humility in which the individuals recognize limitations and imperfections, accurately self-assess, and are open to understanding the experiences of others (Worthington et al., 2017). Watkins et al. (2019a) expand on this concept, outlining four components of humility focused repair: (a) identify the activating (rupture) event, (b) identify the type of humility needed for rupture repair (i.e., posture of curiosity, compassion, seeking to understand, sensitivity, relational communication, immediacy, and management of assumptions), (c) identify the corresponding comfort, and (d) seizing the opportunity to address the rupture repair. For play therapy supervisors, attending to rupture and repair with humility while applying the conceptualizations of ACMS holds especially powerful opportunities for modeling, integrating attachment, and emphasizing the importance of the supervisory relationship. These principles may be especially critical when there is potential for the supervisee to experience difficult emotions in accepting feedback and evaluation.

Evaluation of Multicultural Orientation Framework

The integration of an attachment conceptualization and orientation in supervisory work cannot be fully applied without the supervisor's awareness of and sensitivity toward the cross-cultural interactions taking place within the supervisory relationship. Supervisors must be prepared to integrate a multicultural orientation into their supervision practice as well as assess the play therapy supervisee's cultural practices in the playroom and with client families, and beginning January 1, 2023, RPT™ supervisors must attest to supervisee's overall multicultural orientation. According to Davis et al. (2018), the "multicultural orientation frame[work] articulates a 'way of being' in session for therapists (e.g., cultural humility), a way of identifying and responding to therapeutic cultural markers in sessions (e.g., cultural opportunities), and a way of understanding the self in these moments (e.g., cultural comfort)" (p. 90). In addition to the stance suggested by Davis et al. (2018), supervisors must also pay mindful attention to the complex issues surrounding intersectionality that influence all aspects of the supervisory relationship. Intersectionality is described as overlapping domains of diversity with consideration for the influence of power, privilege, marginalization, and oppression (Green & Flasch, 2019).

With these concepts in mind, play therapists must examine their own way of being within cultural dynamics and adopt an *orientation* through which to conceptualize and view the clients' world contextually. In other words, cultural and social diversity considerations should be foundational to the extent that they supersede one's theoretical orientation. Thus, building competency toward cultural and social diversity in the context of play therapy extends beyond merely having a diverse representation of toys. Instead, play therapists should strive for equity and inclusion in all aspects of professional practice (Gil, 2021). For play-therapists-in-training, this translates to conceptualizing the myriad of social, cultural, and relational lived experiences of children and their families (as outlined by the play therapy competencies) through the lens of social justice and advocacy (see Gil & Drewes, 2021, for more comprehensive information). Of significance, Davis et al. (2018) emphasize that therapists cannot become fully "competent" in matters related to social and cultural diversity because doing so would indicate a finite endpoint, impossible in an ever-evolving society. As a result, the Association for Play Therapy expanded the original competencies to include *ongoing knowledge* of social and cultural diversity in Competencies 2 and 3 and added specific continuing education related to social and cultural diversity to its credentialing program. Therefore, play therapists must commit to a career-long pursuit to understand the complex evolving landscape of cultural identities and experiences.

Considering the tenets outlined by Davis et al. (2018), a multicultural orientation mandates that play therapists examine their own way of being within cultural dynamics, and, in the context of supervision, the supervisor must also be self-aware and maintain an ongoing posture of cultural humility. From this perspective, the supervisor must integrate the complex landscape of various cultural perspectives, values, norms, rituals, and beliefs about many of the core themes surrounding problems, outcomes, relationships, and the therapeutic process for themselves (as the supervisor), the supervisee, the identified client (child), family, and cultural and social contexts in which all these components overlap. Unfortunately, discussions with this degree of complexity tend to promote a power differential whereby the supervisor is in a one-up position. In response to these power differences, the supervisor should remain intentionally aware of power, privilege, oppression, and marginalization and strive to work collaboratively with supervisees, especially in the context of feedback and evaluation. Supervisors should also solicit feedback from the supervisee regarding the supervisee's experience during evaluation and feedback and listen for potential relational ruptures in conjunction with a multicultural lens.

With a multicultural orientation in mind, supervisors should ask themselves:

- How do I consider the influence of power, privilege, oppression, and marginalization in all aspects of the supervisee's development as a person and professional?
- How do I identify cultural markers that arise during supervision sessions and attend to them in such a way that increases the understanding and awareness of the supervisee and myself?
- How are my own cultural values and norms informing my beliefs about evaluation and the way I communicate feedback?

- How am I considering and integrating the supervisee's cultural values and norms into my understanding of their clinical performance, demonstration of play therapy competencies, relational interactions in supervision, and reactions/responses to evaluative feedback?
- How am I demonstrating cultural humility and considering my power/privilege in the delivery of my feedback/evaluations?

Practical Application of Concepts in Evaluation

Evaluation of Play Therapy Competencies

The play therapy competencies and theoretical models in supervision, such as the IDM and the ACMS, provide the conceptual scaffolding upon which play therapy supervisors can apply practical principles for evaluation in the supervisory process. Beginning with the play therapy competencies, supervisors must formally evaluate supervisees across APT's three phases and measure growth toward each of the core play therapy competencies and associated indicators. The competencies articulate key points to assess play therapist knowledge, skills, and professional orientation and elicit measurable progress, while still allowing supervisors to individually tailor education and supervision to match the supervisees' developmental needs. Supervisors must translate these ideas into an objective and operational method for evaluation.

Competency 1: Knowledge and Understanding of Play Therapy

The play therapy competencies (Turner et al., 2020) were developed by a panel of expert RPT-Ss™ from varied backgrounds, theoretical orientations, and experiences. The competency indicators are intentionally left "open-ended" so as to be universally applicable for play therapy supervisors and supervisees from all mental health disciplines, graduate education levels, and professional settings and theoretical orientations. This is both a strength and a limitation of the competencies as the indicators can seem non-specific and vague. Perhaps the most ambiguous competency domain to assess is Competency 1: Knowledge and Understanding of Play Therapy and its associated indicators. Therefore, the first task for the supervisor is to operationally define and identify the benchmarks related to each indicator specific to their style and scope of supervision while also considering the composition of each unique supervisee. For example, one supervisor may operationally define Competency 1.k., which refers to knowledge of assessment in play therapy, as a supervisee's competence in identifying possible play themes within child-centered play therapy while another supervisor may operationally define this indicator as the supervisee's competence in understanding the purpose and results of directive assessment instruments integrated in a play-based format. By more precisely defining the indicators, the supervisor can communicate clear expectations to the supervisee and can listen for specific indicators of play therapy knowledge as the supervisee discusses a recent workshop, assigned reading, or demonstrates a specific component of knowledge (e.g., documentation, diagnosis, impact of trauma, family and systems theory) in case conceptualization.

Group supervision facilitates dynamic opportunities to discuss many of the indicators outlined in Competency 1 and to observe the supervisee's ability to articulate knowledge *and* demonstrate integrated understanding. Creative methods such as sandtray, role play, and creative enactments further illustrate knowledge while simultaneously enhancing supervisee comfort with more complex play therapy methods. For instance, supervisees can participate in a family sculpting activity to gain perspective of family members' lived experiences of family dynamics. However, experiences simply for the purpose of experience do not develop competent play therapists. Supervisors should note the degree of teaching affiliated with Competency 1, particularly if supervisees lack formal, university-based play therapy training and intentionally connect creative experiences to knowledge and practice. In the example provided, a follow-up discussion of family sculpting as it relates to family dynamics, theory, and treatment planning, ensures interventions do not occur in a vacuum, which reduces the likelihood that supervisees will adopt a play therapy practice full of techniques but void of theory. Integration of knowledge is vital to supervisees scaffolding into Competency 2.

Competency 2: Clinical Play Therapy Skills

Evaluating Competency 2: Clinical Play Therapy Skills can be difficult until the supervisee identifies a primary theoretical orientation. For this reason, meaningful assessment in this competency area requires the supervisor to possess a broad understanding of play therapy theories, even beyond their primary theoretical orientation, in order to guide the supervisee toward a theoretical orientation congruent with their personality and view of change. In Phase One, evaluation of basic or primary play therapy skills is underscored; however, in Phases Two and Three, the emphasis shifts to the evaluation of applied skills congruent with the supervisee's primary theoretical orientation. Supervisors can use assessment tools associated with specific theoretical models such as the Play Therapy Skills Checklist (Ray, 2004) for a child-centered orientation and the Adlerian Play Therapy Skills Checklist (Dillman Taylor & Kottman, 2019) paired with video observations to further assess indicators in Competency 2. Other tools, such as the Group Play Therapy Skills Checklist (Garza et al., 2014), can measure skills for specific populations such as Adlerian play therapy groups.

Beyond the theoretical application of play therapy, Competency 2 also encompasses other vital skills related to conceptualization, play themes and dynamics, and treatment planning and documentation. Discussions of the therapeutic powers of play support the evaluation of supervisees' applied understanding of clients' diagnosis/presenting problem and progress toward play therapy treatment goals. Another point evaluation is the use of role-plays which offer direct opportunities for informal assessment while building primary and theory-specific play therapy skills. Likewise, utilizing case analysis synthesizes the comprehensive components of developmental considerations, systemic context and factors, stages of play, theory-based play therapy treatment plans, and play therapy documentation. The supervisor may consider a checklist or self-rating forms (Likert scaling) to quantify skill growth.

Competency 3: Professional Engagement in Play Therapy

Indicators encompassed in Competency 3: Professional Engagement in Play Therapy are geared toward the supervisees' orientation to the field and development of a play therapist professional identity. The supervisor can structure goals within this domain to orient the supervisee to their growing professional identity as a play therapist by creating a personal mission/philosophy statement or crafting long-term plans for involvement in their professional play therapy community post-supervision.

While some indicators in this domain seem straightforward, the hallmark features of this phase are the *integration* of knowledge and *demonstration* of ethical practice, which can be more difficult to assess. Because many of the indicators are difficult to quantify, the supervisor should employ a combination of creative and practical evaluation methods. For example, the supervisor may present an ethical dilemma exercise in play therapy utilizing APT's key documents (Play Therapy Best Practices and the Paper on Touch) for the supervisee to consider. When applied in group play therapy supervision, supervisees are afforded the opportunity to learn from fellow supervisees across different developmental stages and from varied theoretical orientations. However, other indicators, such as practicing self-care to maintain quality play therapy services (competency indicator 3.g.), are undoubtedly important, yet difficult to assess. In these cases, applying creative, expressive approaches for evaluation facilitates layered and integrated possibilities for parallel growth. When symptoms of burnout impact the supervisee's ability to track themes or remain present in play therapy sessions (Turner, 2019), the supervisor may suggest that the supervisee construct a sand tray in which half of the tray represents the ideal self and the other side represents the current self. Keeping the IDM and ACMS in mind, the supervisor's careful and facilitative processing helps the supervisee identify personal needs and to explore emerging person-of-therapist issues.

Evaluation per Phase

Phase 1 Play Therapist Supervisees

The IDM proposes that supervisees change and evolve as professionals over the course of the supervisory process, and each of these three levels is characterized by developmental patterns in the supervisee and the supervisory relationship. Effective supervisors are attuned to these developmental differences across stages; thus, supervisors are better able to recognize developmental norms in supervisees and tailor evaluation standards and practices to meet these developmental needs. The IDM's Level 1 supervisees parallel play therapists-in-training in Phase 1 of the RPT™ credentialing process, and this stage represents supervisees who are just beginning in the play therapy education and clinical practice journey. Typical of this developmental stage, Phase 1 supervisees frequently experience significant evaluation anxiety, confusion about the supervision process and expectations, significant dependency on the supervisor, and require a much higher level of structure to supervision in order to quell the supervisee's feelings of anxiety (Huhra et al., 2008). The supervisor can attend to these developmental needs by carefully explaining the supervision process, slowly and carefully reviewing and discussing the formal and informal methods of evaluation that will be used, establishing collaborated goals linked with specific play therapy competencies as targeted areas of focus, emphasizing the supervisee's internal locus of control, and providing verbal and written summative feedback, which should include both the supervisee's strengths and points for growth.

The supervisor should anticipate that Phase 1 supervisees can become easily discouraged with evaluative feedback, overly personalize perceived criticisms, and eagerly seek the supervisor's praise and approval (Ray, 2011). Developmentally, supervisees at this stage are highly concerned with mastering the basic play therapy skills and demonstrating these skills in the "right" way (Campbell, 2006, Purswell & Stulmaker, 2015). Effective supervisors can utilize this developmental stage of the play-therapist-in-training as a powerful opportunity to help supervisees relate and empathize with the feelings some children may experience when they come to the playroom seeking praise and affirmation from the play therapist. With these developmental characteristics in mind, congruent evaluations at this stage focus on assessing the supervisee's basic play therapy skills, the supervisee's understanding and application of a play therapy theory, and the supervisee's integration of unique ethical components of play therapy practice.

Phase 2 Play Therapist Supervisees

During IDM's level 2 (Phase 2 of the RPT™ credentialing process), supervisees experience an increase in feelings of professional self-efficacy, which facilitates a shift in the supervisee's perspective from a self-oriented focus to a client-oriented focus (Ray, 2011). At this developmental stage, supervisees are more eager to explore aspects concerning the client. As such, supervisors will likely discover that supervisees are more receptive to evaluations that integrate a client-orientation, such as multicultural competence, methods of play therapy assessment of the client and family system, play themes and stages, and skills in case conceptualization. Phase 2 is very much the "adolescence" of supervisee development in which the supervisee is less dependent on the supervisor but vacillates between strong feelings of confidence and the imposter syndrome characterized by self-doubt (Campbell, 2006). With an increased desire for independence, supervisors should expect that this stage of supervision often brings a normative aspect of relational tension as the supervisee pushes back or challenges the supervisor's perspective or evaluative conclusions. Applying the ACMS and attachment framework, supervisors need to redefine how the supervisory safe-haven relationship functions for supervisees at this point in their growth. Just as children utilize attachment differently over time, so do supervisees. At this stage, effective supervisors honor the supervisee's growing desire for autonomy by allowing them to "muddle through" complex issues a bit more on their own, consider advanced dynamics in the play therapy process, and utilize peers for a more active role in feedback in group supervision.

Evaluations in Phase 2 must also integrate any aspects of remediation in areas in which the supervisee is experiencing gaps in learning and/or play therapy skills. At this point in professional development, the supervisee is roughly midway through the credentialing process, and the supervisor is ethically obligated to provide honest, objective, and direct feedback about the supervisee's growth as a play therapist. A play therapy remediation plan should highlight specific play therapy competencies of focus, explain the methods for how these competencies will be addressed and assessed in the next phase, describe the supervisor's role in aiding the supervisee with these targeted goals, and provide a very detailed description of what is expected for the supervisee's growth.

Phase 3 Play Therapist Supervisees

In the final stage, Level 3 (Phase 3 of RPT™ credentialing process), supervisees have settled comfortably in their role as a play therapist, which is accompanied by a growing sense of professional identity, personal style, strong connection with a play therapy theory, and an awareness of their own strengths and ongoing areas for growth (Ray, 2011). Supervisors in this stage aim to facilitate increased self-awareness for the supervisee in order to build skills to self-supervise as the formal supervision process comes to an end (Campbell, 2006; Purswell & Stulmaker, 2015). At this stage, evaluations are summative and aim to assess whether the supervisee has adequately met expectations in regard to the play therapy competencies.

At the close of Phase 3, the supervisor assesses and evaluates the supervisee's competence as a play therapist, revisits any aspects targeted in a remediation plan, and then provides the final and most critical evaluation: endorsement for the supervisee as a Registered Play Therapist. When endorsement cannot be ethically provided due to the supervisee's inadequate benchmark of competence across all indicators of the play therapy competencies or the incompletion of a remediation plan, gatekeeping must be applied. Simply completing the play therapy education, experience, and supervision hours does not entitle a supervisee to RPT™ credentialing; the supervisor is responsible for the professional assessment and evaluation of the supervisee alongside the standards of competence in play therapy. Supervisors are encouraged to consult with others in gatekeeping situations to ensure that supervisor bias or unrealistic expectations are not present. Supervisors must keep open and honest communication with supervisees about gatekeeping and evaluation across the span of supervision so that the final evaluation is not shocking or unexpected to the supervisee. Supervisors can remind supervisees to return to the supervision contract, which should carefully describe the role of gatekeeping, the supervisor's non-obligation to endorse a supervisee if the supervisee does not meet the standards of competence, and the methods for remediation for this type of scenario.

Methods for Formal and Informal Evaluation

Opportunities for assessment and evaluation present themselves at varied and specific points during the supervisory relationship. As previously outlined, progression through the phases establishes clear intervals for summative feedback in which formal measures of evaluation can be easily applied. Using the competencies, the supervisor can evaluate progress using a Likert scale (1: Underdeveloped to 5: Highly Developed) and set goals to target learning and growth. This method supports ownership of competence rather than placing the supervisee in a passive, power-down position. Feedback, both summative and incremental, can be provided utilizing the sandwich method (one strength, one point for growth, one strength), and supervisors should provide written feedback outlining specific strengths, emerging areas of competence, and specific goals for the remainder of supervision that support emerging growth.

Session Observations

The credentialing standards for RPTs™ indicate that supervisors must observe (either live or through video recording) a minimum of five play therapy sessions, divided across phases (APT Professional Credential Program, 2021). Existing literature supports the use of recorded session review to increase self-perception and self-awareness as the supervisee evaluates themself alongside the supervisor (Huhra et al., 2008). As Guttman (2020) states, "supervision exists at the intersection between the demand to perform and the demand to be vulnerable" (p. 68). In the context of play therapy, video review creates an active opportunity for feedback and evaluation of progress toward play therapy competencies. Moreover, some competencies are best observed through the concrete review that recorded sessions provide. For example, components such as play therapy skills and theoretical application can be difficult to ascertain through self-report and developmental awareness alone.

   Scaled self-rating paired with video review supports supervisee growth toward accurately appraising strengths and opportunities for growth which promote professional development. From the perspective of the IDM, the practice of self-rating can help the Phase 1 supervisee to identify primary skills (Ray, 2004), the Phase 2 supervisee to gain confidence and autonomy (when supported with a relational framework), and the Phase 3 supervisee to recognize areas for refinement and advanced training. When used in tandem with a full case conceptualization, video review also allows the supervisor and the supervisee to collaboratively explore play behaviors and emerging play themes so as to deepen understanding of the child and the play therapy process. Session review also invites discussions related to the vulnerable aspects of play therapist development, including the emerging person of the play therapist, subtle countertransference issues, and cultural humility. In these moments, supervisors may consider using intentional self-disclosure about their own professional experiences and co-constructing meaning, which are hallmarks of the relational approach to supervision (Rasmussen & Mishna, 2018).

Despite the strengths of video review as the method for observation, supervisee anxiety may be heightened both during recorded sessions and during session playback, thus impacting the supervisee's performance and ability to receive feedback. Huhra et al. (2008) suggests that supervisors provide supervisee feedback with consideration for their developmental level. This means that the supervisor may need to choose the highest priority of topics for feedback and focus on these one or two goals rather than barrage the supervisee with an exhaustive list of points for growth. Relatedly, Gnilka et al. (2016) identify the relationship between supervisee attachment style and level of defensiveness. Filtering feedback through the attachment model of supervision and the IDM may provide the necessary cushion for the supervisee to tolerate the associated vulnerability. To attend to these feelings of vulnerability, the supervisor may discuss the supervisee's emotional and somatic experiences related to anticipating feedback using grounding, imagery, or sandtray figures immediately prior to the video review. Facilitating an embodied, relational experience not only strengthens the supervisory alliance but also offers an invaluable parallel that the supervisee can call to mind when providing feedback to caregivers.

Gatekeeping

From a developmental perspective, supervisors recognize that clinicians continue to develop as they progress in their careers, thus supervisors must acknowledge the difference between competence, mastery, and expertise. However, supervisors act as gatekeepers to ensure the basic standard of competence is demonstrated by the supervisee. As the highest ethical and defining characteristic of the supervisory role, gatekeeping is implemented in order to ensure supervisee competency before entering the field (Miller & Koerin, 2001) and to reduce the potential for harm to the public (Rust et al., 2013). In the case of the RPT™ credential, supervisees are interfacing with the children, one of the most vulnerable populations, thus gatekeeping within the field of play therapy is even more pressing. When the supervisor identifies a concern regarding the supervisee's skills or issues related to impairment, the supervisor is ethically responsible for providing a clear, measurable remediation plan with ongoing evaluation of progress within the plan. The spirit of remediation is not to block the supervisee from earning the RPT™ credential but rather the goal is to support the supervisee's growth in a structured, quantifiable manner. Remedial methods to support play therapy supervisees may include assigning additional reading, requiring additional training in content areas to address specific competencies, watching additional sessions, or requiring personal therapy to address significant countertransference, boundary concerns, or other problematic interpersonal issues.

Conclusion

The RPT-S™ has the extraordinary opportunity to aid in the growth and development of the next generation of play therapists and thereby invest in a multitude of children on their healing journey. The task of supervision is not a simple one, however, and evaluation plays one of the most central, critical, and helpful functions in the process of the supervisee's personal and professional growth and development. By maintaining a superior understanding of the key concepts related to evaluation in play therapy, implementing a developmentally and attachment-sensitive model, maintaining a multicultural orientation, and applying clear and effective methods for evaluation, supervisors are positioned to be some of the most facilitative figures in the field of play therapy and its ongoing growth for the future.

References

APT Professional Credentialing Program. (2021, May). *Credentialing standards for the Registered Play Therapist*. Association for Play Therapy, Inc. https://cdn.ymaws.com/www.a4pt .org/resource/resmgr/credentials/2021_credentials/rpt_standards_2021_version.pdf

Axline, V. M. (1964). *Dibs in search of self*. Ballantine Books.

Bennett, S., & Saks, L. (2006). A conceptual application of attachment theory and research to the social work student-field instructor supervisory relationship. *Journal of Social Work Education, 42*(3), 157–169.

Bernard, J. M., & Goodyear, R. K. (2014). *Fundamentals of clinical supervision* (5th ed.). Pearson.

Bowlby, J. (1969). *Attachment and loss, 1. Attachment*. Basic Books.

Campbell, J. M. (2006). *Essentials of clinical supervision*. John Wiley & Sons, Inc.

Davis, D. E., DeBlaere, C., Owen, J., Hook, J. N., Rivera, D. P., Choe, E., Van Tongeren, D. R., Worthington, E. L., & Placeres, V. (2018). The multicultural orientation framework: A narrative review. *Psychotherapy, 1*(1), 89–100. http://doi.org/10.1037/ pst0000160

Dillman Taylor, D., & Kottman, T. (2019). Assessing the utility and fidelity of the Adlerian play therapy skills checklist using qualitative content analysis. *International Journal of Play Therapy, 28*(1), 13–21. http://doi.org/10.1037/pla0000082

Falender, C. A. (2018). Clinical supervision—The missing ingredient. *American Psychologist, 73*(9), 1240–1250.

Fitch, J., Pistole, M. C., & Gunn, J. (2010). The bonds of development: An attachment-caregiving model of supervision. *Clinical Supervisor, 29*(1), 20–34. https://doi.org/10 .1080/07325221003730319

Garza, Y., Kinsworthy, S., & Morrison Bennett, M. (2014). Supervision in group play therapy: A skills checklist. *Journal of Individual Psychology, 70*(1). https://doi.org/10.1353 /jip.2014.0008

Gil, E. (2021). White privilege, anti-racism, and promoting positive change in play therapy. In E. Gil & A. A. Drewes (Eds.), *Cultural issues in play therapy* (2nd ed., pp. 32–57). Guilford.

Gil, E., & Drewes, A. A. (2021). *Cultural issues in play therapy* (2nd ed.). Guilford.

Gnilka, P. B., Rice, K. G., Ashby, J. S., & Moate, R. M. (2016). Adult attachment, multidimensional perfectionism, and the alliances among counselor supervisees. *Journal of Counseling and Development, 94*(3), 285.

Greene, J. H., & Flasch, P. S. (2019). Integrating intersectionality into clinical supervision: A developmental model addressing broader definitions of multicultural competence. *Journal of Counselor Preparation & Supervision, 12*(4), 1–29.

Guttman, L. E. (2020). Disclosure and felt security in clinical supervision. *Journal of Psychotherapy Integration, 30*(1), 67–75. https://doi.org/10.1037/int0000176

Hill, E. W. (1992). Marital and family therapy supervision: A relational-attachment model. *Contemporary Family Therapy, 14*(2), 115–125.

Huhra, R. L., Yamokoski-Maynhart, C. A., & Prieto, L. R. (2008). Reviewing videotape in supervision: A developmental approach. *Journal of Counseling and Development, 86*(4), 412–418.

Miller, J., & Koerin, B. B. (2001). Gatekeeping in the practicum: What field instructors need to know. *Clinical Supervisor, 20*, 1–18.

Pistole, C., & Watkins, C. E., Jr. (1995). Attachment theory, counseling process, and supervision. *Counseling Psychologist, 23*(3), 457–478.

Purswell, K. E., & Stulmaker, H. L. (2015). Expressive arts in supervision: Choosing developmentally appropriate interventions. *International Journal of Play Therapy, 24*(2), 103–117. https://doi.org/10.1037/a0039134

Rasmussen, B., & Mishna, F. (2018). The process of facilitating case formulations in relational clinical supervision. *Clinical Social Work Journal, 46*(4), 281–288. https://doi .org/10.1007/s10615-018-0662-9

Ray, D. (2004). Supervision of basic and advanced skills in play therapy. *Journal of Professional Counseling: Practice, Theory and Research, 32*(2), 28–41. https://doi.org/10.1080/15566382 .2004.12033805

Ray, D. C. (2011). *Advanced play therapy: Essential conditions, knowledge, and skills for child practice.* Routledge.

Rust, J. P., Raskin, J. D., & Hill, M. S. (2013). Problems of professional competence among counselor trainees: Programmatic issues and guidelines. *Counselor Education and Supervision, 52*(1), 30–42. https://doi.org/10.1002/j.1556-6978.2013.00026.x

Stoltenberg, C. D., McNeill, B. W., & Delworth, U. (1998). *IDM: An integrated developmental model for supervising counselors and therapists.* Jossey-baas.

Turner, R. (2019). Play heals us, too! *Play Therapy, 14*(2), 32–35.

Turner, R., Schoeneberg, C., Ray, D., & Lin, Y. (2020). Establishing play therapy competencies: A Delphi study. *International Journal of Play Therapy, 29*(4), 177–190. https://doi.org/10.1037/pla0000138

Watkins, C. E., Hook, J. N., DeBlaere, C., Davis, D. E., Van Tongeren, D. R., Owen, J., & Callahan, J. L. (2019a). Humility, ruptures, and rupture repair in clinical supervision: A simple conceptual clarification and extension. *Clinical Supervisor, 38*(2), 281–300. https://doi.org/10.1080/07325223.2019.1624996

Watkins, C. E., Hook, J. N., Mosher, D. K., & Callahan, J. L. (2019b). Humility in clinical supervision: Fundamental, foundational, and transformational. *Clinical Supervisor, 38*(1), 58–78. https://doi.org/10.1080/07325223.2018.1487355

Watkins, C. E., Jr. (1995). Pathological attachment styles in psychotherapy supervision. *Psychotherapy, 32*(2), 333–340.

Worthington, E. L., Davis, D. E., & Hook, J. N. (Eds.). (2017). *Handbook of humility: Theory, research, and applications.* Taylor & Francis.

8 Play Therapy Issues in Supervision

Rebekah Byrd and Yumiko Ogawa

Play Therapy Issues in Supervision

Quality supervision is needed to monitor and support play therapists' professional development, clinical skills, and practice (VanderGast & Hinkle, 2015). Research has noted the support and development of play therapy supervision (VanderGast & Hinkle, 2015, Peabody, 2014, Penn & Post, 2012). This chapter will cover essential components for consideration in play therapy supervision. Readers will gain strategies to avoid and address issues in the supervisory environment and supervision relationship. This chapter will explore the purpose of clinical supervision and information specific to play therapy supervision. Topics covered include ethical considerations of supervisors, confidentiality, dual relationships, gatekeeping, technology in play therapy supervision, burnout, self-care, self-compassion and wellness, and the supervisory relationship termination.

History and Literature

Purpose of Clinical Supervision

Corey et al. (2010) defined clinical supervision as a process in which consistent and reliable observation and appraisal of the therapeutic process is provided by a knowledgeable, skilled, trained, and experienced professional. Bernard and Goodyear offer this working definition of supervision that has been informally adopted as the standard in the United States:

> Supervision is an intervention provided by a more senior member of a profession to a more junior colleague or colleagues who typically (but not always) are members of that same profession. This relationship is evaluative and hierarchical, extends over time, and has the simultaneous purposes of enhancing the professional functioning of the more junior person(s); monitoring the quality of professional services offered to the clients that she, her, or they see; and serving as gatekeeper for the particular profession the supervisee seeks to enter.
>
> (Bernard & Goodyear, 1992 as cited in Bernard & Goodyear, 2018, p. 9)

DOI: 10.4324/9781003196075-10

Further, Corey at al. explains that this supervisor is understanding and competent in the specific knowledge areas and skills essential for professional growth and development. Corey et al. (2010) also noted that supervision as a field has grown and advanced with increased attention to matters such as competence, legal and ethical considerations, accountability and documentation, technology considerations, social justice, and multicultural matters, crisis supervision, and discussing spirituality/religious considerations within the supervision relationship, some of which are addressed in this chapter. Additionally, it is important to note that effective supervision is necessary to the growth and development of supervisees' competence (Bernard & Goodyear, 2018).

Supervision is used in disciplines of the helping profession to assist clinicians in developing, honing, and growing clinical skills necessary to serve a diverse clientele. While all students in licensure prep programs (social work, counseling, psychology etc.) will be involved in a detailed and thorough supervision process as a supervisee, some will also go on to become supervisors in their agencies and workplaces. Doctoral education, educational specialists' degrees, and many states require advanced training and continued education in supervision specifically to supervise in their respective areas, as does the field of play therapy. However, not all individuals come to supervision with the same knowledge, awareness, and skills.

The Play Therapy Supervisor

Anyone aspiring to become a Registered Play Therapist™ (RPT™) requires supervision. While one of the central purposes of supervision is to foster supervisees' personal and professional development, another essential responsibility of supervisors is to ensure supervisees' clients welfare by monitoring and evaluating supervisees, which serves as a gatekeeping tool for the helping profession. Further, play therapy–specific supervision focuses on the child's experience and the child's point of view. Play therapy supervisors must consider that most adults are accustomed to viewing things from the adult point of view, therefore, play therapy supervisees may struggle to shift it to the children's point of view of experience and world (Purswell & Stulmaker, 2015).

Play therapy supervisors may also benefit from understanding research identifying factors that predict supervisee satisfaction. For example, VanderGast and Hinkle (2015) reported that the two distinct variables that led to higher levels of supervision satisfaction based on supervisees' survey result were supervisor's professional identity as a play therapist and supervisee years of experience. As the field of play therapy continues to grow, so do the needs for competent and effective play therapy supervisors (Donald et al., 2015).

The Association for Play Therapy (APT) (2019) noted that play therapists providing supervision must be specifically trained to offer such services including more play therapy experience, knowledge and skills in supervision in general and in play therapy, and understanding the responsibility to clients (including gatekeeping issues). Further, as described by APT (2019), a clinical supervision contractual agreement between supervisor and supervisee must outline details such as adherence to APT Best Practices, professional liability insurance, state board requirements and regulations, relevant state laws, applicable codes of ethics, dual relationships, responsibilities of both supervisee and supervisor, conclusion and termination of supervision, consultation, informed consent, billing, and records information.

Ethical Duty of Play Therapy Supervisors

Confidentiality

One of the common misunderstandings of confidentiality among clinicians in training is that confidentiality in psychotherapy is a single straightforward issue and common sense. Then, as clinicians in training gain more experience, they soon learned that managing confidentiality is often fraught with conflicts and ethical quandaries. Becoming play therapists adds more complexity to it because play therapists have to balance the legitimate right of the legal guardians to obtain their children's information and the child's right to privacy in establishing and preserving the trust in the therapeutic relationship with a child client (APT, 2019; Ashby et al., 2017; Carmichael, 2006). Further, the issue of confidentiality can become a complex challenge when serving as a play therapy supervisor because it involves a twofold issue: confidentiality related to both the supervisee's child clients and the play therapy supervisees.

The multiple layers of confidentiality that play therapy supervisors have to navigate also increase the risk of breaching confidentiality. Play therapy supervisors are mandated reporters, and they hold a legal and ethical responsibility to breach confidentiality when there is a threat of harm to play therapy supervisees' child clients. Play therapy supervisors will assist supervisees in navigating the mandated reporting process when harm is inflicted by a third party. In rare situations, play therapy supervisees can be the cause of harm to their child clients. For instance, a supervisee may refuse to report child abuse to the Child Protective Service because of the fear of making a report or their disagreement with the decision made by a supervisor. In such cases, play therapy supervisors also have to fulfill the legal and ethical responsibility to protect the child's safety by making a report to appropriate authorities.

Any play that a child engages in during a play therapy session can be considered confidential material because play is deemed to be a child's language. This belief, coupled with the murkiness of the child-client's right to privacy in psychotherapy, can contribute to a more relaxed attitude and commitment to confidentiality among play therapists, which functions to their detriment. To avoid such pitfalls, the conversation of confidentiality should take place regularly in play therapy supervision. For example, a supervisor can make it a routine practice to explore how a supervisee can share the information from the therapy sessions with a caregiver without breaching a child's confidentiality.

Dual Relationships

Dual relationships in the mental health field refer to relationships in which a clinician has a professional role with a person and another role or relationship with the same person or with a person closely associated with the same person (Moleski & Kiselica, 2005). Typically, dual relationships are classified into two types: sexual or nonsexual. The codes of ethics of all professional helping organizations clearly prohibit sexual relationships with current clients or supervisees. It is abusive, exploitative, and damages the therapeutic relationship. On the other hand, the nonsexual relationship can contain complexity and ambiguity. For the remainder of this discussion, the authors will only be referring to nonsexual dual relationships by using the term *dual relationships*. Mental health clinicians are now more aware of the complexity of dual relationships due to the increased recognition of more culturally inclusive therapeutic approaches. The current American Counseling Association (ACA) code of ethics (2014) no longer uses the phrase "dual relationship"; instead, it established a section entitled "Managing and Maintaining Boundaries and Professional Relationships," indicating a nuanced understanding of the complexities of boundary issues in counseling. Specific to the play therapy field, the most current, "The Play Therapy Best Practices," issued by APT (2019), states:

> Play therapists are alert to and guard against inappropriate multiple-role relationships with current or former clients, their families, and their significant others, including, but not limited to, socializing and business arrangements, with the recognition that such relationships could impair professional judgment, increase the risk of harm to the client or exploit the client through personal, social, organizational, business, political, or religious relationship.
>
> (p. 5)

If a play therapy supervisor approaches dual relationships as a black-and-white matter, and simply avoids any dual relationships without examining their nature, they may be depriving supervisees of an opportunity to provide culturally responsive play therapy services. Such knee-jerk reactions toward any dual relationships may indicate a lack of multicultural consideration. In addition to the layered nature endemic to supervision, the factors such as systemic approaches in play therapy (involving caregivers, teachers, and other significant people in a child's life) and play therapy as a distinctly specialized field contribute to the probability of a play therapy supervisor having dual relationships with their supervisees or their clients.

Play therapy supervisors are encouraged to welcome the ambiguity in the prospective dual relationships with a potential supervisee and thoroughly examine and assess them. The literature is scarce regarding dual relationships in supervision, let alone in play therapy supervision. Supervisors must familiarize themselves with the codes of ethics for their affiliated professional organizations pertaining to multiple relationships in both clinical and supervisory settings. In addition, the rules and regulations issued by a state licensing board and the guidelines for best practice issued by credentialing bodies are essential documents for supervisors to be acquainted with.

Assessing where the potential dual relationship can fall on a continuum ranging from destructive and harmful to understanding and therapeutic, supervisors should familiarize themselves with an existing ethical decision-making model to determine the appropriate course of action (Heaton & Black, 2005 e.g. Forester-Miller & Davis, 2016; Luke et al., 2013; Cottone, 2001). When a play therapy supervisor is entering into a dual relationship, either by choice or by chance, it may be helpful to visualize the relationship's proximity and possible impact (see Figures 8.1 and 8.2). This visualization is not to draw any conclusion or decision on the potential dual relationship but rather to bring awareness to its potential risks and caution before utilizing ethical decision-making models. This visualization tool applies to a dual-relationship situation between supervisor and supervisee. Comparing figures, one for therapist and client and another for supervisor and supervisee, may help play therapy supervisors avoid minimizing the potential risks submerged in a dual relationship with their supervisees.

Play therapy supervisors may occasionally touch on something personal, idiosyncratic, and emotional if they determine that processing such an issue may unleash supervisees' capabilities, potentials, and tendencies for congruence to provide more effective play therapy (Ray, 2011). For example, Blanco et al. (2014)

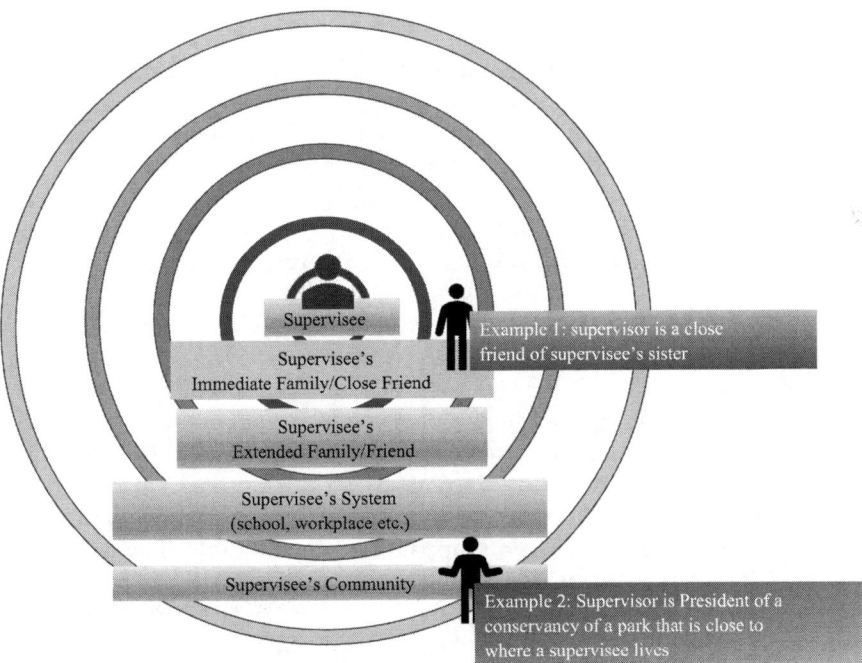

Figure 8.1 Visualization tool for dual relationship: supervisor and supervisee

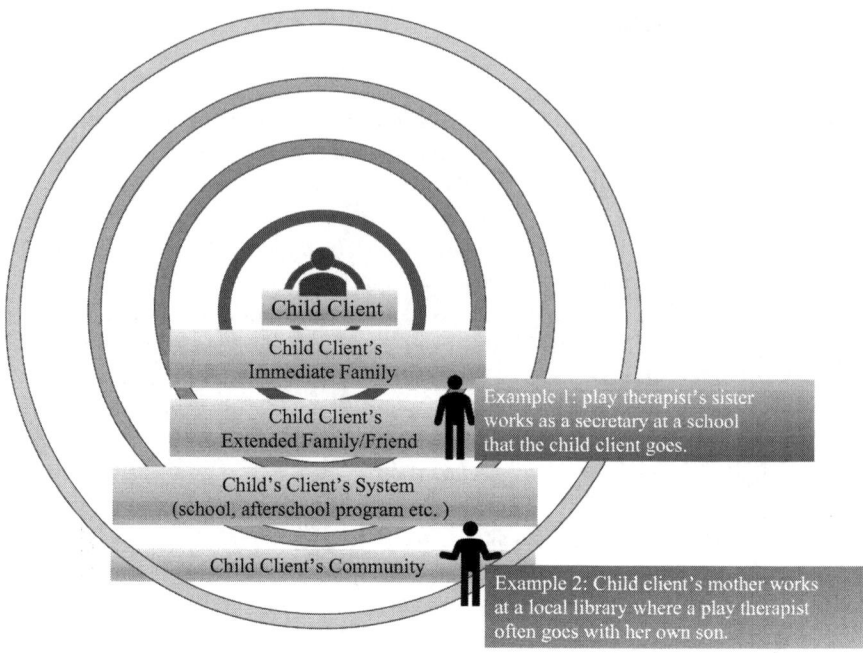

Figure 8.2 Visualization tool for dual relationship: child-client and play therapist

discussed the importance of facilitating the professional and personal growth of novice child-centered play therapists through the acquisition of skills and the development of genuineness. Gil and Rubin (2005) discussed the nature of working with young clients that is potentially evocative of countertransference and shared the creative ways to process it in supervision. In such supervision, the relationship between a supervisor and supervisee plays a paramount role, and a lack of careful assessment of a dual relationship will impair meaningful work in play therapy supervision.

To add more complexity to the dual relationship in supervision, the supervisor is vicariously responsible for the clients of their supervisees. Therefore, the supervisor's relationship to the client of the supervisees is similar to that of the counselor. Supervisors are expected to manage the boundaries with the supervisees' clients in a very similar way to the process used in navigating the boundaries between a counselor and a client (Ashby et al., 2017).

Lastly, supervisors have a responsibility to model appropriate boundaries in the supervisory relationship. Having a transparent discussion of potential boundary-crossing between play therapy supervisor and supervisee and going through the examination process together with a supervisee (identifying potential dilemma, referring to codes of ethics and guidelines for best practices, and going through ethical decision-making models) can be a great learning experience for a supervisee to deal with future dual relationship situations with their clients.

Gatekeeping

Gatekeeping in Play Therapy

When you hear the word "gatekeeping," what kind of image comes to your mind? The authors imagine a castle guard standing at the gate. A guard's responsibility is to make sure that every person who passes the gate is a trusted individual so that they do not bring any harm to the inside community. Their responsibility is to keep the community safe and unharmed. And if the guards can keep the community safe, its residents can work productively, collaboratively, peacefully, and creatively. In the field of play therapy, this guard is a play therapy supervisor whose responsibility includes ensuring that everybody who is coming into the field is equipped with the requisite knowledge, skills, and values for professional practice.

In the mental health field, the term gatekeeping, in general, is defined as "the ongoing responsibility of faculty members and clinical supervisors to monitor trainee progress and appropriateness to enter professional practice" (Homrich, 2018, p. 1). The two primary purposes of gatekeeping are (1) to protect the welfare and prevent harm to future clients of clinicians and (2) to protect the integrity of the clinical professions (Brear et al., 2008). Specific to play therapy supervision, APT states:

> APT believes that RPT-Ss providing supervision to credentialing applicants serve in a gatekeeping capacity. We believe it is supervisors' obligation to identify gaps in knowledge and/or skill sets to provide recommendations for remediation when necessary and to protect the integrity of the play therapy field and the vulnerable children and families play therapists serve.
>
> (APT, n/d, supervision section)

The play therapy supervisor's responsibility for gatekeeping cannot be discussed without referring to the play therapy competencies. APT has identified three broad play therapy competency areas: knowledge and understanding of play therapy, clinical play therapy skills, and professional engagement in play therapy (APT, 2019). Research on play therapy competencies is scarce, yet some researchers have been attempting to identify the specific indicators of these three domains of play therapy competencies to ensure comprehensive education and supervision and enrich the professional identity of play therapists (Turner et al., 2020). Based on existing information on best practices and competencies, play therapy supervisors should develop a comprehensive plan on what, how, and when to assess the supervisee's competency as a foundational work for gatekeeping.

Gateopening

The authors also associated "gated community" with the word "gatekeeping": a community where only the identified and trusted could enter. At first, it seemed there was a discrepancy between an image of a gated community and a humble field of helping professionals involved in play therapy. Yet, being a play therapist is indeed a privilege. Going to a graduate program, obtaining additional training to be a play therapist, and maintaining the licensure, certification, and credential is a privilege. Some may have had a relatively easier way to enter into this "gated community," and others may have experienced a rocky and winding road to get there. However, this community remains challenged in its ability to diversify its profession.

In 2020, as a step to tackling this issue with diversity, APT established the Inclusion, Diversity, and Equity Awareness (IDEA) Team. Ceballos et al. (2021) urged play therapists to address multiculturalism and social justice advocacy in their work to respond to societies that will continue to be diversified and globalized. For play therapy supervisors, this ethical desire to engage in multiculturalism and social justice advocacy work should be extended to their clients and their supervisees. If all mental health professions have the obligation of gatekeeping, the same professions should have another ethical obligation of "gateopening"; to open the gate and invite and support potentially competent clinicians who can contribute to the advancement of mental health among clients, particularly those who do not have an easy access to mental health services. Play therapy supervisors may consider creative ways to open the gate of the play therapy community to those who do not have adequate resources and support to become play therapists. Some of such ideas to open the gate may include low-cost or pro-bono supervision to facilitate equitable distribution of resources to future play therapists and to provide mentorship to high school and undergraduate students with marginalized backgrounds.

Technology in Play Therapy Supervision

Although a comprehensive overview of technology in supervision is addressed in another chapter in this volume, we thought it necessary to mention a few things here. APT (2019) notes specifics for using technology in the play therapy session. Just as understanding how to use play therapy with the client is important, supervisors must think about how/if to effectively use technology in supervision. RPS-Ss need to be very aware of their own level of competence in providing play therapy tele-supervision. The following information is adapted from Play Therapy Best Practices. In its original format it discussed technology use in play therapy sessions with clients. Below, these concepts have been adapted for supervisors to contemplate usage with supervisees:

Play therapy supervisors ensure that:

1. The supervisee is at a place in their level of professional development to benefit from the technology,
2. The technology meets the needs of the supervisee and is culturally appropriate,
3. The supervisee understands the purpose and operation of the technology,
4. The use of the technology is consistent with the supervision goals,
5. The supervisor and supervisee fully understand the potential benefits and limitations of the technology,

6. All possible efforts are made to protect the supervisee and client's identity that may otherwise be compromised through the use of the technology,
7. Confidentiality issues and applicable state and/or federal guidelines, and/or legal and ethical code of their professional organization regarding the use of technology in supervision is carefully reviewed with supervisees and clients (and families) being addressed in supervision,
8. When utilizing technology for supervision or consultation, the supervisor will provide the supervisee with a written informed consent, including the benefits and or limitations of the technology being utilized (p.19).

The play therapy supervisor must also understand HIPPA, state guidelines, laws, and ethics pertaining to using technology in supervision (APT, 2019).

Burnout

Burnout "is the result of a decreased ability to attach with the next client because of the emotional depletion accumulated over a period of caring for others" (Skovholt et al., 2001, p.171). Since play therapists experience stress in many ways, it is important for RPT-Ss to assist supervisees in understanding how stress manifests in unique ways for each individual. Supervision can help manage stress before it leads to distress, burnout, and/or impairment. "Play therapy is difficult work and depends on supervision for the professional growth necessary to prevent counselor burnout and to increase the knowledge, skill, and dispositions of this vital clinical profession" (Fall et al., 2007, p. 142). Since burnout can often be undetected (Lee et al., 2007), it is imperative for RPT-Ss to have these conversations in supervision.

Self-Care, Self-Compassion, and Wellness

Self-care is noted as a key component of wellness. This topic has received increased attention in the helping profession in the past decade (Meany-Walen et al., 2018) and is certainly an important consideration and personal practice for play thera-pists to develop. Self-care is defined as what individuals engage in to take care of self physically, mentally, and emotionally (Michael, 2016). Self-care is also an important ethical imperative (Meany-Walen et al., 2018) as noted in many ethical codes (ACA, 2014; APA, 2017; ASCA, 2016; NASW, 2021) and accreditation standards for clinical training programs (CACREP, 2015). However, little infor-mation exists on how to integrate this into play therapy supervision.

Self-care practices for play therapists have received little to no attention in the field of play therapy research (Meany-Walen et al., 2018). Additionally, due to being inundated with high expectations on a clinician's abilities, time, and resources (Osborn, 2004), self-care is often challenging, burdensome, or seem-ingly unattainable (Byrd & Luke, 2021). Meany-Walden et al. (2018) published the first study to examine play therapists' perceptions of wellness and self-care practices. In their study, one play therapist noted, "I would recommend having a plan and having others you trust who can support and promote wellness and hold you accountable for self-care" (p. 181). This, of course, is something an RPT-S™ can do in supervision. They may find the following assessment useful to assess self-care practices, grow this needed area, and hold supervisees accountable to these practices. Supervisors are encouraged to take this assessment themselves to see where you stand with your current self-care practices to be better suited to model self-care practices and encourage these in your supervisory relationship

Self-Care Assessment

This assessment suggestions a summary of methods that are effective in encouraging self-care. Complete the assessment in its entirety and then indicate one item from each main area that you will commit to improving.

Using the following scale, rate the areas regarding frequency:

5 = Frequently
4 = Occasionally
3 = Rarely
2 = Never
1 = It never occurred to me

Physical Self-Care

_____ Eat regularly (e.g., breakfast, lunch, and dinner)
_____ Eat healthy, healing, and wholesome foods
_____ Exercise/move body actively and intentionally
_____ Seek regular medical/wellness care services for prevention (doctor, chiropractic care, acupuncture, etc.)
_____ Seek care when needed for sickness or injury
_____ Take time off/personal days when needed
_____ Receive massages, chiropractic care, or acupuncture
_____ Dance, swim, walk, run, hike, play sports, sing, or do some other physical activity that is fun and enjoyable
_____ Take time to be sexual – with yourself, with a partner
_____ Get enough sleep
_____ Wear clothes that make you feel good, confident, and comfortable
_____ Take vacations
_____ Take day trips or mini-vacations
_____ Make time away from phones, computers, and other devices
_____ Other:

Psychological Self-Care

_____ Make time for self-reflection and self-awareness
_____ Have your own personal counseling/therapy
_____ Write in a journal or meditate

_____ Read literature that is unrelated to work
_____ Do something at which you are not expert or in charge
_____ Work to decrease stress in your life
_____ Let others know different aspects of you
_____ Notice your inner experience – take note of your thoughts, judgments, beliefs, attitudes, and feelings
_____ Engage your intelligence in a new area, e.g., go to an art museum, history exhibit, sports event, auction, theater performance
_____ Practice receiving from others
_____ Be curious
_____ Say "no" or "not right now" to extra responsibilities
_____ Other:

Emotional Self-Care

_____ Spend time with others whose company you enjoy and who support and encourage you
_____ Stay in contact with important people in your life
_____ Give yourself affirmations, encourage yourself and be compassionate with yourself
_____ Love yourself
_____ Re-read favorite books, re-watch favorite movies or shows
_____ Identify comforting activities, objects, people, relationships, places, and seek them out often
_____ Allow yourself to feel your feelings and to cry
_____ Find things that make you laugh and smile
_____ Express your outrage in social justice and advocacy, letters and donations, marches, protests
_____ Play with children and animals
_____ Other:

Spiritual Self-Care

_____ Make time for reflection and self-awareness
_____ Spend time in and with nature
_____ Find a spiritual connection or community
_____ Be open to what inspires you
_____ Cherish your optimism and hope
_____ Be aware of nonmaterial aspects of life
_____ Try at times to not be in charge or the expert
_____ Be open to not knowing
_____ Identify what is meaningful to you and notice its place in your life
_____ Meditate
_____ Pray
_____ Sing

_____ Spend time with children and animals
_____ Have experiences of awe
_____ Contribute to causes in which you believe
_____ Read inspirational literature (podcasts, music, etc.)
_____ Other:

Workplace or Professional Self-Care

_____ Take a break during the workday (e.g. lunch)
_____ Take time to converse with co-workers
_____ Make quiet time to complete tasks
_____ Identify projects or tasks that are exciting or rewarding
_____ Set boundaries and limits with your clients and colleagues
_____ Balance your caseload so that no one or part of a day is "too much"
_____ Arrange your workspace so it is comfortable, comforting, and feels restorative
_____ Get regular supervision or consultation
_____ Ask and negotiate for your needs (benefits, pay rise)
_____ Have a peer support group
_____ Develop a non-trauma area of professional interest
_____ Other:

Balance

_____ Strive for balance within your work-life and workday
_____ Strive for balance among work, family, relationships, play, and rest

(As cited in Byrd & Luke, 2021 adapted from
Saakvitne & Pearlman, 1996, pp. 61–66, 93–95)

RPT-Ss could use the assessment to gain insight into areas of growth for supervisee and guide additional supervision goals. Interesting to note is that this assessment encourages play in self-care practices, which is very fitting for supervision in play therapy.

Recently there has been increased attention on including self-compassion in our self-care practices (Coaston, 2017; Nelson et al., 2017). Neff (2003) theorizes that self-compassion entails three main components: (a) self-kindness – being kind and understanding toward oneself in instances of pain or failure rather than being harshly self-critical, (b) common humanity – perceiving one's experiences as part of the larger human experience rather than seeing them as separating and isolating, and (c) mindfulness – holding painful thoughts and feelings in balanced awareness rather than over-identifying with them. Moreover, "self-compassion is generally considered the foundation for compassion towards others" (Morgan et al., 2013, p. 87). Skovholt et al. (2001) outlined a developmental framework for career counselors to avoid empathy and caring burnout. This article discussed six paths for counselor personal and professional self-care: "(a) maximizing professional success; (b) creating and sustaining an active, individually designed development method; (c) increasing professional self-understanding; (d) creating a professional greenhouse at work; (e) minimizing ambiguous professional loss; and (f) focusing on one's own need for balanced wellness" (p. 171). This model can certainly be applied to play therapy supervision.

As increased evidence proposes, self-compassion is an essential component of change in therapeutic work and is negatively correlated with both depression and anxiety (Barnard & Curry, 2011). Additionally, self-compassion can assist in reducing symptoms of psychopathology and even improve mental and emotional well-being (Germer & Neff, 2013). Often, beginning play therapists doubt the process and their skills and abilities. As they have grown in confidence in supervision, RPT-Ss can use self-compassion that can aid in helping supervisees recognize ways to take care and be kind to self, even in the middle of the self-doubt, criticism, uncertainty, and even pain (Morgan et al., 2013). Just like self-care, self-compassion involves intention and practice. Self-compassion is also important for RPT-Ss to understand and model for supervisees as they may look to their supervisors as the first to model professional identity (VanderGast & Hinkle, 2015) and ethical behavior specific to play therapy. Thankfully, this volume includes an entire chapter dedicated to self-compassion (please see Chapter 13).

Supervisory Relationship Termination

The termination of clinical supervision is rarely discussed or studied empirically. However, Levendosky and Hopwood (2017) mention that research on parallel process in psychotherapy and clinical supervision suggests that the experience of supervisee in the termination of clinical supervision provides a guiding framework for navigating termination with their own clients. Gil and Crenshaw (2016) state, "in parallel relationships of all kinds (partners/spouses, supervisors/supervisees, employers/employees, friends, etc.), when endings are left without closure, after abrupt or neglected ending, the result can be much unfinished emotional business" (p. 2). Play therapy supervisors should have a clear plan for when termination of supervision best occurs, such as when a supervisee satisfies all credentialing requirements or completes a specific phase and communicate the end goals and timing to their potential supervisees before the initiation of the supervisory relationship.

Depending on a play therapy supervisor's theoretical orientation and both supervisees' and supervisors' interpersonal styles, how to terminate play therapy supervision may vary. However, there is some consensus on the goals of termination of supervision such as consolidation of supervisee's growth and development as the last gatekeeping checkpoint, discussion on authentic feelings associated with termination, and modeling how to process a meaningful good-bye. Those goals are often not met in one session. Therefore, akin to the play therapy termination process, play therapy supervisors might engage in a countdown process toward termination with their supervisees.

Play therapy supervisors can utilize many expressive art activities used for play therapy termination in their supervision termination. For example, "Therapy

Mountain" (Gil & Crenshaw, 2016) can be a great expressive art termination activity as "Supervision Mountain." In the "Therapy Mountain" activity, a therapist asks a child client to compare their therapy experience to climbing a mountain trail by reflecting back their own experience. Once a child client has an image of their "therapy mountain," a therapist will ask them to draw the mountain and the trail up. A therapist may ask some prompting questions such as "Would the trail be steep, or gently wind around the mountain with the climb easy and gentle?" Would you have plenty of room on the trail, or would you be walking on the edge?" (Gil & Crenshaw, 2016, p. 151). In the "Supervision Mountain" as a modified version of "Therapy Mountain," a supervisor can ask prompting questions of their supervisee such as: "What kind of things that you are carrying in your backpack helped you get through the trail?"; "Did you find any good tools during the trail that helped you finish the trail?"; "Now that you are at the top of this mountain, what kind of view are you seeing?"

In addition, sandtray activity prompts such as "create a tray of your experience of supervision" or "create a world of yourself as a credentialed play therapist" can produce materials to process supervisee's supervision termination experience in depth.

Lastly, play therapy supervisors may offer an option for play therapy consultation after the termination of play therapy supervision. When licensed and credentialed in play therapy, the play therapy supervisee will be identified as a play therapy consultee. In general, the consultee is practicing within the bounds of competence and is seeking additional mentorship, guidance, expertise, and perspective on their cases from a more senior clinician. Therefore, generally speaking, the consultant does not have the role of evaluator and is not responsible for the consultee's actions with their cases. Play therapy supervisors should be aware of the distinctions between the roles of play therapy supervisor and play therapy consultant and of the ethical obligations that accompany each role (Ashby et al., 2017).

Conclusion

The complex ethical duties of play therapy supervisors reflect the substantial responsibilities in guiding somebody to be a play therapist. Yet, at the same time, a play therapy supervisor is a rewarding role to take. One of the crucial ways to grow as an effective play therapist is to be supervised by an excellent play therapy supervisor. Being on the receiving end of memorable supervisory experiences impacts and guides how we supervise in the future, and in that sense, the supervision we offer has a generational impact. This idea of leaving your footprint as an excellent supervisor to future play therapists will inspire you to engage in aspirational ethics and the highest standards of practices.

Key Readings and Resources

ACA code of ethics. https://www.counseling.org/docs/default-source/default-document -library/2014-code-of-ethics-finaladdress.pdf

APA ethical principles of psychologist and code of conduct. https://www.apa.org/ethics/ code/ethics-code-2017.pdf

APT play therapy best practices: Clinical, professional and ethical issues. https://cdn
.ymaws.com/www.a4pt.org/resource/resmgr/publications/best_practices_-_sept
_2019.pdf
ASCA ethical standards for school counselors. https://www.schoolcounselor.org/getmedia
/f041cbd0-7004-47a5-ba01-3a5d657c6743/Ethical-Standards.pdf
NASW code of ethics of the national association of social workers. https://www
.socialworkers.org/About/Ethics/Code-of-Ethics/Code-of-Ethics-English

References

American Counseling Association. (2014). ACA code of ethics. https://www.counseling.org
/docs/default-source/default-document-library/2014-code-of-ethics-finaladdress.pdf
American Psychological Association. (2017). Ethical principles of psychologist and code
of conduct (2002, amended effective June 1, 2010, and January 1, 2017). https://www
.apa.org/ethics/code/ethics-code-2017.pdf
American School Counseling Association. (2016). ASCA ethical standards for school
counselors. https://www.schoolcounselor.org/getmedia/f041cbd0-7004-47a5-ba01
-3a5d657c6743/Ethical-Standards.pdf
Ashby, J. S., Wood, L., & Kiperman, S. (2017). Chapter 12: Ethics in play therapy
consultation and supervision. In R. L. Steen (Ed.), *Emerging research in play therapy, child
counseling, and consultation* (pp. 214–231). IGI Global.
Association for Play Therapy. (2019). Play therapy best practices: Clinical, professional &
ethical issues. https://cdn.ymaws.com/www.a4pt.org/resource/resmgr/publications/
best_practices_-_sept_2019.pdf
Association for Play Therapy. (n.d.). Important credentialing announcement: Registered
play Therapist™ (RPT™) & registered play Therapist-Supervisor™ (RPT-S™).
https://www.a4pt.org/page/SpecialAnnouncement
Barnard, L. K., & Curry, J. F. (2011). Self-compassion: Conceptualizations, correlates,
& interventions. *Review of General Psychology*, *15*(4), 289–303. https://doi.org/10.1037/
a0025754
Bernard, J. M., & Goodyear, R. K. (1992). *Fundamentals of clinical supervision*. Allyn &
Bacon.
Bernard, J. M., & Goodyear, R. K. (2018). *Fundamentals of clinical supervision* (6th ed.).
Pearson.
Blanco, P. J., Muro, J. H., & Stickley, V. K. (2014). Understanding the concept of
genuineness in play therapy: Implications for the supervision and teaching of beginning
play therapists. *International Journal of Play Therapy*, *23*(1), 44–54. https://doi.org/10
.1037/a0035478
Brear, P., Dorrian, J., & Luscri, G. (2008). Preparing our future counseling professionals:
Gatekeeping and the implications for research. *Counseling and Psychotherapy Research*, *8*(2),
93–101. https://doi.org/10.1080/14733140802007855
Byrd, R., & Luke, C. (2021). *Counseling children and adolescents: Cultivating empathic connection*.
Routledge.
Carmichael, K. D. (2006). Legal and ethical issues in play therapy. *International Journal of
Play Therapy*, *15*(2), 83–99. https://doi.org/10.1037/h0088916
Ceballos, P., Post, P., & Rodriguez, M. (2021). Practicing child-centered play therapy from
multicultural and social justice framework. In E. Gil & A. A. Drews (Eds.), *Cultural issues
in play therapy* (pp. 13–31). The Guilford Press.

Coaston, S. C. (2017). Self-care through self-compassion: A balm for burnout. *Professional Counselor, 7*(3), 285–297. https://doi.org/10.15241/scc.7.3.285

Corey, G., Haynes, R., Moulton, P., & Muratori, M. (2010). *Clinical supervision in the helping professions: A practical guide* (2nd ed.). American Counseling Association.

Cottone, R. R. (2001). A social constructivism model of ethical decision making in counseling. *Journal of Counseling and Development, 79*(1), 39–45. https://doi.org/10.1002/j.1556-6676.2001.tb01941.x

Council for Accreditation of Counseling and Related Education Programs. (2015). *2016 CACREP standards.* www.cacrep.org/wp-content/uploads/2017/08/2016-Standards -with-citations.pdf

Donald, E. J., Culbreth, J. R., & Carter, A. W. (2015). Play therapy supervision: A review of the literature. *International Journal of Play Therapy, 24*(2), 59–77. https://doi.org/10.1037/a0039104

Fall, M., Drew, D., Chute, A., & More, A. (2007). The voices of registered play therapists as supervisors. *International Journal of Play Therapy, 16*(2), 133–146. https://doi.org/10.1037/1555-6824.16.2.133

Forester-Miller, H., & Davis, T. E. (2016). *Practitioner's guide to ethical decision making* (Rev. ed.). http://www.counseling.org/docs/default-source/ethics/practioner's-guide-toethical -decision-making.pdf

Germer, C. K., & Neff, K. D. (2013). Self-compassion in clinical practice. *Journal of Clinical Psychology: In Session, 69*(8), 856–867. https://doi.org/10.1002/jclp.22021

Gil, E., & Crenshaw, D. A. (2016). *Termination challenges in child psychotherapy.* The Guildford Press.

Gil, E., & Rubin, L. (2005). Countertransference play: Informing and enhancing therapist self-awareness through play. *International Journal of Play Therapy, 14*(2), 87–102.

Heaton, K. J., & Black, L. L. (2005). I knew you when: A case study of managing preexisting nonamorous relationships in counseling. *Family Journal, 17*(2), 134–138. https://doi.org/10.1177/1066480709332854

Homrich, A. M. (2018). Chapter 1. Introduction to gatekeeping. In A. M. Homrich & K. L. Henderson (Eds.), *Gatekeeping in the mental health professions* (pp. 1–24). Wiley.

Lee, S. M., Baker, C. R., Cho, S. H., Heckathorn, D. E., Holland, M. W., Newgent, R. A., Ogle, N. T., Powell, M. L., Quinn, J. J., Wallace, S. L., & Yu, K. (2007). Development and initial psychometrics of the counselor burnout inventory (Report). *Measurement and Evaluation in Counseling and Development, 40*(3), 142–154. https://doi.org/10.1017/jgc.2018.3

Levendosky, A. A., & Hopwood, C. J. (2017). Terminating supervision. *Psychotherapy, 54*(1), 37–46. https://doi.org/10.1037/pst0000096

Luke, M., Goodrich, K. M., & Gilbride, D. D. (2013). Intercultural model of ethical decision making: Addressing worldview dilemmas in school counseling. *Counseling and Values, 58*(2), 177–194. https://doi.org/10.1002/j.2161-007X.2013.00032.x

Meany-Walen, K. K., Cobie-Nuss, A., Eittreim, E., Teeling, S., Wilson, S., & Xander, C. (2018). Play therapists' perceptions of wellness and self-care practices. *International Journal of Play Therapy, 27*(3), 176–186. https://doi.org/10.1037/pla0000067

Michael, R. (2016). What self-care is – And what it isn't. *Psych. Central.* https://psychcentral.com/blog/what-self-care-is-and-what-it-isnt-2/

Moleski, S. M., & Kiselica, M. S. (2005). Dual relationships: A continuum ranging from the destructive to the therapeutic. *Journal of Counseling and Development, 83*(1), 3–11. https://doi.org/10.1002/j.1556-6678.2005.tb00574.x

Morgan, W. D., Morgan, S. T., & Germer, C. K. (2013). Cultivating attention and compassion. In C. K. Germer, R. D. Siegel, & P. R. Fulton (Eds.), *Mindfulness and psychotherapy* (2nd ed., pp. 76–93). The Guilford Press.

NASW. (2021). Code of ethics of the national association of social workers. https://www.socialworkers.org/About/Ethics/Code-of-Ethics/Code-of-Ethics-English

Neff, K. (2003). Self-compassion: An alternative conceptualization of a healthy attitude toward oneself. *Self and Identity, 2*(2), 85–101. https://doi.org/10.1080/15298860309032

Nelson, J. R., Hall, B. S., Anderson, J. L., Birtles, C., & Hemming, L. (2017). Self – Compassion as self-care: A simple and effective tool for counselor educators and counseling students. *Journal of Creativity in Mental Health.* https://doi.org/10.1080/15401383.2017.1328292

Osborn, C. (2004). Seven salutary suggestions for counselor stamina. *Journal of Counseling and Development, 82*(3), 319–328. https://doi.org/10.1002/j.1556-6678.2004.tb00317.x

Peabody, M. A. (2014). Exploring dimensions of administrative support for play therapy in schools. *International Journal of Play Therapy, 23*(3), 161–172. https://doi.org/10.1037/a0037319

Penn, S. L., & Post, P. B. (2012). Investigating various dimensions of play therapists' self-reported multicultural counseling competence. *International Journal of Play Therapy, 21*(1), 14–29. https://doi.org/10.1037/a0026894

Purswell, K. E., & Stulmaker, H. L. (2015). Expressive arts in supervision: Choosing developmentally appropriate interventions. *International Journal of Play Therapy, 24*(2), 103–117. https://doi.org/10.1037/a0039134

Ray, D. C. (2011). *Advanced play therapy: Essential conditions, knowledge, and skills for child practice.* Routledge.

Saakvitne, K. W., Pearlman, L. A., & Traumatic Stress Inst, Ctr for Adult & Adolescent Psychotherapy, LLC. (1996). *Transforming the pain: A workbook on vicarious traumatization.* W W Norton & Co.

Skovholt, T. M., Grier, T. L., & Hanson, M. R. (2001). Career counseling for longevity: Self-care and burnout prevention strategies for counselor resilience. *Journal of Career Development, 27*(3), 167–176. https://doi.org/10.1023/A:1007830908587

Turner, R., Schoeneberg, C., Ray, D., & Lin, Y. W. (2020). Establishing play therapy competencies: A Delphi study. *International Journal of Play Therapy, 29*(4), 177–190. https://doi.org/10.1037/pla0000138

VanderGast, T. S., & Hinkle, M. S. (2015). So happy together? Predictors of satisfaction with supervision for play therapist supervisees. *International Journal of Play Therapy, 24*(2), 92–102. https://doi.org/10.1037/a0039105

Section 3

Special Topics

9 Technology in Play Therapy Supervision

Edward (Franc) Hudspeth

Technology in Play Therapy Supervision

On July 1, 2019, the Association for Play Therapy (APT) released its updated credentialing standards for individuals seeking the Registered Play Therapist™ (RPT™) credential. Within the updated credentialing standards was a change of who could supervise those working toward the RPT™ credential. Before this update, supervision could be provided by any mental health practitioner that was licensed for independent practice and who had received some supervision training. After the effective date of the updated standards, only supervised experience, conducted by a Registered Play Therapist-Supervisor™ (RPT-S™), would be accepted. This significant shift further defined play therapy as a specialized practice requiring supervision by someone trained and credentialed in this practice and trained as a supervisor.

APT offers guidance for play therapists and play therapy supervisors through its Play Therapy Best Practices: Clinical, Professional, & Ethical Issues (APT, 2020). APT is an association representing mental health practitioners from all branches of mental health. These best practice guidelines were developed and are updated based on the codes of ethics and practice guidelines, as well as any updates, of multiple national associations. These practice guidelines do not take the place of or negate the need to follow the ethical codes of an individual's mental health practice. Instead, an RPT™ or RPT-S™ must follow their ethical codes of their mental health practice and the practice guidelines set forth by APT.

APT was an early adopter of distance supervision. In the early days of the association, quality supervision was limited, especially if seeking supervision from an RPT-S™. For many years, there were few RPT-Ss™ in some states. Even if a state had an RPT-S™, it was common for them to live in areas clustered around universities that offered play therapy education, making it difficult for those not in those areas to gain supervision. Therefore, distance play therapy supervision was approved and encouraged to motivate play-therapists-in-training to seek supervision from an RPT-S™.

This chapter is an attempt to demonstrate how an RPT-S™ can be a well-informed supervisor capable of practicing within their branch of mental health's ethical codes, practice guidelines, and the guidelines set forth by APT. It intends

DOI: 10.4324/9781003196075-12

to summarize the ethical codes and practice guidelines of distance supervision for multiple branches of mental health. The overarching goal is to provide supervisors with a comprehensive overview of the necessary components of quality distance supervision and how it works.

Technology Use in Supervision

For those under supervision and those doing supervision, the use of technology can present unique opportunities and challenges. When guidelines for telemental health and distance supervision are incorporated into routine supervision, potential ethical dilemmas, practice issues, and supervision conundrums can be mitigated. Distance supervision and telemental health are rapidly growing practices spanning many mental health disciplines. After the COVID-19 pandemic, distance supervision and telemental health were quickly propelled into the offices of counselors and homes of clients.

Research on the Use of Technology Use in Play Therapy Supervision

Currently, there is no research specifically related to the use of technology in play therapy supervision. However, there are a handful of conceptual articles about the use of technology in play therapy supervision (Davis & Hudspeth, 2014; Hudspeth & Davis, 2015, 2016) and others related to the use of technology in play therapy (Altvater et al., 2017, 2018; Autry, 2017; Hull, 2016; Lamb et al., 2018; McNary et al., 2018; Snow et al., 2012; Stauffer, 2018; Stone, 2020). Considering this, readers must extrapolate findings from research about the use of technology in the practice and supervision of other forms of psychotherapy (see Bernhard & Camins, 2020; Butler & Constantine, 2006; Chapman et al., 2011; Marino et al., 2015; Reese et al., 2009; Rousmaniere et al., 2014; Tarlow et al., 2020; Woo et al., 2020). This research illuminates benefits and limitations of distance supervision.

The Potential Benefits of Distance Supervision

There are numerous reasons for increased demand and need for distance supervision. From a practical standpoint, distance supervision offers convenience and flexibility that may not exist in traditional, in-person supervision. Some of the benefits noted include:

- Increased accessibility of psychotherapy training, especially for clinicians in rural or remote areas (Renfro-Michel et al., 2016, p. 3; Rousmaniere et al., 2014)
- Reduced cost for travel and improved flexibility of scheduling (Dudding & Justice, 2004; Renfro-Michel et al., 2016, p. 3)
- Increased access for peer consultation (in small groups via teleconference or large groups via electronic mailing lists and Web forums) (Renfro-Michel et al., 2016, p. 3)

- Potentially enhanced diversity in trainees due to improved accessibility of training (Renfro-Michel et al., 2016, p. 3)
- Increased ease in recording and documenting supervision and training (Rousmaniere, 2014)
- Improved comfort with using technology (Dudding & Justice, 2004)
- Trainees and supervisors reported preparing more thoroughly for videoconference supervision (Sørlie et al., 1999)
- Web-based supervision may enhance the quality of play therapy supervision because supervisees will have access to a larger pool of potential supervisors (Davis & Hudspeth, 2014, p. 7)

Renfro-Michel et al. (2016) included "enhanced diversity in trainees." Still, they failed to recognize that distance supervision offers access to diverse supervisors with diverse experience that would not normally be accessible if supervision were done solely in person.

The Potential Drawbacks of Distance Supervision

As with telemental health and the development of a therapeutic relationship, some have expressed concern about limitations of the supervisor–supervisee relationship when engaging via technology (see Deane et al., 2015; Jordan & Shearer, 2019; Munchel, 2015). Specific concerns and drawbacks include:

- Potential impaired ability of supervisors to provide help from a distance because of unfamiliarity with local laws and regulations (Abbass et al., 2011)
- Potential reduced accuracy or depth of communication because of the visual constraints and visual cues that may be limited during a videoconference (Kanz, 2001).
- Existing variations in technology proficiency between digital natives and digital immigrants (Perry, 2012; Rousmaniere, 2014)
- Security and confidentiality concerns (Rousmaniere et al., 2014)
- Concerns related to ethics and regulations (Rousmaniere, 2014)
- Possible prohibitions and/or limitations set by state boards against using technology to provide clinical supervision (Barton et al., 2016)

However, these challenges can be mitigated if a sound supervision contract is developed before beginning supervision. When well planned, the process can be as beneficial as traditional face-to-face supervision.

Legal and Ethical Considerations for Distance Supervision

In many ways, distance supervision is like face-to-face supervision. However, engaging in it does require more training and understanding of how laws and ethics guide it. Using technology and accomplishing the task of supervision across a distance is a complicated endeavor.

Federal Laws Regarding Distance Supervision

When considering federal laws and how these impact distance supervision, the primary components of these laws relate to technology's use in the provision of services and collection transmission of data. Specifically, privacy, security, confidentiality, and potential information breaches are covered under these laws. The laws to review and consider are:

- The Health Insurance Portability and Accountability Act 1196 (HIPAA), see HIPAA Administrative Simplification Statute and Rules (U.S. Department of Health and Human Services, 2021)
- The Health Information Technology for Economic and Clinical Health Act of 2009 (HITECH), see Omnibus HIPAA rulemaking (U.S. Department of Health and Human Services, 2013)
- The Family Educational Rights and Privacy Act of 1974 (FERPA), see Part 99-Family Educational and Rights of Privacy (U.S. Department of Education, 2021)

State Laws Regarding Distance Supervision

Most states have rules and regulations that guide the use of technology in supervision (Barton et al., 2016). For those that had not formally addressed distance supervision as part of the licensure process, the coronavirus pandemic forced them to consider and address it. A review of each state's licensure rules and regulation across all mental health branches should now yield statements, rules, and regulations about distance supervision. Some states included, in these statements, updated rules and minimum training standards for those conducting distance supervision. For a comprehensive overview of resources related to state telemental health laws, see the Telehealth Certification Institute's (TCI) State's Rules and Regulations (TCI, 2021) resource page and the Health Resources & Services Administration's (HRSA) Telehealth Licensing Requirements and Interstate Compacts (HRSA, 2021)

Professional Association Ethical Codes and Distance Supervision

Multiple associations, in their codes of ethics and supervision best practices, describe the necessary considerations when using technology in supervision. These include the following:

(a) American Academy of Child & Adolescent Psychiatry (AACAP), Code of Ethics (2014)

(b) American Art Therapy Association (AATA), Ethical Principles for Art Therapists (2013)

(c) American Association for Marriage and Family Therapy (AAMFT), Code of Ethics (2015)

(d) American Counseling Association (ACA), Code of Ethics (2014)

(e) American Mental Health Counselors Association (AMHCA), Code of Ethics (2020)

(f) American Psychological Association (APA), Ethical Principles of Psychologists and Code of Conduct (2017)

(g) American Psychological Association (APA), Guidelines for the Practice of Telepsychology (2013)

(h) American School Counselors Association (ASCA), Ethical Standards for School

Counselors (2016)

(i) Association for Play Therapy (APT), Play Therapy Best Practices: Clinical, Professional, & Ethical Issues (2020)

(j) National Association of Alcoholism and Drug Abuse Counselors (NAADAC) and National Certification Commission for Addiction Professionals (NCCAP), Code of Ethics (2021)

(k) National Association for Social Workers (NASW), Code of Ethics (2021)

(l) National Association for Social Workers (NASW) and Association of Social Work Boards (ASWB), Best Practice Standards in Social Work Supervision (2013)

(m) National Association of Social Workers (NASW), Association of Social Work Boards (ASWB), Council on Social Work Education (CSWE), & Clinical Social Work Associations (CSWA), Standards for Technology in Social Work Practice (2017)

(n) National Board for Certified Counselors (NBCC), Code of Ethics (2016a)

(o) National Board for Certified Counselors (NBCC) Policy Regarding the Provision OF Distance Professional Services (2016b).

Play therapists are not excluded and should be aware of legal and ethical mandates for technology applications within their practice. See Table 9.1 for a summary of codes of ethics and standards of practice related to the use of technology in supervision.

Across these codes and guidelines, readers will find codes and guidelines related to the use of technology and informed consent, communications, record-keeping, confidentiality, and competency. From this, some potential, hypothetical, ethical dilemmas of distance supervision begin to emerge. Although there is a potential for many ethical dilemmas that occur during in-person supervision to also occur during distance supervision, three could be more prominent in distance supervision. These include (a) maintaining confidentiality and privacy, (b) competency, and (c) dealing with crisis situations. Confidentiality and privacy concerns can

Table 9.1 Ethical Codes and Practice Guidelines for Use of Technology in Supervision

APT Best Practices (2020)	ACA Code of Ethics (2014)	AMHCA Code of Ethics (2020)	NASW Supervision (2013) NASW Technology (2017)	APA Telepsychology (2013)	AAMFT Code of Ethics (2015)	ASCA Code of Ethics (2016)	NAADAC Code of Ethics (2021)	AATA Code of Ethics (2013)	AACAP Code of Ethics (2014)
J.5 Use of Telemental Health in Play Therapy (p. 20)	Section E: Evaluation, Assessment, and Interpretation (p. 11) E.2. Competence to Use and Interpret Assessment Instruments (p. 11) E.2.a. Limits of Competence (p. 11)	B. Counseling Process (p. 4) 6. The Use of Technology Supported Counseling and Communications (TSCC) (p. 6) Standard d. (p. 6)	NASW & ASWB (2013) Best Practice Standards in Social Work Supervision Standard 5. Technology (p. 23) Distance Supervision (p. 24) Risk Management (p. 24)	Competence of the Psychologist Guideline 1 (p. 4)	Standard VI: Technology-Assisted Professional Services (p. 7) 6.1 Technology Assisted Services (p. 8)	D. School Counseling Intern Site Supervisors (p. 8) Field/intern site supervisors: Standards f. and g. (p. 8)	Principle VI: E-Therapy, E-Supervision, and Social Media (p. 13) VI-1 Introduction (p. 14) VI-1 Definition (p. 14) VI-3 Informed Consent (p. 14) VI 6 Licensing Laws (p. 15) VI-14 Capability (p. 16) IV-14 Missing Cues (p. 16)	15.0 Professional Use of the Internet, Social Networking Sites and Other Electronic or Digital Technology (p. 14) Standards 15.2 (p. 14)	Principle X: Legal Considerations (p. 16)
J.6 Distance and Online Supervision (see also section H, Supervision/ Consultation) (p. 21)	Section F: Supervision, Training, and Teaching (p. 12) F.2. Counselor Supervision Competence (p. 13) F.2.c. Online Supervision (p. 13)		NASW, ASWB, CSWE, & CSWA (2017) Standards for Technology in Social Work Practice Introduction (p. 8)						

be mitigated by using a HIPAA/HITECH compliant telemental health platform and controlling the setting/location for distance supervision. Issues of competency can be alleviated by adequate technical training of supervisors, supervisees, and clients. Handling crisis situations can be addressed by having clear policies and plans in place.

Technology and Platforms for Distance Supervision

In general, mental health professionals seek the best practices guidelines and compliant platforms to offer safe and effective services to their clients, as should play therapists. When considering the use of technology in supervision, one should explore the technology required to engage in distance supervision and the ethical and legal consideration for adhering to HIPAA, HITECH, and FERPA laws (Hudspeth & Davis, 2015, 2016). Multiple platforms can meet the necessary privacy, security, and confidentiality requirements. Some useful resources include the websites Telemental Health Software Comparisons (Telemental Health Comparisons, 2020) and HIPAA Compliant Video Conferencing Requirements after COVID (Maheu, 2020).

From an individual or agency perspective, when contemplating which telemental health platform to use, internal questions to ask are (a) Is the platform HIPAA/HITECH compliant? (b) Is the platform user-friendly? (c) What tools are integrated into the platform?, and (d) What is the cost? To be more specific about what a telemental health platform should include and/or guarantee, according to Telemental Health Software Comparisons (Telemental Health Comparisons, 2020), all the following statements should be true, documented, and verifiable:

1. Documentation of the platform states that it is HIPAA compliant
2. Documentation of the platform includes 256-bit encryption and describes the type (e.g., asymmetric, TLS and SSL, HTTPS, cryptography, or IPSec)
3. Documentation of the platform describes the encryption of data *in motion* (data that is moving between locations/computers [e.g., the video conferencing that is happening between a counselor/supervisor and client/supervisee]).
4. Documentation of the platform describes the encryption of data *at rest* (data that is stored; potentially in cloud storage or within the platform's app or software on a computer [e.g., client records, supervision logs, etc.]).
5. Documentation of the platform describes the administrative, physical, and technical controls necessary to meet the security standards required by HIPAA
6. Regarding the encryption of data *at rest* and data *in motion*, documentation of the platform states that it has tools/options for and encrypts not only video conferencing but also emails, texts, chats, and Voice over Internet Protocol (VoIP) calls.
7. The company (platform owner) will sign a Business Associate Agreement with any/all covered entity

8. The company (platform owner) has a routine process of testing for vulner-abilities within the system
9. The company (platform owner) does a yearly risk assessment

Other considerations related to preference, functionality, and usability of platforms might include:

1. The platform offers counselor/supervisor/clients tools such as journals, blogs, assessments/surveys, whiteboards, media/file/screen sharing, etc.
2. User requirements are defined and clear, which might include (a) is there software to download and (b) are multiple operating systems supported (PC, Mac, Android)?
3. User controls and options are listed, which might include (a) room access controls and mute options, (b) the platform allows for computer, tablet, and/or phone access, and (c) mobile access is possible
4. Technical support is available, and if there are multiple options, each is listed

Supervision Theories and Distance Supervision

This volume contains many chapters that cover various supervision theories and models. Therefore, for this chapter, a few have been reviewed and mentioned here because they have been specifically applied to distance supervision. This is not to say that all theoretical frameworks for supervision can be utilized during distance supervision; rather, it is to note that research on application has not been accomplished. Dawson et al. (2011) describe the application of the Discrimination Model (Bernard, 1997) in distance supervision by connecting and adapting the tenets of the model to distance supervision. Dubi et al. (2012) consider a transtheoretical model with five phases: Presenting Problem, Issues, Dynamics, Interventions, and Bridge (PIDIB; Raggi et al., 2008). Finally, Miller et al. (2003) used telehealth as the model for application to distance supervision. In their article, and as in many parts of this chapter, tenets of telehealth are applied to distance supervision.

Use of Experiential Activities in Distance Supervision

As with face-to-face supervision, distance supervision allows for the use of experiential activities that support the supervisee's development. Experiential activities are not a substitute for supervision theory and methods; instead, they can be used as tools for the supervisor and the supervisee to gain perspective, insight, and awareness. Like many areas of distance supervision, experiential activities in play therapy supervision have not been researched, and little has been written about them. Zeng et al. (2020) describe narrative, reflective activities for use in online group supervision. Villarreal-Davis et al. (2021) describe three experiential activities that can be used in online group supervision. Included are (a) Phoenix-Out of the Ashes, an art-based activity; (b) Digital Creative Writing Collage; and (c)

Pictured Miniatures and Mindfulness, a sandtray activity. For each, the authors describe the activity and how to implement it, and provide a case example.

Though these are the only articles found, many experiential and expressive activities can be adapted and utilized in distance supervision. As used in the Pictured Miniatures and Mindfulness activity described by Villarreal-Davis et al. (2021), sandtray can be adapted for distance supervision. Online Sand Tray (Fried, 2021) is a free, virtual sandtray that supervisors can use with supervisees. Sandtray can be used to allow supervisee to reflect on their growth and process reactions to client situations. Google's Jamboard (Google, n.d.), a virtual whiteboard, provides an opportunity for supervisor(s) and supervisee(s) to work synchronously and collaboratively. Mural, a digital canvas, can be used for brainstorming and art activities (Mural, n.d.).

Assessment in Distance Play Therapy Supervision

Regardless of the method of supervision, assessment should be a regular part of the process. On a routine basis, supervisors should be assessing the supervision process, the progress of the supervisee, and the supervisee's development of autonomy and movement toward competent independent practice. This requires the assessment of the supervisor, supervisee, and supervisory relationship. If the supervisee is a student in a master's degree program, the program will likely require some type of assessment. Also, some state licensure boards require assessment of supervisees as they work toward their independent practice license. In the case of a post-master's supervisee working toward licensure, it is important to check with and know the evaluation requirements of the licensure board.

Suppose assessment of the supervisee is not mandated. In that case, it is good practice to incorporate routine assessment to (a) demonstrate competency of the supervisor, (b) demonstrate growth and competency of the supervisee, and (c) evaluate the supervisory relationship and outcome of the relationship. Below are examples of assessments that can be utilized. When reviewing and reading about the assessments mentioned, readers will note that these assessments were developed and originate in multiple branches of mental health.

Assessment of the Supervisor

- Supervisor Competency Self-Assessment (Falender et al., 2016) allows the supervisor to identify their strengths as well as those areas in which you can develop greater supervisor competence through continued professional learning and practice
- Psychotherapy Supervisory Inventory (Shanfield et al., 1989) is used to rate the behaviors of the supervisor

Assessment of Supervisees

- Supervisee Levels Questionnaire-Revised (Stoltenberg et al., 1998) allows the supervisor to assess the therapist's competency

- Counseling Competencies Scale-Revised (Lambie et al., 2018) allows the supervisor – or, as a self-assessment, the supervisee – to assess the skills, dispositions, and professional behaviors of supervisees
- Professional Counselor Performance Evaluation (Kerl et al., 2002) allows the supervisor – or, as a self-assessment, the supervisee – to assess the skills, dispositions, and professional behaviors of supervisees
- Postgraduate Competency Document (Storm et al., 1997) is used by supervisors to assess supervisees on seven areas of competency
- Basic Skills Evaluation (Nelson & Johnson, 1999) is used by supervisors to assess supervisee proficiencies and professional growth on 20 core competencies

Assessment of the Supervisory Relationship

- Supervisory Relationship Questionnaire (Palomo et al., 2010) allows the supervisee to evaluate the supervisory relationship
- Relational Behavior Scale (Shaffer & Friedlander, 2015) allows the supervisee to assess relational elements of the supervisory relationship
- Supervisor Relating Style Inventory (Lizzio et al., 2009) assesses the supervisees perceptions of the supervisory relationship process
- Supervision Evaluation and Supervisory Competence Scale (Gonsalvez et al., 2017) allows the supervisee to assess the supervisory competency
- Supervisory Satisfaction Questionnaire (Ladany et al., 1996) is used to assess the supervisees satisfaction of supervision
- Collaborative Supervision Behaviors Scale (Rousmaniere & Ellis, 2013) allows the supervisee to assess supervision from the perspective of collaboration
- Barrett-Lennard Relationship Inventory for Supervisory Relationships (Schacht et al., 1988) allows the supervisee to assess their experience of the facilitative conditions in the supervisory relationship
- Evaluation Process Within Supervision Inventory (Lehrman-Waterman & Ladany, 2001) is used to assess the evaluation process within supervision and measures supervisee experience of the evaluations
- Working Alliance Inventory of Supervisory Relationships (Smith et al., 2002) is completed by the supervisee to explore how a supervisory relationship develops and matures over time
- Working Alliance Inventory Trainee Form (Bahrick, 1990) is completed by the supervisor and supervisee to assess the strength of the working alliance in supervision as perceived by both supervisors and supervisees
- Supervisory Working Alliance Inventory (Efstation et al., 1990) is completed by the supervisor and supervisee to assess the relationship in supervision
- Brief Supervisory Alliance Scale (Rønnestad & Lundquist, 2009) allows the supervisor to assess the supervisory alliance
- Supervisory Relationship Measure (Pearce et al., 2013) assesses the supervisor's perspectives of the supervisory relationship
- Supervisory Styles Inventory (Friedlander & Ward, 1984) is completed by the supervisor and supervisee to assess and evaluate the match of supervisor's

distinctive manner of approaching and responding to trainees and of implementing supervision

Best Practice Guidelines for Distance Supervision

Barton et al. (2016), in their Technology-Based Clinical Supervision Guidelines, provide an overview of distance supervision research and recommendations for licensure boards that exist. While this document was intended as a rationale for distance supervision in substance use disorder work, it provides a sound set of guidelines that can be adapted across licensure boards or used as a set of guidelines for those considering engaging in distance supervision. These guidelines, according to Barton et al. (2016, p. 5) for technology-based clinical supervision (TBCS), should include:

- Develop clinical supervisor's TBCS knowledge and skills through evidence-informed training
- Integrate training on TBCS into clinical supervision training curricula
- Develop processes through which clinical supervisors can determine the appropriateness of TBCS for supervisees and their patients
- Demonstrate competency with the technologies selected for conducting clinical supervision
- Demonstrate knowledge and practices that adhere to privacy/security and confidentiality
- Protections related to conducting clinical supervision using technologies
- Ensure adherence to ethical guidelines and relevant laws and codes specific to supervision of clinical services using technologies
- Develop written agreements with supervisees that include parameters and structure for TBCS.
- Implement clinical practices that include informing patients verbally and in writing about clinical supervision services being delivered through technology platforms

In many cases, professional associations have not created specific guidelines related to distance supervision. However, all have ethical codes related to distance counseling, which can be adapted for use in distance supervision. Some associations also have standards of practice and practice guidelines that specifically mention technology in supervision. For counselors, the AMHCA Standards for the Practice of Clinical Mental Health Counseling (AMHCA, 2021) provide guidelines related to Technology Supported Counseling and Communications (TSCC). Also, NBCC's Policy Regarding the Provision of Distance Professional Services (NBCC, 2016b) provides specific guidelines related to all distance services. Psychologists can refer to the Guidelines for the Practice of Telepsychology (APA, 2013). For social workers, one can refer to Technology in Social Work Practice (NASW/ASWB/SCWE/CSWA, 2017) for guidelines on distance services. Play therapists can look to APT for distance supervision guidelines (APT, 2020; Dugan et al., 2020). The American Telemedicine Association provides a comprehensive set of practice guidelines for distance mental health services (Turvey et al., 2013). Finally, other useful resources include the text Technology in Mental Health: Applications in Practice, Supervision, and Training (Goss et al., 2016) and Martin et al.'s (2017) article Effective Use of Technology in Clinical Supervision.

Bringing It All together

From the information presented in this chapter, it is obvious that distance supervision in play therapy has benefits and limitations. Additionally, distance supervision in play therapy is guided by multiple ethical codes and practice guidelines and requires specific knowledge and training. The complexities in distance supervision, related to competency and confidentiality (which includes security and privacy), can be overwhelming. However, if planned well, distance supervision can become a routine part of a supervisor's practice. Part of the planning requires delineating the responsibilities of the supervisor, supervisee, and those shared by both. Below, is a list of responsibilities that incorporate established supervision practice guidelines with added guidelines related to distance play therapy supervision.

Responsibilities of Supervisor

- In some cases, the supervisor solely supervises the training, utilization, and application of play therapy skills and techniques
- The supervisor will follow the ethical guidelines set forth by the state in which they live, their professional associations, and any other applicable professional bodies
- The supervisor will have, maintain, and provide proof of liability insurance
- The supervisor will have adequate training in supervision and be certified, registered, and/or licensed to provide such supervision. The supervisor must be able to provide proof of their training and credentials if requested
- The supervisor will be available, within reason, to provide the negotiated supervision. The supervisor must provide supervisee(s) with contact information where they may be reached
- The supervisor will provide timely feedback to supervisee(s) through phone, emails, and/or written reports
- The supervisor will return all materials submitted by the supervisee(s) such as videotapes, reports, art products, and/or sandtray photos to the supervisee(s) after review. The supervisor must properly store these materials until they have been returned to supervisee(s)
- The supervisor will maintain a copy of the record/log of dates and hours of supervision given to supervisee(s). This record will also include a copy of any form of written feedback that is offered to supervisee(s)
- The supervisor will periodically review the supervision file of supervisee(s) to ensure they are on track for certification, registration, and/or licensure

- The supervisor will immediately contact supervisee(s) if they believe that the contents of a session indicate an obligation to make a report to any authorities

Responsibilities of Supervisee

- The supervisee must be eligible to provide mental health services as delineated under their state mental health professional code(s) as independent or supervised practitioners working toward a mental health license
- A supervisee that is not licensed to practice independently and working toward licensure will provide documentation of their immediate supervisor's (site supervisor's) awareness of and permission for, receiving supervision of play therapy experience
- The supervisee will obtain the appropriate consents (both client/guardian and site of practice) before discussing, recording, and sending any case-sensitive information. All identifying information must be removed from all case-related material to safeguard client confidentiality. Recorded sessions will contain only the supervisee's name and the date of the session
- The supervisee will follow the ethical guidelines set forth by the state in which they live, their professional associations, and any other applicable professional bodies
- The supervisee will attend all scheduled supervision sessions. The supervisee and supervisor may mutually negotiate a make-up of missed hours and any additional hours of supervision that may be requested
- The supervisee will have, maintain, and provide proof of liability insurance
- The supervisee is required to maintain a record/log of dates and hours of supervision received. The record will also include a copy of any form of written feedback that the supervisor offers
- The supervisee is responsible for keeping and/or destruction of materials submitted for supervision, then returned by the supervisor
- The supervisee is encouraged to seek psychotherapy if personal issues arise that cannot be resolved within the supervision relationship
- The supervisee will contact the supervisor immediately and inform him of any grievances, sanctions, or lawsuits filed against the supervisee

In addition to the supervisor and supervisee responsibilities listed above, other responsibilities exist when engaging in distance supervision.

Responsibilities of Supervisor When Providing Distance Supervision

- Supervisor qualifications with technological competency
- Knowing what technology and platforms are suited for distance supervision
- Determining who is a good candidate for distance supervision
- Informed consent
- Documentation of supervision and security of the supervisory record
- Confidentiality and security of information discussed during supervision

Responsibilities of Supervisee in Distance Supervision

- Choosing a competent supervisor (one that has appropriate training is distance supervision)
- Being trained and competent in using the chosen technological platform
- Documentation of supervision
- Confidentiality and security of information discussed during supervision
- Acknowledging, through informed consent with clients, the risks, and limitations of the supervisee's distance supervision

Responsibilities Shared by Supervisor and Supervisee in Distance Supervision

- Supervisors must have written procedures for determining the identity of the supervisee and vice versa for the supervisee of the supervisor
- The supervisor and supervisee should determine, before beginning distance supervision, a backup means of communication should there be technical issues with the primary means of communication
- The supervisor and supervisee should discuss appropriate locations to engage in distance supervision (e.g., a work or home office rather than a communal conference room or coffee shop)
- Supervisors and supervisees should discuss appropriate hardware for supervision. A desktop computer or laptop would be the most appropriate, whereas a mobile device such as a smartphone would be less appropriate. Regardless of the hardware chosen, the supervisor and the supervisee must make sure that (a) the device's operating system is up-to-date, (b) usernames and passwords are not shared, (c) when using wireless and wired Internet access, there are firewalls in place to prevent unauthorized access to the supervisor and supervisee's network, and (d) the platform for distance supervision is encrypted and meets HIPPA, HITECH, and FERPA security guidelines
- When recording client sessions for observation during supervision, the device utilized to record should not be a wireless device (e.g., smartphone or tablet)

Conclusion

This chapter provides several guidelines and resources that can help those new to distance play therapy supervision find their footing. Distance play therapy supervision provides supervisees with opportunities that they would not normally have. Via technology, supervisees can have access to supervisors with a range of experiences across numerous populations. The technology aspect of distance play therapy supervision can be daunting; however, with training, planning, and practice, concerns can be managed. As supervisees benefit from these new opportunities, so will their clients.

References

Abbass, A., Arthey, S., Elliott, J., Fedak, T., Nowoweiski, D., Markovski, J., & Nowoweiski, S. (2011). Web-conference supervision for advanced psychotherapy training: A practical guide. *Psychotherapy*, *48*(2), 109–118. https://doi.org/10.1037/a0022427

Altvater, R. A., Singer, R. R., & Gil, E. (2017). Part 1: Modern trends in the playroom—Preferences and interactions with tradition and innovation. *International Journal of Play Therapy*, *26*(4), 239–249. https://doi.org/10.1037/pla0000058

Altvater, R. A., Singer, R. R., & Gil, E. (2018). Part 2: A qualitative examination of play therapy and technology training and ethics. *International Journal of Play Therapy*, *27*(1), 46–55. https://doi.org/10.1037/pla0000057

American Academy of Child & Adolescent Psychiatry. (2014). *Code of ethics*. https://www.aacap.org/App_Themes/AACAP/docs/about_us/transparency_portal/aacap_code_of_ethics_2012.pdf

American Art Therapy Association. (2013). *Ethical principles for art therapists*. https://arttherapy.org/wp-content/uploads/2017/06/Ethical-Principles-for-Art-Therapists.pdf

American Association for Marriage and Family Therapy. (2015). *Code of ethics*. https://www.aamft.org/Legal_Ethics/Code_of_Ethics.aspx

American Counseling Association. (2014). *2014 ACA code of ethics*. https://www.counseling.org/Resources/aca-code-of-ethics.pdf

American Mental Health Counselors Association. (2020). *Code of ethics* (Revised 2015, 2020). https://www.amhca.org/HigherLogic/System/DownloadDocumentFile.ashx?DocumentFileKey=24a27502-196e-b763-ff57-490a12f7edb1&forceDialog=0

American Mental Health Counselors Association. (2021). *AMHCA standards for the practice of clinical mental health counseling*. https://www.amhca.org/HigherLogic/System/DownloadDocumentFile.ashx?DocumentFileKey=cea86111-9bdb-984a-c14f-8528a3b3d83f&forceDialog=0

American Psychological Association. (2013). Guidelines for the practice of telepsychology. *American Psychologist*, *68*(9), 791–800. https://www.apa.org/pubs/journals/features/amp-a0035001.pdf

American Psychological Association. (2017). *Ethical principles of psychologists and code of conduct* (2002, amended effective June 1, 2010, and January 1, 2017). https://www.apa.org/ethics/code/ethics-code-2017.pdf

American School Counselors Association. (2016). *ASCA ethical standards for school counselors* (1984, revised 1992, 1998, 2004, 2010, and 2016). https://www.schoolcounselor.org/getmedia/f041cbd0-7004-47a5-ba01-3a5d657c6743/Ethical-Standards.pdf

Association for Play Therapy. (2020). *Play therapy best practices: Clinical, professional, & ethical issues*. https://cdn.ymaws.com/www.a4pt.org/resource/resmgr/publications/apt_best_practices_-_june_20.pdf

Autry, L. L. (2017). Creativity in play therapy using technology. In E. S. Leggett & J. N. Boswell (Eds.), *Directive play therapy: Theories and techniques* (pp. 163–183). Springer Publishing Company.

Bahrick, A. S. (1990). Role induction for counselor trainees: Effects on the supervisory working alliance. *Dissertation Abstracts International*, *51*, 1484–1484 (Abstract No. 1991-51645).

Barton, T., Roget, N., & Hartje, J. (2016). *Technology-based clinical supervision: Guidelines for licensing and certification boards*. National Frontier and Rural Addiction Technology

Transfer Center, University of Nevada, Reno. https://indd.adobe.com/view/9057ec2d
-94b1-4619-b1d0-a8a272b61e11

Bernard, J. M. (1997). The discrimination model. In C. E. Watkins, Jr. (Ed.), *Handbook of psychotherapy supervision* (pp. 310–327). John Wiley & Sons, Inc.

Bernhard, P. A., & Camins, J. S. (2020, May). Supervision from afar: Trainees' perspectives on telesupervision. *Counseling Psychology Quarterly*, 1–10. https://doi.org/10.1080 /09515070.2020.1770697

Butler, S. K., & Constantine, M. G. (2006). Web-based peer supervision, collective self-esteem, and case conceptualization ability in school counselor trainees. *Professional School Counseling, 10*(2), 146–152. https://doi.org/10.1177/2156759X0601000205

Chapman, R. A., Bake, S. B., Nassar-McMillan, S. C., & Gerler, E. R. (2011). Cybersupervision: Further examinations of synchronous and asynchronous modalities in counseling practicum supervision. *Counselor Education and Supervision, 50*(5), 298–313. https://doi.org/10.1002/j.1556-6978.2011.tb01917.x

Davis, P. S., & Hudspeth, E. F. (2014). Web-based play therapy supervision: Why, what, how, and who. *Play Therapy, 9*(4), 6–10.

Dawson, L., Harpster, A., Hoffman, G., & Phelan, K. (2011). A new approach to distance counseling skill development: Applying a discrimination model of supervision. *Vistas* (Article 46). https://www.counseling.org/docs/default-source/vistas/vistas_2011 _article_46.pdf?sfvrsn=8faf7ec1_11

Deane, F. P., Gonsalvez, C., Blackman, R. J., Saffioti, D., & Andresen, R. (2015). Issues in the development of e-supervision in professional psychology: A review. *Australian Psychologist, 50*(3), 241–247. https://core.ac.uk/download/pdf/37028789.pdf

Dubi, M., Raggi, M., & Reynolds, J. (2012). Distance supervision: The PIDIB model. *Vistas* (Article 82). https://www.counseling.org/docs/default-source/vistas/vistas_2012 _article_82.pdf

Dudding, C. C., & Justice, L. M. (2004). An e-supervision model: Videoconferencing as a clinical training tool. *Communication Disorders Quarterly, 25*(3), 145–151. https://doi.org /10.1177/15257401040250030501

Dugan, E., Ray, D. C., & Kenney-Noziska, S. (2020). *Ethical considerations for implementing telemental health in play therapy: A reflective exercise for play therapists based on the Association for play therapy's best practice guidelines.* Association for Play Therapy. https://cdn.ymaws.com /www.a4pt.org/resource/resmgr/telehealth/Dugan_Ray_SKN_-_Telemental_H.pdf

Efstation, J. F., Patton, M. J., & Kardash, C. M. (1990). Measuring the working alliance in counselor supervision. *Journal of Counseling Psychology, 37*(3), 322–329. https://doi.org /10.1037/0022-0167.37.3.322

Falender, C. A., Grus, C., McCutcheon, S., D., Goodyear, R., Ellis, M. V., Doll, B., & Kaslow, N. (2016). Guidelines for clinical supervision in health service psychology: Evidence and implementation strategies. *Psychotherapy Bulletin, 51*(3), 6–18. https://soc ietyforpsychotherapy.org/wp-content/uploads/2014/11/Bulletin51-3_OnlineVer.pdf

Fried, K. (2021). Online sand tray. *Oaklander Training.* https://onlinesandtray.com/

Friedlander, M. L., & Ward, L. G. (1984). Development and validation of the supervisory styles inventory. *Journal of Counseling Psychology, 31*(4), 541–557. https://doi.org/10.1037 /0022-0167.31.4.541

Gonsalvez, C. J., Hamid, G., Savage, N. M., & Livni, D. (2017). The supervision evaluation and supervisory competence scale: Psychometric validation. *Australian Psychologist, 52*(2), 94–103. https://doi.org/10.1111/ap.12269

Google. (n.d.). *Bringing learning to life with Jamboard.* https://edu.google.com/intl/ALL_us/ products/jamboard/

Goss, S., Anthony, K., Stretch, L. S., & Nagel, D. M. (2016). *Technology in mental health: Applications in practice, supervision, and training* (2nd ed.). Charles C. Thomas Publisher, Ltd.

Health Resources & Services Administration. (2021, January 28). *Telehealth licensing requirements and interstate compacts.* https://telehealth.hhs.gov/providers/policy-changes-during-the-covid-19-public-health-emergency/telehealth-licensing-requirements-and-interstate-compacts/

Hudspeth, E. F., & Davis, P. S. (2015). Ethical web-based play therapy supervision. *Play Therapy, 10*(2), 16–20.

Hudspeth, E. F., & Davis, P. S. (2016). Creating an informed consent and contract for web-based supervision. *Play Therapy, 11*(1), 12–17.

Hull, K. B. (2016). Technology in the playroom. In K. J. O'Connor, C. E. Schaefer, & L. D. Braverman (Eds.), *Handbook of play therapy* (pp. 613–627). John Wiley & Sons, Inc.

Jordan, S. E., & Shearer, E. M. (2019). An exploration of supervision delivered via clinical video telehealth (CVT). *Training and Education in Professional Psychology, 13*(4), 323–330. https://doi.org/10.1037/tep0000245

Kanz, J. E. (2001). Clinical-supervision.com: Issues in the provision of online supervision. *Professional Psychology: Research and Practice, 32*(4), 415–420. https://doi.org/10.1037/0735-7028.32.4.415

Kerl, S. B., Garcia, J. L., McCullough, S., & Maxwell, M. E. (2002). Systematic evaluation of professional performance: Legally supported procedure and process. *Counselor Education and Supervision, 41*(4), 321–334. https://doi.org/10.1002/j.1556-6978.2002.tb01294.x

Ladany, N., Hill, C. E., Corbett, M. M., & Nutt, E. A. (1996). Nature, extent, and importance of what psychotherapy trainees do not disclose to their supervisors. *Journal of Counseling Psychology, 43*(1), 10–24. https://doi.org/10.1037/0022-0167.43.1.10

Lamb, R., Etopio, E., & Lamb, R. E. (2018). Virtual reality in play therapy. *Play Therapy, 13*(1), 22–25.

Lambie, G. W., Mullen, P. R., Swank, J. M., & Blount, A. (2018). The counseling competencies scale: Validation and refinement. *Measurement and Evaluation in Counseling and Development, 51*(1), 1–15. https://doi.org/10.1080/07481756.2017.1358964

Lehrman-Waterman, D., & Ladany, N. (2001). Development and validation of the evaluation process within supervision inventory. *Journal of Counseling Psychology, 48*(2), 168–177. https://doi.org/10.1037/0022-0167.48.2.168

Lizzio, A., Wilson, K., & Que, J. (2009). Relationship dimensions in the professional supervision of psychology graduates: Supervisee perceptions of processes and outcome. *Studies in Continuing Education, 31*(2), 127–140. https://doi.org/10.1080/01580370902927451

Maheu, M. (2020). *HIPAA compliant video conferencing requirements after COVID.* https://telehealth.org/hipaa-compliant-video-conferencing-2/

Marino, R. C., Fazio-Griffith, L. J., Williams, J. M., David, J. C., & Esmaeili, A. N. (2015). The advanced use of technology to enhance personal and professional growth during the supervision process for graduate students in counselor education programs. *Vistas* (Article 3). https://www.counseling.org/docs/default-source/vistas/the-advanced-use-of-technology-to-enhance-personal-and-professional-growth-during-the-supervision-process-for-graduate-students-in-counselor-education-programs.pdf?sfvrsn=f6417f2c_8

Martin, P., Kumar, S., & Lizarondo, L. (2017). Effective use of technology in clinical supervision. *Internet Interventions, 8*, 35–39. https://doi.org/10.1016/j.invent.2017.03.001

McNary, T., Mason, E. C. M., & Tobin, G. (2018). The unexpected purpose of technology in the playroom: Catharsis. *Play Therapy*, *13*(3), 4–7.

Miller, T. W., Miller, J. M., Burton, D., Sprang, R., & Adams, J. (2003). Telehealth: A model for clinical supervision in allied health. *Internet Journal of Allied Health Sciences and Practice*, *1*(2), 1–8. https://nsuworks.nova.edu/cgi/viewcontent.cgi?article=1016&context=ijahsp

Munchel, B. F. (2015). *Exploratory study of counseling professionals' attitudes toward distance clinical supervision* [Dissertation, University of South Florida]. Graduate Theses and Dissertations. http://scholarcommons.usf.edu/etd/5997

Mural. (n.d.). *Free your teams imagination.* https://start.mural.co/free-forever?utm_medium =paid-search&utm_source=adwords&utm_campaign=sitelink-extensions-Get -MURAL-Free&utm_medium=paid-search&utm_source=adwords&utm_campaign =201020-Whiteboard&utm_adgroup=Online_Whiteboard&utm_campaign _id=11416478157&utm_content=collaborative%20drawing%20software&utm_ adgroupid=111145311265&gclid=CjwKCAiAh_GNBhAHEiwAjOh3ZIRm8IzRJO MOH5X90dZRZf5dkqYVwODmiPYh3nz8ojnYHq5mL7YSZxoCw54QAvD_BwE

NAADAC, The Association for Addiction Professionals. (2021). *NAADAC/NCC AP code of ethics.* NAADAC. https://www.naadac.org/assets/2416/naadac_code_of_ethics _112021.pdf

National Association for Social Workers (2021). *Code of ethics of the National Association of Social Workers.* https://www.socialworkers.org/About/Ethics/Code-of-Ethics/Code-of -Ethics-English

National Association for Social Workers, & Association of Social Work Boards. (2013). *Best practice standards in social work supervision.* National Association for Social Workers. https://www.socialworkers.org/LinkClick.aspx?fileticket=GBrLbl4BuwI%3D &portalid=0

National Board for Certified Counselors. (2016a). *Code of ethics.* https://www.nbcc.org/ Assets/Ethics/NBCCCodeofEthics.pdf

National Board for Certified Counselors. (2016b). *Policy regarding the provision of distance professional services.* https://www.nbcc.org/Assets/Ethics/NBCCPolicyRegardingPrac ticeofDistanceCounselingBoard.pdf

Nelson, T., & Johnson, L. (1999). The basic skills evaluation device. *Journal of Marital and Family Therapy*, *25*(1), 15–30. https://doi.org/10.1111/j.1752-0606.1999.tb01107.x

Palomo, M., Beinart, H., & Cooper, M. (2010). Development and validation of the supervisory relationship questionnaire (SRQ) in UK trainee clinical psychologists. *British Journal of Clinical Psychology*, *49*(Pt 2), 131–149. Https://doi.org/10.1348/014466509X4 41033

Pearce, N., Beinart, H., Clohessy, S., & Cooper, M. (2013). Development and validation of the supervisory relationship measure: A self-report questionnaire for use with supervisors. *British Journal of Clinical Psychology*, *52*(3), 249–268. https://doi.org/10.1111 /bjc.12012

Perry, C. W. (2012). Constructing professional identity in an online graduate clinical training program: Possibilities for online supervision. *Journal of Systemic Therapies*, *31*(3), 53–67. https://doi.org/10.1521/jsyt.2012.31.3.53

Raggi, M., Dubi, M., & Reynolds, J. W. (2008). The use of a pantheoretical case note format as a clinical tool. *New Jersey Journal of Professional Counseling*, *60*, 5–11.

Reese, R. J., Aldarondo, F., Anderson, C. R., Lee, S.-J., Miller, T. W., & Burton, D. (2009). Telehealth in clinical supervision: A comparison of supervision formats. *Journal of Telemedicine and Telecare*, *15*(7), 356–361. https://doi.org/10.1258/jtt.2009.090401

Renfro-Michel, E., Rousmaniere, T., & Spinella, L. (2016). Technological innovations in clinical supervision: Promises and challenges. In T. Rousmaniere & E. Renfro-Michel (Eds.), *Using technology to enhance clinical supervision* (pp. 3–18). American Counseling Association.

Rønnestad, M. H., & Lundquist, K. (2009). *The brief supervisory alliance scale*. Unpublished manuscript, Department of Psychology, Oslo, Norway.

Rousmaniere, T. (2014). Using technology to enhance clinical supervision and training. In C. E. Watkins & D. Milne (Eds.), *International handbook of clinical supervision* (pp. 204–237). Wiley.

Rousmaniere, T., Abbass, A., & Frederickson, J. (2014). New developments in technology-assisted supervision and training: A practical overview. *Journal of Clinical Psychology, 70*(11), 1082–1093. https://doi.org/10.1002/jclp.22129

Rousmaniere, T. G., & Ellis, M. V. (2013). Developing the construct and measure of collaborative clinical supervision: The supervisee's perspective. *Training and Education in Professional Psychology, 7*(4), 300–308. https://doi.org/10.1037/a0033796

Schacht, A. J., Howe, H. E., & Berman, J. J. (1988). A short form of the Barrett-Lennard Relationship Inventory for Supervisory Relationships. *Psychological Reports, 63*(3), 699–706. https://doi.org/10.2466/pr0.1988.63.3.699

Shaffer, K. S., & Friedlander, M. L. (2015). What do "interpersonally sensitive" supervisors do and how do supervisees experience a relational approach to supervision? *Psychotherapy Research, 27*(2), 167–178. https://doi.org/10.1080/10503307.2015.1080877

Shanfield, S. B., Mohl, P. C., Matthews, K., & Hetherly, V. (1989). A reliability assessment of the psychotherapy supervisory inventory. *American Journal of Psychiatry, 146*(11), 1447–1450. https://doi.org/10.1176/ajp.146.11.1447

Smith, T. R., Younes, L. K., & Lichtenberg, J. W. (2002, August). Examining the working alliance in supervisory relationships: The development of the working alliance inventory of supervisory relationships. Paper presented at the meeting of the American Psychological Association, Chicago, IL.

Snow, M. S., Winburn, A., Crumrine, L., Jackson, E., & Killian, T. (2012). The iPad playroom: A therapeutic technique. *Play Therapy, 7*, 16–19.

National Association of Social Workers, Association of Social Work Boards, Council on Social Work Education, & Clinical Social Work Associations. (2017). *NASW, ASWB, SCWE, & CSWA Standards for technology in social work practice*. National Association of Social Workers. https://www.socialworkers.org/LinkClick.aspx?fileticket=lcTcdsHUcng%3D&portalid=0

Sørlie, T., Gammon, D., Bergvik, S., & Sexton, H. (1999). Psychotherapy supervision face-to-face and by videoconferencing: A comparative study. *British Journal of Psychotherapy, 15*(4), 452–462. https://doi.org/10.1111/j.1752-0118.1999.tb00475.x

Stauffer, S. D. (2018). Technology in play therapy: A collegial debate between seven veteran play therapist. *Play Therapy, 13*(3), 20–23.

Stoltenberg, C., McNeill, B., & Delworth, U. (1998). *IDM supervision*. Jossey-Bass Inc.

Stone, J. (2020). *Digital play therapy: A clinician's guide to comfort and competence*. Routledge.

Storm, C., York, C., Vincent, R., McDowell, T., & Lewis, R. (1997). The postgraduate competency document (PGCD). The reasonably complete systemic supervisor resource guide, 195–202.

Storm, C. L., Todd, T. C., Sprenkle, D. H., & Morgan, M. M. (2001). Gaps between MFT supervision assumptions and common practice: Suggested best practices. *Journal of Marital and Family Therapy, 27*(2), 227–239. https://doi.org/10.1111/j.1752-0606.2001.tb01159.x

Tarlow, K. R., McCord, C. E., Nelon, J. L., & Bernhard, P. A. (2020). Comparing in-person supervision and telesupervision: A multiple baseline single-case study. *Journal of Psychotherapy Integration, 30*(2), 383–393. https://doi.org/10.1037/int0000210

Telehealth Certification Institute. (2021). *States' rules and regulations*. https://www.telemen talhealthtraining.com/states-rules-and-regulations

Telemental Health Comparisons. (2020). *Telemental health software comparisons*. https://tel ementalhealthcomparisons.com/

Turvey, C., Coleman, M., Dennison, O., Drude, K., Goldenson, M., Hirsch, P., Jueneman, R., Kramer, G. M., Luxton, D. D., Maheu, M. M., Malik, T. S., Mishkind, M. C., Rabinowitz, T., Roberts, L. J., Sheeran, T., Shore, J. H., Shore, P., van Heeswyk, F., Wregglesworth, B., ... Bernard, J. (2013). ATA practice guidelines for video-based online mental health services. *Telemedicine Journal and e-Health, 19*(9), 722–730. https://doi.org/10.1089/tmj.2013.9989

U.S. Department of Education. (2021, August 21). *Part 99-Family educational and rights of privacy*. http://www.ecfr.gov/cgi-bin/text-idx?rgn=div5&node=34:1.1.1.1.33

U.S. Department of Health and Human Services. (2013). Omnibus HIPAA rulemaking. *Federal Register, 78*(17), 5566–5702. http://www.gpo.gov/fdsys/pkg/FR-2013-01-25/pdf/2013-01073.pdf

U.S. Department of Health and Human Services. (2021, May 17). *HIPAA administrative simplification statute and rules*. http://www.hhs.gov/ocr/privacy/hipaa/administrative/index.html

Villarreal-Davis, C., Sartor, T. A., & McLean, L. (2021). Using creativity to foster connection in online counseling supervision. *Journal of Creativity in Mental Health, 16*(2), 244–257. https://doi.org/10.1080/15401383.2020.1754989

Woo, H., Bang, N. M., Lee, J., & Berghuis, K. (2020). A meta-analysis of the counseling literature on technology-assisted distance supervision. *International Journal for the Advancement Counselling, 42*(4), 424–438. https://doi.org/10.1007/s10447-020-09410-0

Zeng, H., Cooper, B., & Heher, M. (2020, October). Expressive and experiential arts in online group supervision. *NBCC Visions, 35*(10). https://nbcc.org/resources/nccs/newsletter/expressive-and-experiential-arts-in-online-group-supervision

10 School-Based Play Therapy Supervision

Amanda Winburn and Kenya G. Bledsoe

School-Based Play Therapy Supervision

Clinical supervision plays a significant role in the play therapy profession. Understanding and exploring the supervisory process can foster the development of play therapists in general and, as an emerging subfield, school-based play therapy. This process will ultimately result in better mental health services for all school-aged children. This chapter will review the specific supervision needs and considerations of school-based play therapy supervision. A brief overview of mental health services within K-12, school-based play therapy, and issues related to supervision in school-based play therapy will be discussed.

Mental Health Services in Schools

At the onset of the 20th century, the United States transitioned from a rural to an industrialized society and found itself at an educational crossroads (Brewer, 1942; Lambie & Williamson, 2004). During the early 1900s, Jesse B. Davis and Frank Parsons, the "Fathers of Guidance," were major counseling influences in these formative years (Brewer, 1942). The 1940s and 1950s saw an increased movement toward developing counseling services in schools (Schmidt, 2014). Rogers' client-centered therapy approach to counseling was instrumental in establishing school-based counselors as mental health professionals. This approach prompted mental health professionals to revisit their counseling philosophies and incorporate a holistic view of the relationship between themselves and their students (Granello & Young, 2012).

Following these shifts in thought, the federal and state legislation also paved the way for transitions in mental health services for K-12 students. For example, the Education for All Handicapped Children Act of 1975 (PL 94-142), which mandated free public education for all students, including exceptional children, expanded school counselors' roles as consultants offering counseling-related services such as parent counseling, program planning, and curriculum monitoring (House & Hayes, 2002; Schmidt, 2002). Additionally, recognized publications such as "A Nation at Risk: The Imperatives for Reform" (The National Commission of Excellence in Education, 1983) highlighted the declining achievement of students

DOI: 10.4324/9781003196075-13

across the United States, prompting the need for educational standards and accountability (Johnson, 2002). This publication incited a similar level of concern as the launching of the Russian satellite, Sputnik, resulting in an increase in accountability across the school community. As a result, students services were increasingly required to assess how they spent their time, how they are delivered, and the impact their programming efforts had on students' outcomes (Gysbers, 2010; Lambie & Williamson, 2004).

Play Therapy in Schools

According to the US Department of Education (2005), school-based therapists should have a comprehensive knowledge and understanding of recognisable barriers to equal educational opportunities for students. These early interventions are critical to a child's success, and school-based play therapists have the clinical skills needed to play an integral part in identifying children's needs and assisting teachers with supporting student development. Professionals trained in play therapy can use the modality to intervene with students at risk of failure. These school-based play therapy interventions can be employed individually or in a small-group setting. For example, school-based play therapy interventions can be instrumental in supporting social emotional learning within a comprehensive school counseling program.

Group-centered play therapy is one approach for school-based play therapists to use when combining group-centered interventions and play therapy for tiered interventions within a multi-tiered support system (MTSS) (Harpine, 2008). MTSS is a process of implementing high-quality evidence-based practices that are identified based upon the students needs, progress, and then making adjustments based upon that student's outcomes. Play-based group interventions can effectively work within an MTSS model to address deficiencies prohibiting students from reaching their full academic potential (Harpine, 2008). In small groups, students can work through behavior and emotional issues while increasing positive peer relationships. According to Swank et al. (2018), group-centered play therapy within schools demonstrates a high level of promise in reducing problem behaviors when compared to psychoeducational group interventions.

Understanding the child's needs is integral to utilizing an approach that encourages progress through play therapy interventions. In addition, this understanding helps the school-based play therapist measure outcomes inside the playroom and, with stakeholders' support, outside of therapy. Whether the behavioral challenges result from defiance, impulsivity, or poor peer relationships, the school-based therapist should consider the best approach for the student. For example, a nondirective approach may be considered if the focus is on using the therapeutic relationship to help students develop healthy communication and expression (Kottman, 2011). This may also be considered for students who have trouble with aggression and poor social skills. If the student needs more structure with attention to specific behavior goals as determined by an intervention plan, such as an Individual Education Plan (IEP), the school-based therapists may consider a directive approach necessary for success. Directive play therapy may be more efficient working within an IEP because tiered interventions are often time-limited and goal-oriented.

School-Based Play Therapy Supervision

Central to this chapter is the notion that supervision is crucial for the development and maintenance of therapeutic skills, professional identity, counselor self-efficacy, and multicultural cultural competence (Bernard & Goodyear, 2019; Bledsoe et al., 2021a; Borders & Brown, 2005; Cashwell & Dooley, 2001; Inman & Deboer, 2013; Tang, 2020). The same is true within the field of play therapy. Supervision is a necessary part of becoming an RPT™ or SB-RPT™ (APT, 2017; APT, 2014), and it is a topic that has received modest attention in the professional literature. This is especially true when we focus specifically on school-based play therapists. While each of the disciplines in which play therapists may have their foundational mental health training and license (e.g., School Counseling, School Psychology, Licensed Professional Counselor, Licensed Clinical Social Worker, and Licensed Marriage and Family Therapist) APT (2017) outlines a need for supervision in their own standards and ethical codes. The primary track for school-based play therapists originates from the school counseling or school psychology profession. Within the field of school counseling, post-master's degree clinical supervision is encouraged but is not mandated by The American School Counseling Association (ASCA, 2016). The ASCA Ethical Standards (2016), Section B.3.h., and ASCA's The School Counselor and School Counselor Supervision position statement (2021) instructs school counselors to seek supervision from school counselors and other professionals knowledgeable about counseling ethics.

Because of the challenges faced by novice counselors, Stickel and Trimmer (1994) suggested participation in some type of formalized reflection (i.e., supervision). This reflection would be utilized to increase self-efficacy concerning problem-solving, decision-making, and establishing skills for complex issues (McMahon & Patton, 2000). Clinical supervision, an intervention provided by a more experienced member of a profession to a more junior colleague or colleagues who typically (but not always) are members of that same profession (Bernard & Goodyear, 2019), has been suggested as a way to support the novice as they work through the challenges faced during the formative years of their career (Borders & Brown, 2005). Early career mental health professionals new to the field may benefit from skill development that extends beyond what they received in counseling training programs (McMahon & Patton, 2000).

Influence of CACREP

The Council for Accreditation of Counseling and Related Educational Programs Standards (CACREP) is the premier specialty accreditation body for counseling programs in the United States and abroad, providing educational standards and competencies that ensure training, supervision experience, and coursework for counselors-in-training. CACREP is a counseling accreditation body that emerged as a significant aspect of counseling in 1981 in response to the American Counseling Association's (formerly the American Personnel and Guidance Association) task force to develop national standards for counseling accreditation (Granello & Young, 2012). CACREP (2016) requires that counselors-in-training receive weekly clinical supervision from site supervisors (i.e., school counselors) and university supervisors (i.e., counselor educators) during the practicum and the internship field placements (CACREP, 2016, Section 3, F, J; Neyland et al., 2019; Oberman & Studer, 2021).

In 2015, the Council on Rehabilitation Education merged with CACREP, making CACREP the exclusive accrediting body of counseling programs. Previously, the CORE accredited rehabilitation counseling programs and was separate from CACREP. These councils recognized the necessity of supervision as a counselor-in-training acquires the necessary skills to provide counseling services and made clinical supervision a mandatory feature of any CACREP accredited counseling program (CACREP, 2016).

Influence of ASCA

Since the primary source of school-based play therapy originates from the field of school counseling, it is relevant to this chapter to better understand the influence of the primary professional association governing the school counseling profession. As part of its mission to advance the school counseling profession, ASCA has published a variety of documents to guide its members, including the ASCA National Model (2019), ASCA Ethical Standards for School Counselors (2016), and The School Counselor and School Counselor Supervision Position Statement (2021). The ASCA National Model *(2019)* recommends that school counselors seek consultation and supervision to guide and support ethical decision-making, incorporate reflection to enhance professional development and growth, and receive in-service instruction and supervision (ASCA, 2019).

The ASCA Ethical Standards for School Counselors (2016) is created to guide the ethical decision-making practices of school counselors, counseling educators, and supervisors/directors of school counseling programs (ASCA, 2016). For this chapter, section B of the ASCA Ethical Standards *(2016)* is the most pertinent section for school-based play therapists originating from a school counseling background. More specifically, attention is given to Section B.3.h. which states, "seek consultation and supervision from school counselors and other professionals who are knowledgeable of the school counselor ethical practices when ethical and professional questions arise" (ASCA, 2016, p. 7). More recently, ASCA published The School Counselor and School Counselor Supervision Position Statement encouraging novice school counselors to participate in counseling supervision (ASCA, 2021).

Influence of the APT

The Association for Play Therapy (APT) established guidelines for mental health professionals seeking to become credentialed as a registered play therapist or school-based play therapist. APT currently offers three different types of credentials: Registered Play Therapist™ (RPT™), School Based-Registered Play Therapist™ (SB-RPT™), and Registered Play Therapist-Supervisor™ (RPT-S™). Credentialing works through a three-phased approach and is fully outlined on their website. These phases outline credentialing criteria in curriculum instruction, clinical experience, and supervision. The criteria for seeking SB-RPT™ does vary slightly from those seeking the RPT™ credential. Future SB-RPTs™ require additional supervision hours along with additional clinical experience. For example, RPTs™ must participate in no less than 35 hours of supervision during their training, while SB-RPTs™ must participate in no less than 50 (Association for Play Therapy, 2019). The clock to work through Phases 1 to 3, which includes curriculum instruction, experience, and supervision, can be no less than 24 months.

Types of Supervision

Graduate Supervision

SB-RPTs™ may or may not have graduated from a CACREP accredited program, therefore it is difficult to assume what type of graduate supervision an individual may or may not have received. For those graduating from a CACREP accredited institution, we can be more certain because CACREP requires extensive clinical supervision of counselors-in-training during graduate programs (CACREP, 2016; Oberman & Studer, 2021). During graduate training, school counselors receive university faculty supervision, along with site supervisors during their practicum and internship experiences. However, after graduation, clinical supervision is often lacking or replaced by administrative supervision once the novice school counselor is employed in their first position as a professional school counselor (Merlin-Knoblich et al., 2018; Moyer, 2011).

For SB-RPTs™ seeking credentialing, APT has established guidelines for the development of clinical skills. APT requires that all SB-RPTs™ in training be supervised by an RPT-S™ for a period of no less than one school year and earn a minimum of 600 direct student-contact hours utilizing play therapy. Additionally, the supervisee should participate in 50 hours of simultaneous play therapy supervision (Association for Play Therapy, 2019). After graduation, additional clinical supervision is not required for license renewal; however, SB-RPTs™ are required to earn continuing education hours for renewal every 36 months. For novice SB-RPTs™ (much like novice school counselors), supervision may be conducted by administrative or program supervisor.

Administrative or Program Supervision

Administrative supervision is different for a registered school-based play therapists employed by a school district compared to a registered play therapist who is in private practice or works for a mental health agency. Within the typical school district (public or private), administrative supervision is readily available and is usually provided by a school administrator (Sutton & Page, 1994). Administrative supervision is designed to benefit the organization as a place of education, not the clinical development of the supervisee (Perera-Diltz & Mason, 2012). While administrative supervision is accessible with an emphasis on compliance and accountability by a school administrator, this supervision is not specific to clinical skills and the administrator does not typically have a mental health background (Sutton & Page, 1994).

Program supervision is another form of readily available supervision and is usually provided by a program coordinator at the district level, assigned to supervise the school-based therapists. Similar to administrative supervision, program supervision is designed to benefit the organization, not the clinical development of the therapists (Perera-Diltz & Mason, 2012). Program supervision does not support or deepen the therapeutic skills of the novice school-based therapist. Administrative and programmatic supervision does not adequately address the professional development needs of novice mental health therapists.

Clinical Supervision

Within the professional literature, clinical supervision is described as an intervention provided by a more experienced member of the profession to a more junior member to enhance professional services offered to clients (Bernard & Goodyear, 2019). When examining supervision through the modality of play therapy, a founding theorist such as Landreth (2012) argues that play therapists should be playful. Mullen et al. (2007) believe that play therapy supervision should include playful components and experiential strategies to support clinical skills and philosophies, model play therapy interventions, and build the supervisees' professional identity. As play therapists, we know that play is a form of communication regardless of age or developmental level. While supervision is serious and fundamental to professional growth, there is room within the relationship to incorporate the key elements of the field, play and playfulness.

Notably, existing literature on play therapy supervision remains limited, mainly conceptual, and more often geared toward novice play therapists (Donald et al., 2015; Hudspeth, 2015; VanderGast et al., 2010). However, there is almost a complete absence of research into clinical supervision experiences of school-based play therapists and how clinical supervision is experienced in a school setting. Additionally, within this diverse application of supervision, many play therapy supervisors are not formally trained within the school setting and rely solely on experience in practice (Falender, 2018). Knowing this, future research in supervision within play therapy must include the school-based play therapist in order to increase understanding of their experiences and professional development.

Ethical and Multicultural Considerations

During the supervision process, it is not uncommon for ethical dilemmas and obstacles to appear. Ensuring that supervision is applied in an ethical, competent, and legal manner is vital to the development of competent mental health professionals (Association for Counselor Education & Supervision, 2011; Herlily et al., 2002). While the Association for Play Therapy outlines in their ethical codes the need for supervision to be grounded in theory for it to be considered competent (2016), they also outline best practices that include ethical and multicultural considerations.

Obstacles to School-Based Supervision

A shortage of trained supervisors is one of many explanations why counselors-in-training receive limited or inadequate supervision (Dollarhide & Miller, 2006). Additionally, a lack of time, financial support, and release-time from school are also obstacles to clinical supervision (Bledsoe et al., 2021b; Perera-Diltz & Mason, 2012). In some instances, access plays a significant role, play therapists who work in rural areas and may simply not have access to a supervisor for clinical supervision (Donald et al., 2015; Ray, 2004).

Professionals transitioning from school counseling to school-based play therapy understand the challenges of seeking post-master's supervision. Ironically, ongoing counseling supervision is encouraged for school-based counselors but not mandated by the ASCA Ethical Standards (2016). The American School Counselor Association's Ethical Standards (2016) instructs school counselors to seek supervision from school counselors and other professionals knowledgeable about counseling ethics when problems emerge (see Section B.3.h.). Supervision is a requirement to become a school-based play therapist; however, if these professionals come from a school setting where clinical supervision is already in short supply, ongoing supervision and support of these early professionals could be even more challenging to access and maintain.

Role stress

Managing large student caseloads in K-12, all while working in isolation or with limited supervision, can be difficult even for the most experienced counselors. This stress is exacerbated for the professionally inexperienced. Rønnestad and Skovholt (2003) suggested that novice therapists' "professional innocence" is most visible when interacting with clients for the first time (p. 46). If role stress is not managed appropriately, it can cause novice professionals is to become overwhelmed early in their careers and lead to performance fatigue, job dissatisfaction, and burnout (Mullen et al., 2017). Additionally, role stress can lead to performance anxiety and self-doubt, two potentially harmful effects on establishing therapeutic relationships (Theriault et al., 2009). According to Randick et al. (2019), training programs should increase wellness-enhancing skills such as taking leadership roles or peer supervision. Additional opportunities for supervision can help support early professions and provide tools necessary for navigating job stress and reduce the likelihood of burnout and low job satisfaction.

Benefits of Supervision

Supervision is a vital component to the future growth and development of SB-RPTs™. Benefits of clinical supervision include professional identity development, self-efficacy, and counselor wellness (Cashwell & Dooley, 2001; Cinotti & Springer, 2016; Crutchfield & Borders, 1997; Dollarhide & Miller, 2006; Herlihy et al., 2002). Not only is supervision beneficial for the supervisee, but also for the student, student development, and student outcomes (Cook et al., 2012).

Professional Identity Development

Professional identity development extends beyond graduating and obtaining licensure and credentialing and encompasses the beliefs, values, traditions, and roles of therapy (Granello & Young, 2012). Clinical supervision provides that missing link to the profession, enabling novice and seasoned professionals to continue clarifying their professional identity and working with administrators and supervisors to redefine their roles within their school setting (Herlihy et al., 2002; Luke & Bernard, 2006). Previous studies have focused on the professional identity of mental health professionals working with children and adolescents. For example, Sutton and Fall's (1995) study revealed that professional identity was impacted by the appropriateness of job responsibilities assigned to the school counselor that aligned with comprehensive models such as the ASCA National Model (2012). Thus, significant efforts have altered school counselor professional identity from an educator with a vocational checklist to a clearly defined mental health professional delivering data-driven, results-oriented counseling programs for school-aged children (Lambie & Williamson, 2004; Schmidt, 2014). Obtaining professional identity development via clinical supervision can help offset role ambiguity (Bledsoe et al., 2021; Granello & Young, 2012). This is especially true for school counselors, who have now been credentialed as registered school-based play therapists. This specialization deepens their knowledge base in play therapy skills, theories, and interventions. Continued supervision and support allow that identification and specialization to continue to grow and solidify.

Self-efficacy

Self-efficacy is the amount of perceived confidence as a result of skill development and the practice of those skill sets (Bandura, 1977, 1982). Confidence in one's abilities as a mental health professional is critical for personal fulfillment, quality job performance, and effective support and services provided to the student. Therefore, with an increase in skills provided by clinical supervision, there is the added benefit of self-efficacy (i.e., practitioners internalize their skill set and become confident in their abilities) to address the myriad of clients' presenting issues (Cashwell & Dooley, 2001). Additionally, increased self-efficacy leads to higher self-concepts, minimal state and trait anxiety, and an increased perception of problem-solving abilities, further proving that clinical supervision enhances positive efficacy for counseling practitioners and counselors-in-training.

The value of clinical supervision and its impact on self-efficacy, therapeutic effectiveness, and confidence has been embedded within the literature (Boyd & Walter, 1975; Cinotti & Springer, 2016; Cook et al., 2012). Supervision yields positive results related to increased effectiveness and accountability, enhanced counseling skills, support for professional development, and boosted self-confidence and job comfort (Benshoff & Paisley, 1996; Bledsoe et al., 2021; Crutchfield & Borders, 1997). Stickel and Trimmer (1994) suggested that novice professionals that participated in some type of formalized reflection (i.e., supervision) increase self-efficacy surrounding problem-solving, decision-making, and establishing skills for handling complex issues. Finally, as Cashwell and Dooley (2001) noted, the ultimate measure of a therapist is confidence in their abilities, which can be positively impacted by clinical supervision. In this way, clinical supervision may assist novice school-based play therapists establish a strong professional identity, the techniques and skills to provide outstanding client care, and the courage to do so.

Wellness and Self-Care

Wellness is "a way of life oriented towards optimal health and well-being in which the individual integrates body, mind, and spirit to live more fully (Myers, Sweeney, & Witmer, 2000, p. 252). It is not uncommon for novice counselors or therapists to feel overwhelmed and experience stress early in their professional careers due largely to lack of confidence in their skill sets and their inability to regulate and express emotions adequately (Orlinsky et al., 2001; Skovholt & Rønnestad, 2003). Unfortunately, novice professionals do not always recognize the value of taking care of themselves to adequately care for their clients, leading to burnout and compassion fatigue (Moyer, 2011; Young & Lambie, 2007).

Scholars have reported that a lack of supervision in combination with difficult and stressful caseloads (McCarthy et al., 2010) increased the demands on school-based therapists and impacted their overall wellness (Lawson, 2007; Young & Lambie, 2007). Therefore, it is important for individuals to take good care of themselves, and engage in clinical supervision which can provide an avenue that permits therapists to reflect and discuss personal concerns that are essential to wellness (McMahon & Patton, 2000). Studies have shown that ongoing clinical supervision can increase counseling skills and offset stress levels, fatigue, and lack of confidence (Cashwell & Dooley, 2001; Crutchfield & Borders, 1997). Clinical supervision provides novice counselors with validation and normalization, both of which are desirable and helpful processes that foster wellness and self-care (Theriault et al., 2009). Potential strategies for supervisors while working with future SB-RPTs™ could include helping these individuals to develop wellness-enhancing changes and interventions within their setting and practice. Maintaining their training and support systems are also key factors to sustaining a high degree of overall wellness.

Conclusion

Supervision in play therapy is a specialized component in the training of future and novice play therapists. Supervisors and supervisees have certain responsibilities within the relationship that contribute to play therapist growth and professionalism and the efficacy of play therapy and services that the client/student receives. Unfortunately, when we evaluate the specific components of play therapy supervision, we know very little about school-based play therapy supervision. While APT has stressed the need for future research on play therapy supervision (Donald et al., 2015), that same call should be extended to look directly at the supervision of school-based therapists to evaluate if any experiences or needs vary between settings. Additional research in this area will help the field develop and provide supervision that supports the growth and development of future school-based play therapists that focus on the K-12 setting.

References

American School Counselor Association (2012). *The ASCA National Model: A framework for school counseling programs*. Alexandria, VA: Author.

American School Counselor Association. (2016). *Ethical standards for school counselors*. Author.

American School Counselor Association. (2019). *The ASCA national model: A framework for school counseling programs* (4th ed.). Author.

American School Counselor Association. (2021). The school counselor and school counseling supervision. https://www.schoolcounselor.org/Standards-Positions/Position-Statements/ASCA-Position-Statements/The-School-Counselor-and-School-Counselor-Supervis

Association for Counselor Education and Supervision. (2011). *Best practices in clinical supervision.* https://acesonline.net/wp-content/uploads/2018/11/ACES-Best-Practices-in-Clinical-Supervision-2011.pdf

Association for Play Therapy. (2014). Credentialing guide: Registered play therapist (RPT) and supervisor (RPT's). http://c.ymcdn.com/sites/www.a4pt.org/resource/resmgr/RPT_and_RPTS_Credentials/RPTS_Guide.pdf

Association for Play Therapy. (2017). *Credentialing guide: School based-registered play therapist (SB-RPT).* https://cdn.ymaws.com/www.a4pt.org/resource/resmgr/credentials/2020_credentials/sb-rpt_guide_master.pdf

Association for Play Therapy. (2019). *Credentialing standards for the registered play therapist: APT professional credentialing program.* https://cdn.ymaws.com/www.a4pt.org/resource/resmgr/credentials/RPT_Standards.pdf

Bandura, A. (1977). Self-efficacy: Toward a unifying theory of behavioral change. *Psychological Review, 84*(2), 191–215.

Bandura, A. (1982). Self-efficacy mechanism in human agency. *American Psychologists, 37*(2), 122–147.

Barzegary, L., & Zamini, S. (2011). The effect of play therapy on children with ADHD. *Procedia-Social and Behavioral Sciences, 30*, 2216–2218.

Benshoff, J. M., & Paisley, P. O. (1996). The structured peer consultation model for school counselors. *Journal of Counseling and Development, 74*(3), 314–318. https://doi.org/10.1002/j.1556-6676.1996.tb01872.x

Bernard, J. M., & Goodyear, R. (2019). *Fundamentals of clinical supervision* (6th ed.). Pearson.

Bledsoe, K. G., Burnham, J. J., Cook, R. M., Clark, M., & Webb, A. L. (2021a). A phenomenological study of early career school counselor clinical supervision experiences. *Professional School Counseling, 25*(1), 2156759X21997143.

Bledsoe, K. G., Burnham, J., Cook, R., Clark, M., & Webb, A. (2021b). Exploring the clinical supervision experiences of early career school counselors. *Professional School Counseling, 25*(1), 1–10. https://doi.org/10.1177/2156759X21007143

Bledsoe, K. G., Logan-McKibben, S., McKibben, B., & Cook, R. (2018). A content analysis of school counseling supervision. *Professional School Counseling, 22*(1), 1–8. https://doi.org/10.1177/2156759X19838454

Borders, L. D., & Brown, L. L. (2005). *The new handbook of counseling supervision.* Routledge.

Boyd, J. D., & Walter, P. B. (1975). The school counselor, the cactus, and supervision.

Brewer, J. M. (1942). *History of vocational guidance: Origins and early development.* Harper & Brothers.

Cashwell, T. H., & Dooley, K. (2001). The impact of supervision on counselor self-efficacy. *Clinical Supervisor, 20*(1), 39–47. https://doi.org/10.1300/J001v20n01_03

Cinotti, D. A., & Springer, S. I. (2016). Examining the impact of non-counseling supervisors on school counselor self-efficacy. *Vistas, 71*, 1–11.

Cook, K., Trepal, H., & Somody, C. (2012). Supervision of school counselors: The SAAFT model. *Journal of School Counseling, 10*

Council for Accreditation of Counseling and Related Educational Programs [CACREP]. (2016). *2016 standards for accreditation.* http://www.cacrep.org/wp-content/uploads/2018/05/2016-Standards-with-Glossary-5.3.2018.pdf

Crutchfield, L. B., & Borders, L. D. (1997). Impact of two clinical peer supervision models on practicing school counselors. *Journal of Counseling and Development, 75*(3), 219–230. https://doi.org/10.1002/j.1556-6676.1997.tb02336.x

Dollarhide, C. T., & Miller, G. M. (2006). Supervision for preparation and practice of school counselors: Pathways to excellence. *Counselor Education and Supervision, 45*(4), 242–252. https://doi.org/10.1002/j.1556-6978.2006.tb00001.x

Donald, E. J., Culbreth, J. R., & Carter, A. W. (2015). Play therapy supervision: A review of the literature. *International Journal of Play Therapy, 24*(2), 59–77. https://doi.org/10.1037/a0039104

Donald, E. J., Culbreth, J. R., & Carter, A. W. (2015). Play therapy supervision: A review of the literature. *International Journal of Play Therapy, 24*(2), 59–77. https://doi.org/10.1037/a0039104

Drewes, A. A., & Mullen, J. A. (2008). *Supervision can be playful: Techniques for child and play therapist supervisors.* Aronson.

Falender, C. A. (2018). Clinical supervision – The missing ingredient. *American Psychologist, 73*(9), 1240–1250. https://doi.org/10.1037/amp0000385

Fall, M., Drew, D., Chute, A., & Moore, A. (2007). The voices of registered play therapists as supervisors. *International Journal of Play Therapy, 16*(2), 133–146.

Granello, D. H., & Young, M. E. (2012). *Counseling today: Foundations of professional identity.* Pearson.

Gysbers, N. C. (2010). *Remembering the past, shaping the future: A history of school counseling.* American School Counseling Association.

Harpine, E. C. (2008). *Group interventions in schools: Promoting mental health for at-risk children and youth.* Springer Science & Business Media.

Herlihy, B., Gray, N., & McCollum, V. (2002). Legal and ethical issues in school counselor supervision. *Professional School Counseling, 6*(1), 55–60.

House, R. M., &Hayes, R. L. (2002). School counselors: Becoming key players in school reform. *Professional School Counseling, 5*, 249–256.

Hudspeth, E. F. (2015). Clinical supervision in play therapy: Research, practice, and application [special issue]. *International Journal of Play Therapy, 24*(2), 55–118. https://doi .org/10.1037/pla0000011

Inman, A. G., & DeBoer Kreider, E. (2013). Multicultural competence: Psychotherapy practice and supervision. *Psychotherapy, 50*(3), 346–350. https://doi.org/10.1037/ a0032029

Johnson, R. S. (2002). *Using data to close the achievement gap: How to measure equity in our schools.* Corwin Press.

Kottman, T. (2011). *Play therapy: Basics and beyond* (2nd ed.). American Counseling Association.

Lambie, G. W., & Williamson, L. L. (2004). The challenge to change from guidance counseling to professional school counseling: A historical proposition. *Professional School Counseling, 8*(2), 124–131.

Landreth, G. L. (2012). *Play therapy: The art of the relationship* (3rd ed.). Routledge.

Lawson, G. (2007). Counselor wellness and impairment: A national survey. *The Journal of Humanistic Counseling, Education and Development, 46*(1), 20–34.

Luke, M., & Bernard, J. M. (2006). The school counseling supervision model: An extension of the discrimination model. *Counselor Education and Supervision, 45*(4), 282–295. https:// doi.org/10.1002/j.1556-6978.2006.tb00004.x

McCarthy, G., Hegarty, J., Savage, E., & Fitzpatrick, J. J. (2010). PhD Away Days: a component of PhD supervision. *International Nursing Review, 57*(4), 415–418.

McMahon, M., & Patton, W. (2000). Conversations on clinical supervision: Benefits perceived by school counsellors. *British Journal of Guidance and Counseling, 28*(3), 339–351. https://doi.org/10.1080/713652301

Merlin-Knoblich, C., Harris, P. N., Chung, S. Y., & Gareis, C. R. (2018). Reported experiences of school counseling site supervisors in a supervision training program. *Journal of School Counseling, 16*(3), n3.

Moyer, M. (2011). Effects of non-guidance activities, supervision, and student-to-counselor ratios on school counselor burnout. *Journal of School Counseling, 9*(5). https://files.eric.ed .gov/fulltext/EJ933171.pdf

Mullen, J. A., Luke, M., & Drewes, A. A. (2007). Supervision can be playful, too: Therapy techniques that enhance supervision. *International Journal of Play Therapy, 16*(1), 69–85. http://dx.doi.org.umiss.idm.oclc.org/10.1037/1555-6824.16.1.69

Mullen, P. R., Blount, A. J., Lambie, G. W., & Chae, N. (2017). School counselors' perceived stress, burnout, and job satisfaction. *Professional School Counseling, 21*(1). https://doi.10.1177/2156759X18782468

Myers, J. E., Sweeney, T. J., & Witmer, J. M. (2000). The wheel of wellness counseling for wellness: A holistic model for treatment planning. *Journal of Counseling and Development, 78*(3), 251–266.

National Commission on Excellence in Education. (1983). *A nation at risk: The imperatives for educational reform.* National Commission on Excellence in Education.

Neyland-Brown, L., Laux, J. M., Reynolds, J. L., Kozlowski, K., & Piazza, N. J. (2019). An exploration of supervision training opportunities for school counselors. *Journal of School Counseling, 17*(1), 1–2. https://files.eric.ed.gov/fulltext/EJ1203244.pdf

Oberman, A. H., & Studer, J. R. (2021). *A guide to practicum and internship for school counselors-in-training.* Routledge.

Orlinsky, D. E., Botermans, J. F., & Rønnestad, M. H. (2001). Towards an empirically grounded model of psychotherapy training: Four thousand therapists rate influences on their development. *Australian Psychologist, 36*(2), 139–148.

168 *Amanda Winburn and Kenya G. Bledsoe*

Perera-Diltz, D. M., & Mason, K. L. (2012). A national survey of school counselor supervision practices: Administrative, clinical, peer, and technology mediated supervision. *Journal of School Counseling, 10*, 1–34. http://www.jsc.montana.edu/articles/v10n4.pdf

Randick, N. M., Dermer, S., & Michel, R. E. (2019). Exploring the job duties that impact school counselor wellness: The role of RAMP, supervision, and support. *Professional School Counseling, 22*(1), 2156759X18820331.

Ray, D. (2004). Supervision of basic and advanced skills in play therapy. *Journal of Professional Counseling: Practice, Theory, and Research, 32*(2), 28–41.

Schmidt, J. J. (2002). *Counseling in the schools: Essential services and comprehensive programs* (4th ed.). Allyn and Bacon.

Schmidt, J. J. (2014). *Counseling in schools: Comprehensive programs of responsible services for all students* (6th ed.). Pearson.

Skovholt, T. M., & Rønnestad, M. H. (2003). Struggles of the novice counselor and therapist. *Journal of Career Development, 30*(1), 45–57.

Stickel, S. A., & Trimmer, K. J. (1994). Knowing in action: A first-year counselor's process of reflection. *Elementary School Guidance and Counseling, 29*, 102–109.

Sutton, J. M., & Page, B. J. (1994). Post-degree clinical supervision of school counselors. *School Counselor, 42*(1), 32–39.

Sutton Jr., J., & Fall, M. (1995). The relationship of school climate factors to counselor self-efficacy. *Journal of Counseling and Development, 73*(3), 331–336.

Swank, J. M., Cheung, C., & Williams, S. A. (2018). Play therapy and psychoeducational school-based group interventions: A comparison of treatment effectiveness. *The Journal for Specialists in Group Work, 43*(3), 230–249.

Tang, A. (2020). The impact of school counseling supervision on practicing school counselors' self-efficacy in building a comprehensive school. *Professional School Counseling, 23*.

Theriault, A., Gazzola, N., & Richardson, B. (2009). Feelings of incompetence in novice therapists: Consequences, coping, and correctives. *Canadian Journal of Counseling, 43*(2), 105–119.

VanderGast, T. S., Culbreth, J. R., & Flowers, C. (2010). An exploration of experiences and preferences in clinical supervision with play therapists. *International Journal of Play Therapy, 19*(3), 174–185. https://doi.org/10.1037/a0018882.

Young, M. E., & Lambie, G. W. (2007). Wellness in school and mental health systems: Organizational influences. *Journal of Humanistic Counseling, Education and Development, 45*(1), 98–113.

US Department of Education, National Center for Education Statistics. (2005). The Condition of Education 2005 (NCES 2005-07). Washington, DC: U.S. Government Printing Office.

11 Touch Considerations in Infant and Early Childhood Play Therapy Reflective Supervision

Janet A. Courtney

Introduction

We may think of receiving supervision as a recent societal phenomenon, but when one considers it, we have always had some type of career overseeing guidance, such as being in an apprenticeship with a more experienced elder. Centuries ago, the Greek philosopher, Aristotle, who lived between 384 and 322 BCE, conceptualized that ethical *Virtue* is about doing the right thing – at the right time – toward the right person – with the right intention – and in the right manner (Aristotle, 1998, adapted, pp. 32–33). He conceptualized that the *right* course of action depended upon the need to contemplate the particular details of each individual circumstance which he labeled *Practical Wisdom* (Hallwell &Aristotle, 1998). Essentially, he considered that every life situation is unique and that it is prudent to understand that the context of a situation can be influenced by many different factors, which need to be carefully thought through to understand the best course of action. This is exactly what happens in supervision. In a modern-day sense, obtaining supervision as a mental health practitioner might be considered a version of "practical wisdom" that is completed within a safe, trusted professional relationship.

This chapter will first review the constructs of reflective supervision from an infant mental health perspective. Next, it will explore touch considerations in play therapy including briefly reviewing the neurobiology of touch, followed by exploring the impact of touch on a supervisee's work with infants/young children and families. Finally, a brief FirstPlay Therapy case vignette conglomerate is presented to demonstrate how issues of touch may arise within a reflective supervisory session.

Reflective Supervision in Infant Mental Health

Reflective supervision emerged in the 1980s within the infant mental health field for practitioners who were experiencing the challenging, emotionally laden nature of working with vulnerable infants and young children and families (Eggbeer et al., 2007; Schafer, 2007). These practitioners needed a style of supervision that provided them an opportunity to step back and reflect on what they were

DOI: 10.4324/9781003196075-14

feeling related to their own emotional responses to the challenges of the work (Weatherston et al., 2010). Of course, we may consider that most mental health and play therapy supervision is designed to be "reflective." However, the hall-mark of reflective supervision within infant mental health is the emphasis on the exploration of the *parallel process* within a safe *holding environment*. In this, special devotion of time is given to explore the thoughts, feelings, actions, and reactions that may arise within all relationships, including that between the supervisee and the infant/young child, between the supervisee and the parent, the supervisee to themselves, and between the supervisee and the supervisor – including addressing the power dynamics of their relationship (Eggbeer et al., 2010; Williams Kapten, 2020). The supervisee seeks to understand how each of these relationships affects the others. Reflective supervisors help to create a safe place where supervisees can feel supported, seen, and heard as they explore their client needs. Creating this holding environment requires supervisors to be fully present and sensitively affirming – not critical or judging – to their supervisees' internal experiences.

At the same time, reflective supervision also gives equal attention to grow-ing self-awareness through examining the multiple dimensions of diversity. This includes a supervisee's need to reflect on their personal cultural attitudes, biases, race, gender, classism, sexism, homophobia, xenophobia, and views about other marginalized identities (Jendrusina & Martinez, 2019; Yeung et al., 2013). In a personal conversation with play therapist and infant mental health specialist Meyleen Velasquez (personal communication, August 15, 2021), she advised that, "One way to examine and address these vast diversity dynamics is by using *cultural humility* to address racial trauma, increase awareness of implicit biases, eradicate microaggressions, and build tools to work with diverse communities." Through cultural humility, supervisees can explore, critique, and actively shift values, beliefs, and experiences that affect their perception and further marginalize com-munities (Liu et al., 2019; Pallato, 2019; Upshaw et al., 2020). Over the years, reflective supervision to enhance self-awareness has grown to be used in a variety of fields, including play therapy (Seymour & Crenshaw, 2015).

Touch Considerations and Understanding the Neurobiology of Touch

Touch is a powerful form of communication. However, while most practitioners would agree that it is of the utmost importance to address the subject of touch in clinical practice, until recently, very little has been written about the topic (Courtney & Nolan, 2017), especially as a focus of attention within clinical play therapy supervision. In an effort to learn more about the attitudes and experiences of play therapists related to touch in child sessions, Courtney and Siu (2018) sur-veyed a sample of play therapists to gain their perspectives. What was discovered in the research was that many play therapists are indeed using touch within ses-sions – such as giving a child a hug – and at the same time, they are very concerned about the liability of the touching for a variety of different reasons including that somehow a child may negatively misconstrue a caring gesture. We know that the issues of touch in sessions for children are very different from issues of touch with adults. Gray et al. (2017) stressed the "practice reality" of working with children: "young children do not participate in the more traditional forms of talking therapy by having a quiet, reflective conversation sitting in a chair across from the therapist. They are on the move and touch will inevitably happen" (p. 217). The answer to the quandary of touch with children is for practitioners to also be trained in the ethical considerations of touch (Association for Play Therapy, 2019; Courtney & Nolan, 2017; Courtney & Siu, 2018; Gray et al., 2017; Reamer, 2017).

Touch is vital to human growth and development, for without it we will not thrive and may even die – even if other areas of need are provided, such as food and hygiene (Ardiel & Rankin, 2010). Long ago, Aristotle, who understood that touch is so crucial to living, wrote, "its absence spells doom to man and all animals" (as summarized by Weber, 1991, p. 18). The importance of touch for a child's development and healing has long been documented (Brazelton & Sparrow, 2006; Field, 2014). Brody (1997) advised, "a child who experiences touch from a capable toucher will grow toward healthy maturity and will heal from earlier trauma and neglect" (p. xiv). Of all our senses, touch has historically been the least researched – although this has changed over the past 20 years (Field, 2014). Through the field of neuroscience, we now understand through the advances of brain imaging that the quality of early human attachment relationships (including *how* they were touched) directly impacts lifelong emotional, physical, relational, and brain development – both positively and negatively (Badenoch, 2008; Siegel, 2015). We now better understand how the circuits of the mind are connected to memory, touch sensations, emotions, attachment, and trauma (van der Kolk, 2014).

From a neurobiological point of view, let's consider what happens in the body in relation to touch. Note, for purposes of this chapter, we are addressing only caring and nurturing forms of touch. Harmful touch, such as hitting, spanking, slapping, and punching can produce different types of chemical reactions within the body, such as the release of cortisol. The answer to the question comprises several multidimensional bodily processes that arise, including *sensory mirror neurons*. These are nerve cells that fire when you watch another person being touched and are linked to our ability to have empathy for another (Ramachandran, 2011). We also know that the parasympathetic nervous system – our rest-and-recovery system – is activated when we receive light pressure to the body – think a relaxing massage. Other essential neurobiological processes are the "feel good" neurotransmitters including oxytocin, serotonin, and dopamine that are released when caring touch is provided. In particular, considerable research attention has been given to the calming and connectivity hormone oxytocin, also coined the "love" attachment-forming hormone (Field, 2014). Research has revealed – and this is very important to understand when facilitating touch between parents and infants/young children – that when caring touch is provided and oxytocin is released, it is shown that cortisol simultaneously lowers in the body. For example, this could be a parent offering their anxious child a warm hug that can lower the cortisol in their body to help them calm – of course, the parent must first be in a regulated place to provide the hug.

Most excitingly is the newly discovered research on touch that comes from the work of Francis McGlone and colleagues from the Liverpool John Moores University related to attachment and bonding. The newly discovered nerves are called C-tactile afferents (CTs) that are activated through gentle-type stroking – the kind a loving mother gives to an infant (Jackson & McGlone, 2020). Found on the hairy part of the skin, the slower-moving unmyelinated nerves that are activated through touch are very different from other types of nerves that are stimulated by other forms of touch such as temperature, pressure, or itch – or what is also referred to as discriminative touch. Most revealing is that the C-tactile afferents travel to the emotional and social part of the brain, while discriminative types of touch travel to the somatosensory cortex. The relevance to the work with infants/young children and parents is that caring touch provides a key role in the development of interpersonal relationships beginning with early attachment and bonding processes. Of course, we have always assumed this to be true, but now, through new advances in neuroscience, we know it is the case. Jackson and McGlone (2020), write that the key point is that "stimulation of CTs is not arbitrary, it is essential for the development of a healthy body and mind – and the science supporting this claim is indisputable" (p. 18).

Considering the Supervisee's Experiences of Touch

Gil and Johnson (1993) write that a therapist's personal history of touch will highly impact the therapeutic encounter. Touch interactions can trigger emotional and physiological memory reactions that a practitioner may not consciously register within the moment (van der Kolk, 2014). These unconscious practitioner processes could activate reactions toward a client in ways that could potentially cause harm or retraumatize a client. Clinical supervision can also play a role in helping practitioners identify potential countertransferences surrounding touch and how these personal reactions can impact professional judgement and behavior (Courtney & Gray, 2014; Gil & Rubin, 2005; VanFleet et al., 2010). Courtney (2017) advocated that "perhaps more than any other area of professional countertransference inquiry, it should be considered a priority that practitioners explore how their own life experiences related to touch can potentially impact their behaviors and actions in their work with children" (p. 12).

Gray et al. (2017, p. 224) advised that it is vital for practitioners to develop self-awareness regarding touch and suggested several areas that can be used as guidelines that supervisors can also explore with supervisees within reflective supervisory play therapy sessions to include:

- The distinction between the child's needs regarding touch as separate from their own needs
- Demonstrate self-awareness regarding comfort and discomfort concerning personal space boundaries related to touch with clients in practice
- Use reflection, self-awareness, and self-regulation to manage personal biases related to touch and to maintain professionalism in practice

- Recognize the link between countertransference(s) and personal history, and reactions related to touch
- Use reflective-oriented supervision and/or consultation to identify personal issues and take action, as needed, for self-care
- Recognize one's own personal biases and cultural, religious, and family norms related to touch

Reflective Supervision within FirstPlay Therapy

FirstPlay Therapy Reflective Supervision: Some Background

FirstPlay Therapy utilizes the reflective supervision infant mental health approach as a supervisory model. Formulated by Janet A. Courtney in the early 2000s, FirstPlay is an infant play therapy model that supports gentle touch interactions through therapeutic storytelling between parents and their infants aged up to 36 months (Courtney, 2020a, 2020b; Courtney & Nowakowski-Sims, 2018; Courtney et al., 2017). With underpinnings in Developmental Play Therapy (Brody, 1997), attachment theory, and research on touch, FirstPlay intervenes at the pre-symbolic level of play to enhance attachment and bonding in the parent–infant relationship. FirstPlay reflective supervision entails initial attendance at the FirstPlay Infant Play Therapy 45-hour intensive training that includes a live parent–infant lab where practitioners assist in facilitating warm and caring touch between an infant and parent dyad in real time. Training also includes a section on the ethics of touch, including practitioner's exploration of their own experiences and self-awareness of touch. Following the training, in order to obtain certification, practitioners need to complete several tasks that are reviewed within reflective supervision sessions, including attendance at group supervision, a review of a parent–infant session video, and by turning in five post-training case session reflective forms.

A Brief FirstPlay Case Vignette of Supervisee Brenda

Brenda works for an agency with a housing unit designed to support homeless pregnant young mothers and their babies after birth. The program assists mothers to find housing, work, and childcare. Brenda introduced a new mother, Marta, to the FirstPlay model and had permission to videotape the session for her FirstPlay reflective supervision requirements. When the video was reviewed during the reflective supervision session in which Brenda was guiding the mother with her baby in the Baby Tree Hug story, it was observed that there was a moment when the infant became uncomfortable with the touch. Prior to that point in the session, the infant was observed to show cues of relaxed enjoyment and connection with her mother in the FirstPlay process. Brenda could be observed in the video pausing the facilitation as she appeared to be contemplating how best to intervene. The video was stopped at that point in the supervision and the FirstPlay Supervisor asked Brenda to share what she was experiencing and feeling at that moment. The following is a process recording of the supervision.

Side note: What we are paying attention to in the FirstPlay reflective supervision process are the thoughts and feelings that arise within the supervisee as they observe their work through watching the video, as well as what they were feeling at the time of facilitation with the client. In the following case process recording, you can see that we are paying attention to three areas: (1) the needs and cues of the infant and monitoring how the infant is responding to the touch, (2) the needs of the parent and how they are giving and responding to the reciprocal touch experience, and (3) the arising needs and parallel process that emerges for the supervisee.

FirstPlay Reflective Supervisor: I noticed the infant was pulling back and her head turned away from the mother at this moment when the mother was touching and moving the baby's legs. And, I noticed you paused at the moment too. Can you share what was happening for you and what you were feeling at the moment?

Brenda: Yes, I was trying to read the cues of the baby at the time, and I could see she was tensing up with the touch, and I was struggling to figure out what to do. I was aware that the baby could not say in words what she was feeling but could only tell us through her body what she was feeling and that we needed to pay attention to that. I did not see that Mom was picking up on the baby's cues at that point.

FirstPlay Reflective Supervisor: Did you notice what was happening with *your* body at that moment.

Brenda: Well, yes, when I was watching the mother touch the baby and the baby began to tense and pull back and looked uncomfortable, I could also feel that my body was tensing up too. I recognize that my body often tenses when I am starting to feel nervous or uncomfortable about something – or when I am not sure what to do about a situation. I can also see in the video that I shifted my body to a new position – I think I was trying to release some of that tension that I was starting to feel too.

FirstPlay Supervisor: Good, so you were also able to connect to how your own body was responding – that's those sensory mirror neurons in action. Good, to be so self-aware at the somatic level, and it seems you automatically adjusted your body to a place of comfort at the time. What else were you experiencing at that moment?

Brenda: I was struggling to think about the best way to address the issue with the mother as I did not want to say anything to her that would cause her to shut down from being open to the process. I was trying to say something that would not be minimizing but rather something meaningful. I was sensitive that this mother had some traumatic experiences surrounding touch in her life growing up. I also wanted to bring some attunement for the mother to her baby, and at the same time, I wanted to give her permission to not do it all as I realized this is a Mom that wants to check all the boxes and do everything asked of her. I had already discussed with Mom upfront that the baby is always in the driver's seat and that we need to follow the lead of the baby. I finally said to her: "I think the baby's body language is telling us that she does not like that activity so much. It's okay not to have to do all the story. You can move on to the next part."

FirstPlay Reflective Supervisor: Yes, I can see in the video that this mother really trusts you and she accepted your guidance in a good way and moved on to the next activity.

Summary of Interaction

Brenda, who had worked toward obtaining a lot of self-awareness about her own experiences with touch, was able to connect to her own somatic discomfort in the moment when she was observing the infant's cues of tension and pulling back from a certain type of touch that the mother was providing. At the same time, Brenda automatically knew what to do to regulate herself in the moment. She was also sensitive that the mother had some traumatic experiences with touch. Brenda was able to caringly intervene to address the infant body language cues of communication, and at the same time she supported the mother to have permission to not have to do it all.

Conclusion

Perhaps of all our varied relationship roles that we engage with over a lifetime, the supervisor and supervisee relationship is unique – especially when it is able to develop over time. This chapter reviewed the constructs of reflective supervision from an infant mental health/infant play therapy perspective. It also examined the clinical issues of touch in practice with infants/young children and parents along with the understanding of the neurobiology of touch. Also highlighted was the potential impact of touch on a supervisee's work with clients that included suggested guidelines that supervisors can use to help assist supervisees to grow self-awareness in play therapy practice. Considering the parallel process, a reflective supervisor can help to support a supervisee to look within to examine any emerging thoughts, feelings, and reactions that may arise during a supervisory session when reviewing client material. This takes great vulnerability on the part of the supervisee as well as a sensitive caring supervisor to help guide the process within a safe holding environment. This chapter also showed how issues of touch can be addressed within infant play therapy reflective supervisory sessions as demonstrated through a FirstPlay Therapy case vignette. Ongoing reflective supervision is a valuable method for supervisees to gain self-awareness and professional growth development.

Recommended Resources

Alliance for the Advancement of Infant Mental Health: https://www.allianceaimh.org/
International Association for the Study of Affective Touch: https://iasat.org/
World Association for Infant Mental Health: https://waimh.org/
Zero to Three: https://www.zerotothree.org/

References

Ardiel, E., & Rankin, C. H. (2010). The importance of touch in development. *Pediatric and Child Health, 15*(3), 153–156.

Association for Play Therapy. (2019). Paper on touch: Clinical, professional, & ethical issues. Retrieved 20 September 2021, from https://cdn.ymaws.com/www.a4pt.org/resource/resmgr/publications/2019/paper_on_touch_2019_-_final.pdf

Badenoch, B. (2008). *Being a brain-wise therapist: A practical guide to interpersonal Neurobiology.* Norton & Co.

Brazelton, T., & Sparrow, J. (2006). *Touchpoints: Birth to three* (2nd ed.). DeCapo Press.

Brody, V. A. (1997). *The dialogue of touch: Developmental play therapy* (2nd ed.). Jason Aronson.

Courtney, J. A. (2017). Overview of touch related to professional ethical and clinical practice with children. In J. A. Courtney & R. D. Nolan (Eds.), *Touch in child counseling and play therapy: An ethical and clinical guide* (pp. 3–17). Routledge.

Courtney, J. A. (2020a). *Healing child and family trauma through expressive and play Therapies: Art, Nature, Storytelling, Body, Mindfulness.* Norton & Co.

Courtney, J. A. (2020b). *Introduction Infant Play Therapy: Foundations, Programs, Models and Practice.* Routledge Publishing.

Courtney, J. A., & Gray, S. W. (2014). Phenomenological inquiry into practitioner experiences of developmental play therapy: Implications for training in touch. *International Journal of Play Therapy, 23*(2), 114–129. http://doi.org/10.1037/a0036366

Courtney, J. A., & Nolan, R. D. (2017). *Touch in child counseling and play therapy: An ethical and clinical guide.* Routledge.

Courtney, J. A., & Nowakowski-Sims, E. (2018). Technology and the threat to secure attachment relationships: What play therapists need to consider. *Play Therapy, 13*(3), 10–14.

Courtney, J. A., & Siu, A. F. Y. (2018). Practitioner experiences of touch in working with children in play therapy. *International Journal of Play Therapy, 27*(2), 92–102. http://doi.org/10.1037/pla0000064

Courtney, J. A., Velasquez, M., & Bakai Toth, V. (2017). FirstPlay® infant massage storytelling: Facilitating corrective touch experiences with a teenage mother and her abused infant. In J. A. Courtney & R. D. Nolan (Eds.), *Touch in child counseling and play therapy: An ethical and clinical guide* (pp. 48–62). Routledge.

Eggbeer, L., Mann, T. L., & Seibel, N. L. (2007). Reflective supervision: Past, present, and future. *Zero to Three, 28*(2), 5–9.

Eggbeer, L., Shahmoon-Shanok, R., & Clark, R. (2010). Reaching toward an evidence base for reflective supervision. *Zero to Three, 31*(2), 39–50.

Field, T. (2014). *Touch* (2nd ed.). The MIT Press.

Gil, E., & Johnson, T. C. (1993). *Sexualized children: Assessment and treatment of sexualized children and children who molest.* Launch Press.

Gil, E., & Rubin, L. (2005). Countertransference play: Informing and enhancing play therapist self awareness through play. *International Journal of Play Therapy, 14*(2), 87–102.

Gray, S. W., Courtney, J. A., & Nolan, R. D. (2017). Competencies and recommendations supporting the ethics of touch in child counseling and play therapy. In J. A. Courtney & R. D. Nolan (Eds.), *Touch in child counseling and play therapy: An ethical and clinical guide* (pp. 217–230). Routledge.

Halliwell, S., & Aristotle, A. (1998). *Aristotle's poetics.* University of Chicago Press.

Jackson, E., & McGlone, F. (2020). The impact of play on the developing social brain: New insights from the neurobiology of touch. In J. A. Courtney & R. D. Nolan (Eds.), *Touch in child counseling and play therapy: An ethical and clinical guide* (pp. 18–36). Routledge.

Jendrusina, A. A., & Martinez, J. H. (2019). Hello from the other side: Student of color perspectives in supervision. *Training and Education in Professional Psychology, 13*(3), 160–166. https://doi.org/10.1037/tep0000255

Liu, M. W., Liu, Z. R., Garrison, Y. L., Kim, J. Y., Chan, L., Ho, Y. C., & Yeung, C. W. (2019). Racial trauma, microaggression, and becoming racially innocuous: The role of acculturation and white supremacist ideology. *American Psychologist, 74*(1), 143–155. https://doi.org/10.1037/amp0000368

Pallato, B. A. (2019). The multicultural guidelines in practice: Cultural humility in clinical training and supervision. *Training and Education in Professional Psychology, 13*(3), 227–232. https://doi.org/10.1037/tep0000253

Ramachandran, V. S. (2011). *The tell-tale brain: A neuroscientist's quest for what makes us human.* Norton & Co.

Reamer, F. (2017). Ethical and risk-management issues in the use of touch. In J. A. Courtney & R. D. Nolan (Eds.), *Touch in child counseling and play therapy: An ethical and clinical guide* (pp. 18–32). Routledge.

Schafer, W. (2007). Models and domains of supervision and their relationship to professional development. *Zero to Three, 28*(2), 10–16.

Seymour, J. W., & Crenshaw, D. A. (2015). Reflective practice in play therapy and supervision. In D. A. Crenshaw & A. L. Stewart (Eds.), *Play therapy: A comprehensive guide to theory and practice* (pp. 483–495). Guilford Press.

Siegel, D. J. (2015). *The developing mind. How relationships and the brain interact to shape who we are* (2nd ed.). Guilford Press.

Upshaw, N. C., Lewis, D. E., Jr., & Nelson, A. L. (2020). Cultural humility in action: Reflective and process-oriented supervision with Black trainees. *Training and Education in Professional Psychology, 14*(4), 277–284. https://doi.org/10.1037/tep0000284

van der Kolk, B. (2014). *The body keeps score.* Viking Books.

VanFleet, R., Sywulak, A. E., & Sniscak, C. C. (2010). *Child-centered play therapy.* Guilford Press.

Weatherston, D., Weigand, R. F., & Weigand, B. (2010). Reflective supervision: Supporting reflection as a cornerstone for competency. *Zero to Three, 31*(2), 22–30.

Weber, R. (1991). A philosophical perspective on touch. In K. E. Barnard & T. B. Brazelton (Eds.), *Touch: The foundation of experience* (pp. 11–43). International Universities Press.

Williams Kapten, S. (2020). Power, powerlessness, and the parallel process. *Journal of Psychotherapy Integration, 30*(1), 147–154. https://doi.org/10.1037/int0000168

Yeung, J., Spanierman, L. B., & Landrum-Brown, J. (2013). "Being white in a multicultural society": Critical whiteness pedagogy in a dialogue course. *Journal of Diversity in Higher Education, 6*(1), 17–32. https://doi.org/10.1037/a0031632

Section 4

Playful Supervision Strategies

12 Sandtray Techniques in Play Therapy Supervision

Crystal Brashear, Donna Hickman, Rebecca Mathews, and Nancy Thomas

Introduction

Sandtray is a projective, expressive counseling modality that provides the opportunity to explore and process material using a tray of sand and a collection of miniature figures (Homeyer & Sweeney, 2017). Through kinesthetic engagement with these humble supplies, people of all ages and developmental stages create and communicate nonverbally. When used with adults, the cultivated tray then serves as a catalyst for verbal processing. Authors increasingly advocate for the use of sandtray in counseling supervision (Hartwig & Bennett, 2017; Niles, 2021; Prasath & Copeland, 2021; Saltis et al., 2019).

This chapter equips readers with an introduction to the modality, complete with a multifaceted rationale for its use in play therapy supervision. A brief session overview includes instructions on setting up the experience, selecting and delivering prompts, processing with supervisees, and documenting the session. Readers will discover how sandtray can integrate two models of supervision, and incorporate Jungian, constructivist, and solution-focused principles. Four case studies apply these concepts to play therapy–specific scenarios. Finally, readers will encounter creative solutions for overcoming challenges in sandtray supervision. Essential resources are provided so that supervisors can help each supervisee reach their full potential.

Sandtray Supervision Session Overview

Sandtray requires only a tray of sand and a collection of miniature figures. The tray can be any shape (e.g., round like a mandala, square, or rectangular so figures can wedge into corners) but must be large enough to accommodate a multiple clusters of figures. Trays can be made of plastic (e.g., potted plant saucer), metal (e.g., cake pan), or thick glass (e.g., pie plate). The sand should feel nice to the touch and should not leave a dusty residue. The figures can be purchased as a set or collected over time. Miniatures should not be breakable if used in play therapy sessions, but for supervision they can be made of glass or another fragile material if desired. Miniatures from the following categories should be represented: people, animals (e.g., dog, dinosaur, large rubber snake), landscape (e.g.,

DOI: 10.4324/9781003196075-16

trees, rocks), dividers (e.g., fencing, bridges), other structures (e.g., house, wishing well), vehicles, and assorted objects (e.g., rug, padlock with key, magnifying glass). Supervisees can project meaning onto any object, so there is little pressure to ensure that every possible item is represented in the miniature collection. The standard protocol for a sandtray supervision session is as follows:

1. The supervisor invites the supervisee to look over the collection of miniatures and create a scene in the sand. The prompt (i.e., the specific type of scene to be built) is motivated by the *benefit* the supervisor hopes the supervisee will experience
2. The supervisor observes the supervisee as they select and arrange the figures, paying special attention to the nonverbal communication of the supervisee
3. The supervisor facilitates the processing of the created tray by asking open-ended questions. Again, the direction of the questions and reflections will be determined by how the supervisor hopes the supervisee will *benefit*. The supervisor avoids touching the miniatures and only uses names/labels that the supervisee first provides
4. The supervisor documents the session by taking a photograph of the tray to accompany the completed supervision session note

Beyond this basic procedure lies limitless variation. The following sections include many suggestions for prompts, as well as examples of processing questions and additional options to further supervisee growth.

Rationale for Sandtray Supervision

Sandtray is a reflective practice to improve supervisee self-awareness and insight (Armstrong, 2008). It leverages the power of metaphor as the supervisee selects figures and projects meaning onto them (Morrison & Homeyer, 2008). The created tray can then be collaboratively explored and expanded upon in ways that traditional talk-based supervision cannot match (Schuck & Wood, 2011). Creative supervision modalities such as sandtray can support the development of supervisee empathy and self-awareness (Prasath & Copeland, 2021). Further, sandtray helps identify and process supervisee incongruences (Purswell & Stulmaker, 2015). The tray highlights supervisee polarity (i.e., ambivalence), which helps the supervisor recognize and resolve tension between counseling delivery methods, client concerns, countertransference issues, or other conflicts that may exist (Armstrong, 2008).

Sandtray is also an experiential modality. Each step in the process requires the supervisee to make decisions, from selecting miniatures, to arranging them in the tray, to choosing a starting point for verbal processing. The visual and kinesthetic qualities of sandtray facilitate a memorable encounter. Because of this, experiential activities such as sandtray improve recall (Purswell & Stulmaker, 2015) and enable supervisees to better integrate practice with theory (Fazio-Griffith et al., 2021). Sandtray supervision strengthens client conceptualization and perspective-taking

(Niles, 2021). Clinical issues can be expressed through sandtray (Niles, 2021). All of this enhances professional and personal competence.

Sandtray can help bypass supervisee defensiveness (Garrett, 2017). Developmentally, supervisees can experience feelings of guilt, shame, or fear (Stoltenberg et al., 2014). A developmental model for understanding and addressing supervisee defensiveness is explored later in this chapter. Sandtray is an ideal medium to support supervisees in identifying and working through this fear (Garrett, 2017). The sensory experience of touching the sand and handling the miniatures can move the supervisee beyond typical defenses to more fully access and experience emotions (Armstrong, 2008). Supervisors create emotional safety by providing alternatives to verbal expression (Kascsak & Silverberg, 2021). The miniatures become the words that supervisees cannot voice (Niles, 2021).

Sandtray can prove especially helpful when supervisees are struggling. At times, supervision sessions may become frustrating or uncomfortable for the supervisee. When this occurs, sandtray work can provide a calming, creative outlet for supervisees to express their feelings and regulate their responses. In addition, sandtray can be used to provide a short break if supervisees are overwhelmed by the intensity of the session (Deaver & Shiflett, 2011). Garrett (2017) provided some recommendations for prompts when a mini-break is needed:

- "Why don't you take a few minutes to create a scene or just play in the sand before we start our session today?"
- "Today has been challenging – how about we take the last ten minutes of our session to create a tray that will help you relax before you go home?"
- "Build a tray showing what you would do if you had a weekend with a completed to-do list and zero deadlines."

Sandtray is a flexible modality that works with a variety of supervisee theoretical approaches (Hartwig & Bennett, 2017; Homeyer & Sweeney, 2017), from Gestalt and Adlerian (Eberts & Homeyer, 2015) to cognitive-behavioral (Sweeney & Homeyer, 2009). Sandtray is also a good fit as a school counseling modality (Richards et al., 2012; Swank & Lenes, 2013). With the burgeoning need for mental health services in schools, school counselors require a developmentally appropriate and culturally sensitive way to work with a wide variety of students (Blalock, 2021). Similar to traditional play therapy, sandtray therapy allows students the opportunity to integrate their experiences and discover their inner resources (Homeyer & Sweeney, 2017).

Additionally, sandtray supports a trauma-informed approach to supervision and enables the supervisee to experience safety (Kascsak & Silverberg, 2021). Within this safety, sandtray offers supervisees an opportunity to grow in self-confidence. They learn to conceptualize client cases innovatively while simultaneously releasing emotion (Anekstein et al., 2014) during the experience. The kinesthetic component of sandtray supports self-regulation as supervisees give voice to deep-seated thoughts and feelings. Sandtray, therefore, has the potential to improve the efficacy of the learning process and the supervisor–supervisee relationship (Anekstein et al., 2014).

Sandtray is also a modality that can address the needs of diverse supervisees and the clients they serve. Multicultural competence is core to counselor training, but it may be vital in contexts where verbal expression is not the only source of meaning. Sandtray ignites the power of nonverbal expression (Homeyer & Sweeney, 2017; Ramsey, 2014), reducing language barriers that might impede supervisee progress. Sometimes, despite sharing a language, thoughts and feelings are misunderstood out of cultural context. Sandtray employs expression through symbols (Morrison & Homeyer, 2008), allowing the supervisee greater flexibility of meaning. Therefore, sandtray can benefit any cultural group (Jeppsen, 2012) and is used in many countries as a therapeutic modality (Ramsey, 2014). Sandtray supervision can help supervisees connect self-understanding with multicultural competence improvement (Paone et al., 2015). Garrett (2017) provides several additional culturally focused sandtray supervision prompts.

- "Select a few items that celebrate the unique cultural makeup of your client."
- "Create a tray depicting your client's underlying cultural aspects."
- "Divide your tray in half and create two parallel scenes: one depicting your own cultural values, and the other depicting your client's cultural values."
- "Select a few items that represent your own cultural background and your client's cultural background and create a tray illustrating how these two worlds interact."

Perhaps most importantly, sandtray and play therapy supervision fit naturally as both rely heavily on developmentally appropriate creative modalities (Carson & Becker, 2004). This is accomplished through parallel play. While the supervisor models essential skills such as creating safety, the supervisee experiences what the client experiences in session (Perryman et al., 2016). Insights from parallel play enable supervisees to be more fully present with their clients (Purswell & Stulmaker, 2015). Supervisees become increasingly adept at utilizing this modality with each scene in the sand. Sandtray can teach supervisees to understand and work with nonverbal cues, a crucial skill when counseling children (Armstrong, 2008). Playful supervision helps build a professional play therapist identity (Niles, 2021; Perryman et al., 2016). In fact, Drewes and Mullen (2008) assert that failure to utilize play in the supervision of play therapists is incongruent.

Integrating Sandtray with Supervision Models and Principles

The best supervisors do more than support; they leverage their understanding of supervision models to focus sessions and make the most of limited time. Two supervision approaches are presented here: the Discrimination Model (Bernard & Goodyear, 2018), which provides the supervisor a framework for making here-and-now directional choices, and the Integrated Developmental Model

(Stoltenberg & McNeill, 2010), which recognizes the different needs that supervisees experience with each stage of growth. Fusing these two models together can provide a comprehensive framework upon which supervisors can rely.

Sandtray with the Discrimination Model

Within the Discrimination Model (Bernard & Goodyear, 2018), supervisors take on three distinct roles – teacher, counselor, and consultant – to explore three supervisee focus areas – process/intervention, conceptualization, and personalization. In the teacher role, supervisors provide education (e.g., process of therapy, purpose of different approaches, how to terminate, etc.) and evaluation (Bernard & Goodyear, 2018). In the counselor role, supervisors provide a safe space to self-examine, with the intended benefit of the supervisee's increased self-awareness. In the consultant role, supervisors take on a more collegial relationship and collaborate with the supervisee. This engenders supervisee self-efficacy and helps the supervisee develop their unique counseling style. The first focus area is process/intervention, in which the supervisee grows in counseling skill competency. The second focus area is conceptualization, in which the supervisee improves in hypothesis-forming and theory application. The third focus area is personalization, in which the supervisee improves themselves. This work renders the supervisee more capable of forming and maintaining strong therapeutic rapport with clients, as well as helps overcome detrimental countertransference with clients. Supervisors can use an infinite number of sandtray directives to address the nine possible combinations of the Discrimination Model (Graham et al., 2014). The supervisor has the freedom to flexibly adjust the sandtray modality to fit the emerging roles and foci (Anekstein et al., 2014). The following prompts provide an example for each focus area.

Intervention:

- "Build a tray depicting what you think your client needs to think/feel/do in order to accomplish their goal"

Conceptualization:

- "Make a scene showing the client and their presenting problem, as you see it"

Personalization:

- "Construct a tray that illustrates how *you* feel when you think about this client"

One important caution must be mentioned here: Sandtray presents the potential for deeper emotional processing, so supervisors must proceed with intentionality when personalization is the focus area. The counselor role is an important part of the discrimination model, but supervisors should tread carefully to avoid broken boundaries and dual relationships (Anekstein et al., 2014).

Sandtray With the Integrative Developmental Model

The Integrative Developmental Model (Stoltenberg & McNeill, 2010) outlines three developmental stages through which supervisees pass: Level 1 (beginner), Level 2 (end of internship/post-graduation), and Level 3 (2–3 years of counseling experience). Sandtray is a useful tool in promoting supervisee growth across all stages of skill development (Graham et al., 2014). The adaptability of sandtray means the supervisor can adjust the level of directiveness based upon the supervisee's needs (Homeyer & Sweeney, 2017). Supervisors can use sandtray to assess the developmental progress of the supervisee (Stark & Frels, 2014). Supervisors can then craft prompts to meet the unique needs present at each level (Perryman et al., 2016). Hartwig and Bennett (2017) suggest four ways that sandtray can be used to support the development of supervisees: modeling sandtray as an intervention, case consultation, building self-awareness, and with groups of supervisees.

The Level 1 supervisee experiences high anxiety; this elicits dependency on the supervisor and motivation to perform well (Stoltenberg & McNeill, 2010). Beginner supervisees may have little insight and be self-focused in session (Stoltenberg et al., 2014). Since Level 1 supervisees can be new to sandtray, prompts at this developmental stage might remain open-ended and straightforward:

- "Create a scene about how you are feeling today"
- "Make a tray that shows what your play therapy session felt like today"

Processing with the Level 1 supervisee can also focus on simple self-reflection. For example, the supervisor may ask the supervisee to share what led them to choose a certain miniature, or how it relates to them as a counselor-in-training (Hartwig & Bennett, 2017).

As they continue to develop, Level 2 supervisees can experience tension between dependence on the supervisor and autonomy. They may demonstrate fluctuating motivation as mistakes increase. They become increasingly likely to take the client's perspective. Prompts at this developmental stage might focus on building self-awareness and setting boundaries:

- "Create a tray that maps your path to becoming a play therapist"
- "Build a scene that depicts the tension you felt with your client in session"
- "Make a scene showing what you would like to get out of our supervision session today"
- "Create a tray illustrating what it is like to set limits for a child in session"

Processing with the Level 2 supervisee can improve their self-trust and ability to elicit and implement feedback. Additionally, the interpersonal tension the supervisee experiences as they transition from dependence to autonomous can be addressed in sandtray (Niles, 2021).

As they further progress and gain a few years of experience, the Level 3 supervisee's motivation and autonomy stabilize. Their professional identity becomes more secure and their reliance on a supervisor lessens (Stoltenberg & McNeill, 2010). Prompts can focus on solidifying this growth:

- "Create a tray that demonstrates who you are as a play therapist"
- "Build a scene about what you want future supervision/consultation to look like"

Processing with the Level 3 supervisee can shift toward a collaborative effort, in which the supervisor increasingly takes on the role of consultant. As Level 3 supervisees complete their supervision requirements, processing can help to launch them as autonomous clinicians.

Jungian Principles in Sandtray Supervision

Jungian sandplay, founded by Dora Kalff, emphasizes spirituality and symbols, self-connection, and the therapeutic relationship (Cunningham, 2013). In sandplay supervision, the supervisor uses countertransference as a vital source of information about the supervisee's inner experience and how that is impacting their work with clients (Cunningham, 2013) Sandplay supervision opens the door to the unconscious (Graham et al., 2014) and can lead to a cathartic experience (Gladding, 2016). These experiences support a supervisee's ability to generate new insight, new solutions, and new perspectives (Bainum et al., 2006; Markos et al., 2008). This is especially important when a supervisee encounters some level of fear or immobility with a client case. The synesthetic experience is a particularly potent component of sandtray (Homeyer & Sweeney, 2017), producing distinct insight into the inner workings of a supervisee (Anekstein et al., 2014; Deaver & Shiflett, 2011). Both the depth and novelty of this inner-world exploration will ameliorate the supervisory relationship and the resulting growth. While much overlaps between sandtray and sandplay, differences are worth noting. One difference is that sandtray focuses on the tray builder's conscious processing, while sandplay focuses more on unconscious processes.

Constructivist Principles in Sandtray Supervision

Sandtray supervision fits within a constructivist pedagogical approach to supervision (Saltis et al., 2019) which posits that "individuals actively create their world as they experience it" (McAuliffe et al., 2010, p. 2). Sandtray supports the supervisee to acknowledge and communicate their reality and make changes within it (Dale & Lyddon, 2000). Miniatures are used as symbols to represent their subjective reality and can be arranged to illustrate their experience (Armstrong, 2008). Through sandtray, supervisees can be empowered to construct future possibilities and solutions (Saltis et al., 2019).

Solution-Focused Principles in Sandtray Supervision

Blending sandtray with solution-focused supervision can help supervisees experience a safe, strengths-based supervision (Stark et al., 2015). Supervisees find that increased awareness of self changes how they approach client concerns. Flaherty (2018) introduced the Jack-in-the-Box technique, in which the supervisor first provides a non-directive prompt. While processing the tray, the supervisor listens for areas of concern or problems the supervisee wants to solve (e.g., feeling more effective in play therapy, having stronger parent consultation, etc.). The supervisee is asked to consider one miniature not in the tray that may help them make progress toward resolving that concern, even if to a small degree. The supervisee then adds this to the tray, which shifts the supervisee from a process to a problem-solving space.

Sandtray Supervision Techniques

Supervisors set the stage for successful sandtray work by forming a strong alliance, thoughtfully selecting a tray, and curating miniatures. Once this has been accomplished, selecting a prompt that fits the supervisee's emerging need becomes more fluid. Processing is best accomplished using curiosity and fervent belief in the supervisee's ability to engage in meaningful self-exploration. With sandtray, documentation can become an opportunity for continued reflection and growth.

Case Study: John

John is a 45-year-old Caucasian male counseling at an inpatient hospital under Amelia's supervision. A wide variety of experiences have helped John grow in self-efficacy over the years. He was recently assigned a young client with a diagnosis of comorbid ADHD, bipolar, and schizophrenia, who is taking several medications to stabilize her mood. John finds that the medications leave his client unable to function, lethargic and unmotivated. He tries to advocate for this client by discussing the case with the psychiatrist on staff, but to no avail. Despite John's vision of potential for this client, he believes she is not benefiting from the therapeutic services offered at the hospital.

John feels stuck and has no idea where to go from here. He presents this case to Amelia, who decides it might be beneficial for John to process his stuckness using sandtray (Armstrong, 2008; Flaherty, 2018). Amelia invites John to build a tray about his journey of becoming a counselor (Figure 12.1). Sandtray helps John process the highs and the lows (the rocks, fences, hurdles, and serpents) of his journey, putting his current struggle into perspective. He explores the difficulty in advocating for his client, the feeling of being stuck (sitting in front of a large rock, surrounded on all sides), and the resulting sadness (depicted by the helpless posture of the figure). John processes his efforts and how he has done everything in his control, remembering the importance of the relationship in therapeutic progress. John returns to work with a renewed sense of purpose and a desire to remain present and empathetic with his client, regardless of the circumstance.

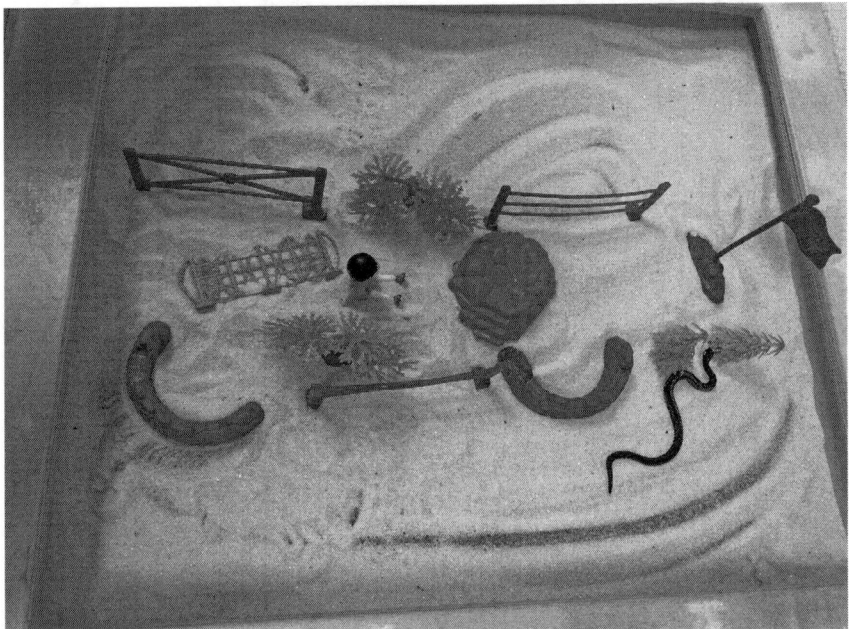

Figure 12.1 John's sand tray

Case Study: Lispeti

Lispeti is a 28-year-old female who has been a Licensed Professional Counselor (LPC) for two years and is receiving supervision towards becoming a Registered Play Therapist™ (RPT™). Her graduate training and internship focused on working with adults from a person-centered theoretical perspective. She has been a quick learner and happily embraced the tenets of play therapy. Lispeti recently began working with 5-year-old Jeremiah, who begins every session by tearing the playroom apart (e.g., sweeping toys off shelves, kicking walls). Lispeti has pondered setting limits, but she wonders whether that is consistent with her person-centered views. She is struggling to know how to maintain safety in session.

Steve, Lispeti's supervisor, can see the tension she is experiencing around setting limits. Additionally, it is evident that her confidence has declined since working with Jeremiah, and she is doubting her abilities with other clients. Though he is well-trained in sandtray, Steve lacks the space for a typical setup in his office. However, Steve knows that sandtray is an adaptable modality that can be accomplished without traditional miniatures (Brashear et al., 2019). Steve invites Lispeti on a nature walk to gather items related to her feelings about setting limits with Jeremiah. Through the creation and processing of her tray (Figure 12.2), Lispeti notices that she has built walls around herself and that the miniatures relating to Jeremiah are all sharp and prickly. Lispeti realizes she is experiencing anxiety because she does not believe Jeremiah will respect her limits, and she does not

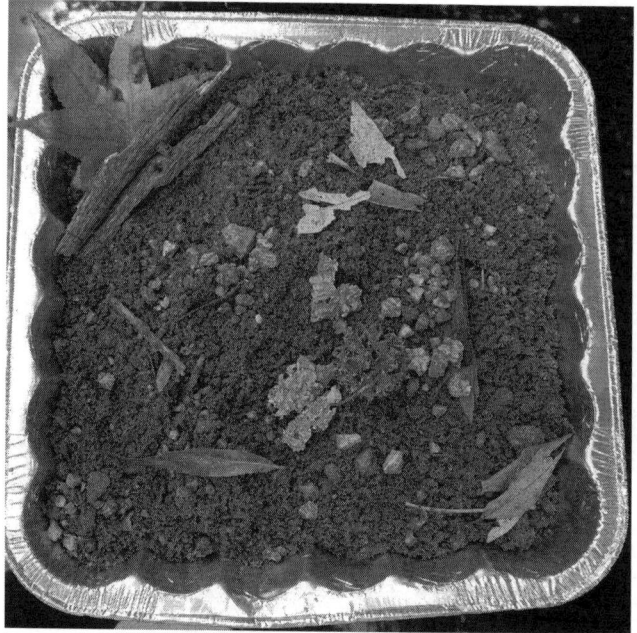

Figure 12.2 Lispeti's sand tray

know how to handle his rejection of them. Steve supports Lispeti by normalizing her apprehension as a common experience. Together they spend time practicing limit-setting, with Lispeti speaking "as" the miniatures and acting out how she expects Jeremiah to respond. Lispeti is delighted to witness the variety of ways Steve models limit-setting, and she returns to session with Jeremiah with increased confidence.

Case Study: Emma

Emma is George's newest counseling intern. She is a 25-year-old African American woman wanting to specialize in working with children who have survived trauma. She is completing her post-graduation licensure hours at George's private practice in a rural town in East Texas. They see primarily middle-class Caucasian individuals and families. One parent was visibly taken aback upon discovering that Emma is her child's counselor. Tension has been building from the very first consultation, in which the client's mother made it very clear that she did not expect to see a counselor who looked like Emma. As weeks have progressed, Emma has continued to maintain empathy and unconditional positive regard for her client. However, during their fifth consultation, her client's mother spent most of the time voicing strong political opinions laced with racial microaggressions. Emma's frustration is boiling, and she is struggling with maintaining cultural sensitivity.

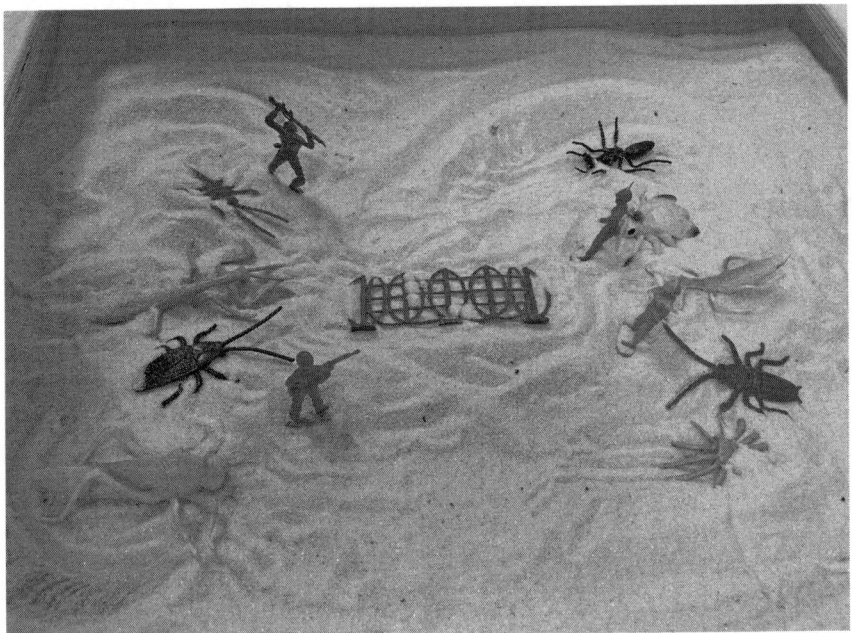

Figure 12.3 Emma's sand tray

A new counselor unsure of herself and her abilities, Emma brings her concern to George. Hearing her frustration, George invites her to process these strong feelings by building a scene in the sand that depicts her experience of diversity (Figure 12.3). Sandtray helps Emma express feelings of frustration (the two sides at war), conceptualize the parent as a unique individual with a unique belief system (seeing both sides, both similarities and differences), and explore symbols to represent her unconditional positive regard and empathy despite differing belief systems (the bridge connecting the sides). Emma feels a weight lifted after the miniatures give voice to her struggle. She returns to work with a renewed counselor identity and a fresh resolve to maintain emotional boundaries for her wellness with her client's parent.

Case Study: Amaya

Amaya has been an elementary school counselor for 12 years. She loves working with her students, but lately she has been feeling burned out at school. She had fantasized about starting her own private practice one day but felt afraid to make such a big career change in her mid-40s. Amaya is passionate about the value of using play therapy with her younger clients, but as a school counselor, she is limited to how much "therapy" she can do with her students. She has been working on her RPT™ credential with her supervisor, Lisa, for the past year.

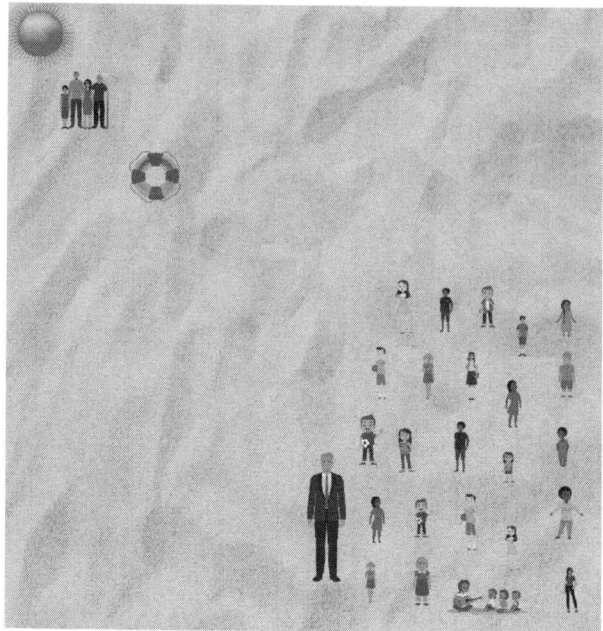

Figure 12.4 Amaya's sand tray

Amaya feels safe with Lisa and looks forward to their supervision sessions each week.

At the beginning of one online session, Amaya fights back her tears while describing how stressed she is at school each day. Lisa says, "I can tell how overwhelmed you are feeling right now. Why don't you take a few minutes to create a sandtray?" Amaya has no idea how to accomplish this, until Lisa sends her a link to a virtual sandtray website. Though initially skeptical, Amaya feels comfortable enough with Lisa to give it a try. She is surprised by how emotional she feels as she creates her scene (Figure 12.4). She talks to Lisa about the paralyzing anxiety she experiences before each school day. As she drags and drops figure after figure into the virtual tray, Amaya experiences the weight of a caseload of 850 students, 60 teachers, and hundreds of parents. While processing her scene with Lisa, Amaya feels that burden lifting. She recognizes that she needs to work on setting better boundaries at school. She commits to leave work each day by 5:00 pm to eat dinner at home with her family. After processing her tray with Lisa, Amaya can finish her supervision session with a renewed focus.

Conclusion

Although sandtray is a desirable modality to help supervisees improve counseling self-efficacy and competency, supervisors need the training to utilize it effectively. A good rule of thumb is that supervisors need to have their own experiences with creating and processing trays before facilitating sandtray with supervisees. Garrett (2017) points to DeDomencio's (1995) rule that challenges mental health professionals to create and process at least 30 to 50 trays before facilitating sandtray with clients. The same rule could be applied to supervisors. Currently, no standardized set of training guidelines exist for sandtray therapists to follow. Thus, play therapy supervisors have an ethical responsibility to model competency and ensure their supervisees are properly trained in sandtray before utilizing it with clients (Hartwig & Bennett, 2017). Supervisors can provide a comprehensive sandtray training experience by combining sandtray supervision sessions with assigned readings, videos, lectures, and written reflections (Warr-Williams, 2012).

Overcoming Challenges in Sandtray Supervision

Play therapy supervision is increasingly offered virtually. Supervisors wishing to utilize sandtray through an online platform have several options. The first is a free website (Fried, n.d.) that allows visitors to drag, drop, resize, and reposition miniature images into a virtual tray. A photograph of the completed tray can be shared through the online platform. Alternatively, Villarreal-Davis et al. (2020) have made a set of printable pdf miniatures and tray available for public use. Supervisees can cut out the images to prepare for the virtual supervision session and then arrange them during session, allowing for kinesthetic engagement. Lastly, supervisees can hunt for a tray and a collection of objects in and around their homes. Dry rice, oatmeal, sugar, salt, or cornmeal make excellent sand substitutions. The hands of a creative supervisee can form a humble paperclip into a meaningful symbol in seconds.

Some play therapy supervisors need to tote their supplies to multiple locations, and/or provide supervision with an entire group of supervisees at once. In this case, supervisors can shrink their setups down to make them more portable. Tiny erasers printed and shaped to resemble food, animals, people, and other objects can be sourced inexpensively. Charms from cheap jewelry also work as minuscule figures. When the "miniatures" are this small, the "tray" size is also greatly reduced. Food storage containers with snap-on lids can be filled with sand and stacked together for maximum portability.

Supervisors who face such challenges must employ cognitive flexibility. They must begin seeing the world around them as children do, with wonder and imagination. The search for sandtray alternatives becomes a treasure hunt of sorts, connecting the supervisor with the creative worlds of the supervisee and the young clients they serve.

Key Readings and Resources for Sandtray Supervision

The following resources may prove helpful for developing a basic understanding of sandtray therapy:

- *Sandtray Therapy: A Practical Manual* (Homeyer & Sweeney, 2017) remains the go-to as the primer offering a basic introduction to sandtray therapy, including lists of crucial figures and color photographs to illustrate important concepts
- *Sandtray Therapy: A Humanistic Approach* (Armstrong, 2008) integrates humanistic principles (e.g., Person-Centered and Gestalt approaches) with sand tray work. It includes a DVD of a full-length sandtray session with an adult female client and an entire chapter on sandtray supervision

The following resources offer supplies for conducting sandtray therapy and supervision:

- Free Online Sandtray (Fried, n.d.) is a website offering the ability to engage in sandtray virtually. Visitors to the site can place a variety of miniatures (seven pages of selections), resize the miniatures, rotate and flip miniatures, copy miniatures to create multiples, and screen-share during teletherapy. Readers can access it at https://onlinesandtray.com/
- Sandtray Therapy Miniatures Trays & More (n.d.) is a website offering a variety of sandtray supplies. Readers can access it at https://www.playtherapysupply.com/sand-tray-therapy

References

Anekstein, A. M., Hoskins, W. J., Astramovich, R. L., Garner, D., & Terry, J. (2014). "Sandtray supervision": Integrating supervision models and sandtray therapy. *Journal of Creativity in Mental Health, 9*(1), 122–134. https://doi.org/10.1080/15401383.2014.876885

Armstrong, S. A. (2008). *Sandtray therapy: A humanistic approach* (1st ed.). Ludic Press.

Bainum, C. R., Schneider, M. F., & Stone, M. H. (2006). An Adlerian model of sandtray therapy. *Journal of Individual Psychology, 62*, 36–46.

Bernard, J. M., & Goodyear, R. K. (2018). *Fundamentals of clinical supervision* (6th ed.). Allyn & Bacon.

Blalock, S. (2021). School-based sandtray counseling on a shoe string. *Journal of Creativity in Mental Health.* https://doi.org/10.1080/15401383.2021.1928575

Brashear, C. A., Mathews, R., & Hickman, D. (2019, December 13). *Nature walk sandtray: Utilizing natural elements as sandtray miniatures* [Experiential Session]. Association for creativity in counseling annual conference, Clearwater Beach, FL.

Carson, D. K., & Becker, K. W. (2004). When lightning strikes: Reexamining creativity in psychotherapy. *Journal of Counseling and Development: JCD, 82*(1), 111–115. http://doi.org.proxy.tamuc.edu/10.1002/j.1556-6678.2004.tb00292.x

Cunningham, L. (2013). *Sandplay and the clinical relationship.* Sempervirens Press.

Dale, M. A., & Lyddon, W. J. (2000). Sandplay: A constructivist strategy for assessment and change. *Journal of Constructivist Psychology, 13*(2), 135. https://doi.org/10.1080/107205300265928

Deaver, S. P., & Shiflett, C. (2011). Art-based supervision techniques. *Clinical Supervisor, 30*(2), 257–276. https://doi.org/10.1080/07325223.2011.619456

DeDomenico, G. S. (1995). *Sandtray world play: A comprehensive guide to the use of sand tray in psychotherapeutic and transformational settings.* Vision Quest Images.

Drewes, A. A., & Mullen, J. A. (2008). *Supervision can be playful: Techniques for child and play therapist supervisors*. Aronson.

Eberts, S., & Homeyer, L. (2015). Processing sand trays from two theoretical perspectives: Gestalt and Adlerian. *International Journal of Play Therapy*, *24*(3), 134–150. https://doi.org /10.1037/a0039392

Fazio-Griffith, L., Marino, R., & IGI Global. (2021). *Techniques and interventions for play therapy and clinical supervision* (Vol. 1–1 online resource (25 PDFs (310 pages))). IGI Global. http:// services.igi-global.com/resolvedoi/resolve.aspx?doi=10.4018/978-1-7998-4628-4

Flaherty, A. (2018, June 27). *Jack in the box technique*. https://vimeo.com/277335052

Fried, K. (n.d.). *Free online sand tray*. Retrieved March 12, 2021, from https://onlinesandtray .com/

Garrett, M. (2017). Enhancing counselor supervision with sandtray interventions. *Journal of Higher Education Theory and Practice*, *17*(5), 39–45.

Gladding, S. T. (2016). *The creative arts in counseling* (5th ed.). American Counseling Association.

Graham, M. A., Scholl, M. B., Smith-Adcock, S., & Wittmann, E. (2014). Three creative approaches to counseling supervision. *Journal of Creativity in Mental Health*, *9*(3), 415–426. https://doi.org/10.1080/15401383.2014.899482

Hartwig, E. K., & Bennett, M. M. (2017). Four approaches to using sandtray in play therapy supervision. *International Journal of Play Therapy*, *26*(4), 230–238. https://doi.org /10.1037/pla0000050

Homeyer, L. E., & Sweeney, D. S. (2017). *Sandtray therapy: A practical manual* (3rd ed.). Routledge.

Jeppsen, M. L. (2012). *Sand tray therapy: Utilizing indigenous objects with traumatized Haitian orphans* [Ph.D., Regent University]. http://search.proquest.com/docview/1037958599 /abstract/C95A1F3052D6407APQ/1

Kascsak, T. M., & Silverberg, S. (2021). A trauma-informed approach to supervision using play therapy and experiential techniques. In L. Fazio-Griffith & R. Marino (Eds.), *Techniques and interventions for play therapy and clinical supervision* (pp. 1–16). IGI Global. https://doi.org/10.4018/978-1-7998-4628-4.ch001

Markos, P. A., Coker, J. K., & Jones, W. P. (2008). Play in supervision: Exploring the sandtray with beginning practicum students. *Journal of Creativity in Mental Health*, *2*(3), 3–15. https://doi.org/10.1300/J456v02n03_02

McAuliffe, G. J., Eriksen, K., & ACES. (2010). *Handbook of counselor preparation: Constructivist, developmental, and experiential approaches*. SAGE Publications. http://ebookcentral.proquest .com/lib/uncg/detail.action?docID=1016390

Morrison, M., & Homeyer, L. E. (2008). Supervision in the sand. In A. A. Drewes & J. A. Mullen (Eds.), *Supervision can be playful: Techniques for child and play therapist supervisors* (pp. 233–248). Jason Aronson/Rowman and Littlefield.

Niles, E. A. (2021). An integrative approach to play therapy supervision using sandtray therapy. In L. Fazio-Griffith & R. Marino (Eds.), *Techniques and Interventions for Play Therapy and Clinical Supervision* (pp. 106–119). IGI Global. https://doi.org/10.4018/978 -1-7998-4628-4.ch007

Paone, T. R., Malott, K. M., Gao, J., & Kinda, G. (2015). Using sandplay to address students' reactions to multicultural counselor training. *International Journal of Play Therapy*, *24*(4), 190–204. https://doi.org/10.1037/a0039813

Perryman, K. L., Moss, R. C., & Anderson, L. (2016). Sandtray supervision: An integrated model for play therapy supervision. *International Journal of Play Therapy*, *25*(4), 186–196. https://doi.org/10.1037/pla0040288

Prasath, P. R., & Copeland, L. (2021). Rationale and benefits of using play therapy and expressive art techniques in supervision. In L. Fazio-Griffith & R. Marino (Eds.), *Techniques and interventions for play therapy and clinical supervision* (pp. 17–37). IGI Global. https://doi.org/10.4018/978-1-7998-4628-4.ch002

Purswell, K. E., & Stulmaker, H. L. (2015). Expressive arts in supervision: Choosing developmentally appropriate interventions. *International Journal of Play Therapy, 24*(2), 103–117. https://doi.org/10.1037/a0039134

Ramsey, L. C. (2014). Windows and bridges of sand: Cross-cultural counseling using sand tray methods. *Procedia - Social and Behavioral Sciences, 159*, 541–545. https://doi.org/10.1016/j.sbspro.2014.12.421

Richards, S. D., Pillay, J., & Fritz, E. (2012). The use of sand tray techniques by school counsellors to assist children with emotional and behavioural problems. *Arts in Psychotherapy, 39*(5), 367–373. https://doi.org/10.1016/j.aip.2012.06.006

Saltis, M. N., Critchlow, C., & Smith, J. A. (2019). Teaching through sand: Creative applications of sandtray within constructivist pedagogy. *Journal of Creativity in Mental Health, 14*(3), 381–390. https://doi.org/10.1080/15401383.2019.1624995

Sandtray Therapy Miniatures Trays & More. (n.d.). *Play therapy supply*. Retrieved March 19, 2021, from https://www.playtherapysupply.com/sand-tray-therapy

Schuck, C., & Wood, J. (2011). *Inspiring creative supervision*. Jessica Kingsley Publishers.

Stark, M. D., & Frels, R. K. (2014). Using sandtray as a collaborative assessment tool for counselor development. *Journal of Creativity in Mental Health, 9*(4), 468–482. https://doi.org/10.1080/15401383.2014.897663

Stark, M. D., Garza, Y., Bruhn, R., & Ane, P. (2015). Student perceptions of sandtray in solution-focused supervision. *Journal of Creativity in Mental Health, 10*(1), 2–17. https://doi.org/10.1080/15401383.2014.917063

Stoltenberg, C. D., Bailey, K. C., Cruzan, C. B., Hart, J. T., & Ukuku, U. (2014). The integrative developmental model of supervision. In C. E. Watkins & D. L. Milne (Eds.), *The Wiley international handbook of clinical supervision*. John Wiley & Sons, Ltd. https://doi-org/10.1002/9781118846360.ch28

Stoltenberg, C. D., & McNeill, B. W. (2010). *IDM supervision: An integrative developmental model for supervising counselors and therapists* (3rd ed.). Taylor and Francis.

Swank, J. M., & Lenes, E. A. (2013). An exploratory inquiry of sandtray group experiences with adolescent females in an alternative school. *Journal for Specialists in Group Work, 38*(4), 330–348. https://doi.org/10.1080/01933922.2013.835013

Sweeney, D. S., & Homeyer, L. E. (2009). Sandtray therapy. In A. A. Drewes (Ed.), *Blending play therapy with cognitive behavioral therapy: Evidence-based and other effective treatments and techniques* (pp. 297–318). John Wiley & Sons, Inc.

Villarreal-Davis, C., Sartor, T. A., & McLean, L. (2020). Utilizing creativity to foster connection in online counseling supervision. *Journal of Creativity in Mental Health*, 1–14. https://doi.org/10.1080/15401383.2020.1754989

Warr-Williams, J. (2012). *Conversations in the sand: Advanced sandplay therapy training curriculum for masters level clinicians* [Dissertation, University of Pennsylvania]. https://repository.upenn.edu/edissertations_sp2/25

13 Supporting Self-Compassion in Play Therapist Supervision

Staci Born and Charlotte Heckmann

Supporting Self-Compassion in Play Therapist Supervision

Play therapist well-being is critical for clients, therapists, supervisors, and organizations. Studies have estimated that between 21% and 67% of mental health professionals are experiencing high levels of burnout (Morse et al., 2012). Play therapy involves therapists' active participation in, or observation of child client's experiences through, play – play that is sometimes aggressive, traumatic, chaotic, and dysregulating. Play therapists draw from their nervous-system activation to help their clients heal, cope, and integrate their challenges (Dion, 2018). Witnessing children play out the adversities they have experienced, paired with an adult's desire to nurture and protect children, places additional emotional complexity upon play therapists (Webb, 2007). The experiential nature of play therapy is incredibly healing and can also position therapists at greater risk for vicarious traumatization, compassion fatigue, and burnout (Meany-Walen et al., 2018).

Self-compassion increases well-being and resilience to stress and trauma and may shield play therapists from burnout. Clinicians who practice self-compassion have stronger therapeutic relationships, reduced compassion fatigue and burnout, and overall greater well-being (Boellinghaus et al., 2014). Experienced counselors have reported that self-compassion was a profound part of personal growth in recoveries from family-of-origin wounds, working more effectively with clients, lowering unrealistic self-expectations, developing effective boundaries, and self-correcting (Patsiopoulos & Buchanan, 2011).

Self-Compassion

More than just looking on the bright side, self-compassion acknowledges our own suffering, treats ourselves kindly when we experience suffering, and recognizes that suffering is a part of human experience (Neff, 2003b, 2012). Rooted in Buddhist philosophical thought and related to the construct of empathy, compassion linguistically means to "suffer with," and self-compassion shifts the direction of compassion toward the self (Germer & Neff, 2019). The term suffering is used to describe the challenges, errors, and setbacks that are a part of the human

DOI: 10.4324/9781003196075-17

condition. Compassion and self-compassion are separate constructs from each other, as well as from empathy. Compassion and self-compassion differ from empathy by taking the concept one step further. They emphasize understanding the suffering of others, *and* feeling compelled to take action to mitigate it.

Understanding the components of the Self-Compassion Scale assists readers in conceptualizing the development of self-compassion skills. Neff (2003a) developed the most widely used measure of self-compassion, the Self-Compassion Scale. When measuring self-compassion, the scale assesses six components: (1) self-kindness – the ability to extend kindness and understanding to oneself when experiencing difficulty; (2) self-criticism – the judgmental and critical self-talk experienced during difficulties; (3) common humanity – the perception that suffering is a part of the human experience; (4) isolation – the perception that suffering makes one separate and isolated from others; (5) mindfulness – the mindful ability to acknowledge pain and suffering in balanced awareness; and (6) over-identification – when one's identity is consumed by pain and suffering (Neff, 2003a).

Self-compassion is the root of well-being. Individuals who have greater self-compassion are less anxious and depressed (Neff et al., 2007) and have more positive feelings about themselves (Leary et al., 2007). While reducing self-criticism is a key tenet of self-compassion, highly self-compassionate people have more than a sunny disposition; they have greater emotional intelligence and a clearer perspective on their problems (Neff, 2003a; Neff et al., 2007). In relationships, those who have greater self-compassion are more emotionally available (Neff & Beretvas, 2013), have a greater ability to compromise in conflict, and report greater authenticity and less turmoil in conflict situations (Yarnell & Neff, 2013). Self-compassion is also positively correlated with intrinsic motivation to learn and grow, and negatively correlated with a desire to perform to enhance self-image (Neff et al., 2007). Self-compassion has physical benefits, too. It is related to an individual's ability to maintain diet, exercise, and smoking cessation programs (Kelly et al., 2010; Magnus et al., 2010; Neff, 2012).

Self-compassion is more than self-care. Self-care is typically the activities we engage in to promote well-being. However, our efforts are diluted if our minds wander to our to-do list or replay a difficult session with a client while engaging in self-care. Self-compassion promotes kindness to ourselves when we encounter our self-criticism; mindful attention to our pain rather than avoidance; and a connection to others because suffering is a part of the human experience (Neff, 2003b). Therefore, practicing self-compassion while engaged in self-care activities is the true origin of well-being.

Self-Compassion and Cultural Humility

Suffering is universal, yet not all suffering is equal (Germer & Neff, 2019). Play therapists' ability to attend to others with empathy and compassion is limited by their ability to recognize common humanity and the context of others' lives.

Attention to self-compassion in supervision is paramount. Personal reflection of our privileges is an important prelude to understanding the experience of others.

This critical reflection creates space for cultural humility (see Chapter 2), compassion, and empathy. Exploring personal privilege and oppression can evoke pain and suffering. Attending to this suffering with acknowledgment of the systems and activities that maintain privilege, and mindful attunement to our reactions to this awareness is the root of compassion and self-compassionate action (Germer, 2019; Germer & Neff, 2019). Fostering self-compassion predicts higher cultural competence (Gottlieb & Shibusawa, 2020). While cross-cultural variation in self-compassion exists, greater self-compassion significantly predicts less depression and greater life satisfaction across cultures (Neff et al., 2008).

Play Therapists and Self-Compassion

Self-compassion is an acquirable skill. Play therapy supervisors can facilitate and teach supervisees self-soothing techniques, mindful awareness, and strategies for challenging self-judgment (Gilbert et al., 2006; Harman & Lee, 2010; Neff et al., 2007). As more is understood about self-compassion, nurturing and practicing self-compassion deserves a front seat in professional-helper training and supervision, especially in play therapy.

Play therapists come from diverse subdisciplines of mental health practice, including counseling, marriage and family therapy, school counseling, psychology, social work, psychiatry, and psychiatric nursing. While wellness practices are frequently examined within subdisciplines of mental health, few examine wellness practices across subdisciplines. Green et al. (2014) surveyed burnout among mental health subdisciplines and found no significant differences, which is important to consider when applying existing literature to play therapists. Wellness and self-care promotion are often a part of mental health professionals' training. However, play therapists report that their academic program provided inadequate or no preparation for wellness and self-care practices (Meany-Walen et al., 2018). Some academic programs infuse wellness workshops for helpers in training which has demonstrated an increase in self-awareness and ability to balance personal and professional demands for trainees (Wolf et al., 2014). However, the maintenance of these wellness practices after graduation is not well understood (Lenz & Smith, 2010).

Time spent in practice and under supervision is a protective factor for new play therapists. Novice play therapy professionals report experiencing lower levels of self-compassion when compared to their peers who have been in the field for more than seven years (Born et al., 2022). These findings reflect what has been observed across mental health subdisciplines, too; more years in practice as a children's mental health professional have been negatively related to emotional exhaustion and depersonalization (Green et al., 2014).

Play therapy supervision plays a critical role in promoting, practicing, and discussing therapist well-being. Supervisors' modeling of self-compassion practices and actively practicing self-compassion during supervision facilitate co-regulation through mindful attention, increase connectedness among and between participants, and promote self-soothing. Self-compassion in supervision enhances parallel processes between the supervisory relationship and supervisees' therapeutic relationships. The desired outcome of self-compassion practices in play therapy supervision protects the supervisee against the ill-effects of compassion fatigue and vicarious traumatization. Self-compassion enhances the healing powers of play therapy.

Self-Compassion and Play Therapist Impairment

Supervisee's professional codes of ethics, as well as the Association for Play Therapy's Best Practices (2020), clearly emphasize the critical role of professional competence by self-monitoring for signs of impairment, seeking assistance when impairment is noted, assisting colleagues in recognizing impairment, and importantly, refraining from providing therapeutic services when impaired. Vicarious traumatization, secondary traumatic stress, compassion fatigue, and burnout are often erroneously used interchangeably in the literature (Newell & MacNeil, 2010) and can significantly impair play therapists' functioning. This chapter briefly introduces and differentiates each phenomenon and describes the relationship of each construct to self-compassion.

Vicarious Traumatization

Vicarious trauma arises when a play therapist experiences affective and cognitive alterations after empathically engaging with a client's trauma. Specifically, the play therapist experiences "significant disruptions in one's sense of meaning, connection, identity, and world view, as well as in one's affect tolerance, psychological needs, beliefs about self and other, interpersonal relationships, and sensory memory" (Pearlman & Saakvitne, 1995, p. 151). Play therapists may be particularly at risk of experiencing vicarious trauma due to the experiential nature of play therapy and witnessing the re-experiencing of traumatic instances through symbols and play (Meany-Walen et al., 2018; Webb, 2007). If not attended to, vicarious traumatization can impair play therapists' professional functioning, pose risks to client welfare, and disturb adherence to ethical responsibilities (Lawson, 2007). Foreman (2018) and Williams et al. (2012) found significant negative correlations between counselor wellness and levels of vicarious trauma, even when accounting for factors associated with supervision working alliance, job satisfaction, and therapists' perception of their workload.

Self-compassion is an important buffer to vicarious traumatization. Emotional pain often accompanies confronting upsetting life situations out of our control (Germer & Neff, 2013). Play therapy supervisors can promote self-compassion by guiding supervisees to direct mindful attention toward their emotional pain and by practicing self-kindness. These skills assist play therapists in approaching their negative affect instead of avoiding it. Additionally, acknowledging the global suffering of all humans creates connection and combats isolation among play therapists.

Secondary Traumatic Stress

Like vicarious traumatization, secondary traumatic stress occurs because of direct exposure to clients who have experienced trauma (Newell & MacNeal, 2010). The major distinction between secondary traumatic stress and vicarious traumatization is that secondary traumatic stress emphasizes the behavioral symptoms that result from exposure to a client's trauma (Figley, 1995; Newell & MacNeil, 2010). The behavioral indications of secondary traumatic stress parallel post-traumatic stress disorder, including re-experiencing content from a client's story and avoiding or numbing toward potential triggers of the traumatic event (Figley, 1995). Self-compassion reduces the occurrence of secondary traumatic stress. Avoidance behaviors and fearful cognitions maintain the perilous impact of secondary traumatic stress (Hotchkiss, 2018). Play therapy supervisors can support supervisees through mindfulness and self-kindness, which counteract negative affect and cognitions.

Compassion Fatigue

Compassion fatigue differs from vicarious traumatization and secondary traumatic stress because it can occur with little or no contact with clients who have experienced trauma (Sansbury et al., 2015). Compassion fatigue is the overall experience of physical and emotional exhaustion that can emerge due to prolonged use of empathy to support clients who are suffering (Figley, 2002; Newell & MacNeil, 2010; Rothschild, 2006). Like burnout (described below), compassion fatigue occurs over time, while vicarious traumatization and secondary traumatic stress can have a more rapid onset (Newell & MacNeil, 2010). Play therapy involves the use of the physical and affective self, therefore play therapists may be at an increased risk for developing compassion fatigue (Meany-Walen et al., 2018). Self-compassion may be vital to preventing compassion fatigue (Upton, 2018). Self-compassion practice presents the opportunity to nurture empathic awareness and compassion toward others and oneself (Siegel & Germer, 2012).

Burnout

Unmediated vicarious traumatization, secondary traumatic stress, or compassion fatigue can develop into burnout (Argentero & Setti, 2011; Sansbury et al., 2015). Burnout is often a gradual and progressive process that results in emotional exhaustion, an inability to depersonalize client experiences, and a decreased sense of accomplishment. Burnout is globally affiliated with prolonged strain at work and a lack of professional support (Maslach & Jackson, 1981). Broadly, self-compassion has been significantly negatively associated with burnout (Richardson et al., 2018). Specifically, counselors have reported that self-compassion development was associated with increased emotional balance, mental clarity, groundedness, openness, wisdom, joy, creativity, freedom, job satisfaction, and burnout prevention (Patsiopoulos & Buchanan, 2011).

Supervision Activities That Support Self-Compassion in Play Therapy

Self-compassion has a critical role in play therapist well-being. Supervisors who choose to incorporate self-compassion in their supervision practices should consider mindful attention to their practice of self-compassion. Authenticity and genuineness are at the core of the supervisory relationship and working alliance. Therefore, genuinely engaging in self-compassion activities are critical to successful use in supervision. Some of the following strategies have been adapted from Germer and Neff's (2019) Teaching the Mindful Self-Compassion Program. This author has adjusted them to demonstrate the application of self-compassion practice in play therapy supervision.

Assessing Self-Compassion

Assessment is a crucial component of effective play therapy supervision (see Chapter 7). Play therapy supervisors can intentionally evaluate the supervisee's self-compassion to understand existing practices that support self-compassion and strategies to improve self-compassion. Neff (2003a) developed the Self-Compassion Scale to measure an individual's self-compassion. This scale, which is freely available on the Internet, allows supervisees and their supervisors to add important knowledge and tools to their play therapy practice. Visit www.self-compassion.org to test how self-compassionate you are. This site includes the assessment and online scoring. This website also contains a pdf version of the Self-Compassion Scale.

Soft Landings

As opposed to crash landings, Soft Landings are broad mindfulness tools that can be used for beginning supervision or transitioning from one topic or case to the next. The purpose of Soft Landings is to allow play therapist supervisees to become present in supervision through a 1- to 2-minute activity. The brevity of the activities demonstrates the potential rapidity and ease of becoming present in professional and personal activities (Germer & Neff, 2019), which is critical, given the demands of play therapy clinical work. This author suggests utilizing a Soft Landing before implementing additional self-compassion activities described in this chapter.

Directing mindful attention to our suffering is courageous work and therefore supporting ourselves through self-compassion is critical. Soft Landings might include brief mindful breathing, offering ourselves words of encouragement, or a quick body scan to notice tension or stress in our body and compassionately melt it away (Germer & Neff, 2019).

Self-Compassion Visualization and Creation

This activity can be done after supervisees complete the Self-Compassion Scale (www.self-compassion.org) or after the supervisee has a foundational knowledge of self-compassion. If the supervisee completes the scale, a set of scores for each subscale of self-compassion will be presented (self-kindness, self-judgment, mindfulness, overidentification, common humanity, isolation). Review the descriptions of the subscales. Then, identify the supervisees self-compassion strengths and opportunities for enhancement.

Invite the supervisee to participate in a guided visualization. The purpose of using imagery is to invite the supervisee to experience self-compassion using images, as these can evoke deeper emotional connections and activate other sensory experiences.

- Start by inviting the supervisee to close their eyes if they feel comfortable, or to cast their gaze downwards
- Notice your breath, do nothing to change it. Just notice the sensations that accompany your breath entering your body, nourishing your body, and exiting your body.
- Next, I will share some prompts and you are to allow whatever enters your mind as an image, to just be – no need to judge ourselves harshly or avoid what arises. Our feelings and thoughts are not facts, they just are – feelings and thoughts.
- First, when you think of compassion, notice what images, thoughts, or feelings arise in you. Just allow whatever comes to you to be there or allow things to come and go as they please
- Allow an image, or multiple images, to arise that represents *self-compassion* for you. Take your time. If nothing comes immediately, that is okay. See what emerges after time. It does not have to be a vivid picture; just a felt sense of an image is ok. If numerous images come up, that's okay too. See which one fits as time goes on
- As you experience what is arising for you:
  - What image holds warm feelings for you?
  - What image understands you, your struggles, your feelings?
  - What image shows kindness, care, and concern for you
  - What image is wise, strong, and supporting of you?
  - What image accepts you as you are?
- Notice if your image is a person or not, real or imagined, an animal or living things in nature, young or old, masculine or feminine. Notice the colors associated with it
  - How does your body feel as you hold this image in your mind?
  - Where do you feel sensations?
  - How does your heart feel as you hold this image in your mind?
  - What facial expressions does this image display toward you?
  - What posture or stature does it convey toward you?
  - How does the image communicate with you? What does it say? What tone does it use?
  - When you feel ready, open your eyes

Supervisees can then be invited to take 5 minutes to jot down important experiences, words, and images they encountered during the visualization. Invite the supervisee to draw or create their self-compassion image using a variety of art supplies like pipe cleaners, clay, feathers, etc. Play therapy supervisees can process their experience of visualizing self-compassion while they create, or after their creation. Questions may include:

- Tell me about your creation
- If you could name your creation, what would it be called?
- What is it particularly good at? How can you tell?
- What does it need? How can you tell?
- If your creation could say something, what would it say?
- If your creation could do something, what would it do?

Many more processing questions may be developed based on preference, theory, and spontaneity. Encourage supervisees to place their self-compassion object in a place that reminds them to practice self-compassion during their day.

Self-Soothing Touch

When stimulated through slow-stroking movement or light pressure touch, C-tactile nerve fibers of the skin signal a parasympathetic response from the brain that typically involves a pleasant sensation, decrease in heart rate, reduction in pain, and reward activation (Croy et al., 2022; Stammers, 2017). For example, in interpersonal relationships, kindness and compassion can be expressed with touch by placing a hand on another person's shoulder, offering a hug, or holding someone's hand. While context and receptivity to touch are critical factors in determining their appropriate use, supervisees who are open to self-soothing touch may find it a reliable and novel strategy for activating regulation and practicing self-compassion.

Upon discerning openness to utilizing self-soothing touch, the play therapy supervisor can invite supervisees to explore the forms of touch they find most soothing. The following is a list of self-soothing gestures. Supervisors should read and demonstrate each gesture with the supervisee. Then, allow about 15 seconds for supervisees to experience each gesture before moving on to the next – holding each posture for at least 15 seconds is important. Supervisors can invite supervisees to close their eyes if they feel comfortable.

- Two hands over the heart
- Cupping one hand over a fist over the heart
- One hand on the belly and one over the heart
- Two hands on the belly
- One hand on a cheek
- Cradling one's face in the hands
- Gently stroking one's arms

- Crossing one's arms and giving a gentle squeeze
- Gently stroking one's chest, either back and forth or in small circles
- Cupping the hands in one's lap (Germer & Neff, 2019)

After moving through the above gestures, play therapy supervisors can invite supervisees to explore other forms of self-touch that may soothe. Allow an additional 30 to 60 seconds to explore or practice a self-soothing touch. Encourage supervisees to notice how their bodies respond to their preferred soothing touch. Following the self-soothing touch, ask supervisees what touch they preferred and did not prefer. Supervisees may also notice that they engaged in self-judgment while practicing soothing touch. Supervisors can help supervisees become aware of this and consciously shift back to self-kindness and self-soothing touch (Germer & Neff, 2019). Self-soothing touch is a powerful self-compassion tool as it can be implemented in many spaces and serve as grounding comfort for play therapist supervisees.

Offering Self-Compassion During Suffering

Use this activity after introducing self-soothing touch. This is an opportunity for supervisees to practice mindful reflection while unpacking stressful clients, sessions, or another professional suffering. In this activity, supervisors instruct supervisees to:

1. Think of a difficult situation in your work life that is causing you stress
2. As you think about the situation, use your senses to feel your way into the problem until you notice some discomfort in your body. Notice where in your body you feel the discomfort most
3. Next, slowly say to yourself, "This is a moment of suffering." This is you practicing mindfulness by being present and not avoiding the pain. You might also say, "This hurts," "Ouch!" or "This does not feel good"
4. Then, say to yourself slowly, "Suffering is a part of living." This is you practicing common humanity. You might also say, "Others would feel just like me," "I'm not alone," or "Me too"
5. After, place your hands in a self-soothing touch you enjoyed. Feel the warmth of your hands and the support you can provide yourself. Say to yourself slowly, "May I be kind to myself." "May I give me what I need." This is you practicing self-kindness. Sometimes it can be hard to find the right words without offering advice. Think of what you would say to a friend who is having the same difficulty as you. Offer those words to yourself. (Germer & Neff, 2019, pp 262).

Pause and allow supervisees to experience the moment. Follow-up questions might explore what supervisees noticed about the experience as they moved into the distress and then implemented self-compassion. Supervisors may inquire about the feelings the play therapist supervisee had toward themselves before, during, and after this self-compassion activity.

Self-Compassion Sandtray

Sandtray in play therapy supervision provides an expressive tool to increase supervisee self-awareness (see Chapter 12 for more on sandtray in play therapy supervision). The following are selected prompts that can facilitate the exploration of self-compassion in play therapist development.

- Create a tray that describes your beliefs, thoughts, or feelings about self-kindness or common humanity or mindfulness (pick one)
- Create a tray about what your life would look like without self-judgment or isolation or overidentification (pick one)
- Create a tray that describes a conflict you are experiencing in your play therapy practice. Once complete, explore the tray, explore the presence/absence of self-compassion, explore what the addition of self-compassion would look like in the tray

Compassionate Movement

Movement in play therapy supervision provides the kinesthetic opportunity to enhance a supervisee's self-awareness (see Chapter 15 for more on movement in play therapy supervision). The purpose of compassionate movement is to "move the body from the inside out, rather than in prescribed ways," (Germer & Neff, 2019, p. 222). Play therapy supervisors can guide supervisees to:

1. If able, stand and notice the soles of your feet on the floor. If standing is not possible, a person may notice their arms against their chair, or their bottom in their seat
2. Rock your feet/arms/bottom forward and backward a little and side to side, anchoring your body in your awareness
3. Scan your whole body for other sensations and notice areas of comfort and areas of tension
4. Focus for a moment on a place in your body where you experience tension. Slowly, begin to move your body in a way that feels good to you. You might gently twist your shoulders, roll your head, or bend over and allow your arms to dangle. Or you might jump, shake your arms, or move your feet rapidly. Most importantly, do what feels right for you. Listen to your body and give your body the movement it needs
5. Return your body to stillness and feel your body in the present moment. Notice any changes since you began to move in this way

(Germer & Neff, 2019, p. 222)

Supervisors can process with supervisees how they encountered listening to their body and if they were able to. Additionally, self-judgments may have arisen in this activity and can be discussed too. Supervisors might repeat this activity and ask the supervisee to hold a challenging case in their mind before enacting the scan and movement.

Self-Compassion Letter

Without mindful attention, we often douse ourselves in self-critical thoughts when we make an error or engage in a behavior we are trying to avoid. Unsurprisingly, self-criticism does not motivate change. Instead, self-criticism can be replaced by motivating ourselves with compassion and encouragement (Germer & Neff, 2019). This is a writing activity; begin by asking supervisees to:

1. Think about a behavior you would like to change in your practice of play therapy. This behavior should be something that you often beat yourself up about and is causing difficulty in your life. Write this behavior down
2. Write down how you internally react when you catch yourself doing this behavior. What do you say to yourself? What is the tone of this voice? Write this down
3. Take a moment to shift your perspective to the part of yourself that feels criticized. Notice how you feel when you receive the critical messages. Offer yourself self-compassion if needed, for how hard it is to be treated so harshly. Notice
4. Turn towards your self-critical voice with interest and curiosity. Reflect on why the criticism has gone on for so long. Perhaps the inner critic is trying to protect you in some way, or keep you safe, or help you. What is motivating this inner critic? Write this down
   a. Some may not be able to find a way that their inner critic is attempting to help. This is okay. Continue to offer yourself self-compassion for how you've suffered from this criticism
   b. If you do identify how your self-critical voice may be trying to help you, try to acknowledge this effort. Let your inner critic know that even though the criticism did not serve you well, you understand it was doing its best
5. Now it is time to allow your inner compassionate voice to be heard. This part of you offers you unconditional love and acceptance. This part of you sees how the behavior you criticize yourself for is causing problems in your life
6. Close your eyes and offer yourself a self-soothing touch. Allow the inner compassionate part of you to emerge. It may appear as an image in your mind or a sensation in your body
7. With your eyes still closed, reflect on the behavior that is causing you difficulty. Your inner compassionate voice would like you to try to make a change because it wants the best for you, not because you are undesirable as you are. Repeat a phrase to yourself that portrays your compassionate voice. [Supervisors can offer examples such as]:
   a. I love you, and I don't want you to suffer.
   b. I care about you, and I want to help you make a change
   c. I don't want you to keep hurting yourself. I can support you.
8. Now, open your eyes and write a letter to yourself using your inner compassionate voice. Address the behavior you would like to change. What words do

you need to hear to make a change? What feelings do you need to experience to make a change?

(Germer & Neff, 2019, pp. 242–246)

Once the letter is complete, supervisees can read the letter to themselves or another person if they choose. Explore with supervisees how they experienced their inner critic and inner compassionate voice. Supervisees may keep the letter to remind themselves of their inner compassionate and inner critic voice.

Conclusion

Self-compassion is a powerful tool in enhancing mental health, interpersonal well-being, and motivation. It also serves as a protective force against vicarious traumatization, secondary traumatic stress, compassion fatigue, and burnout that plagues play therapists. Play therapists must be active in preventing their own burnout, rather than a passive recipient of self-care and stress reduction from outside sources. Play therapist supervisors who employ self-compassion strategies in their personal and/or professional lives provide the opportunity to facilitate self-compassion practices in their supervisory relationship, therefore impacting supervisees and the clients they serve.

Key Readings

Germer, C. K., & Neff, K. D. (2013). Self-compassion in clinical practice. *Journal of Clinical Psychology, 69*(8), 856–867. https://doi.org/10.1002/jclp.22021

Germer, C., & Neff, K. (2019). *Teaching the mindful self-compassion program: A guide for professionals*. The Guilford Press.

Neff, K. D. (2003a). The development and validation of a scale to measure self-compassion. *Self and Identity, 2*(3), 223–250.https://doi.org/10.1080/15298860309027

Neff, K. D. (2003b). Self-compassion: An alternative conceptualization of a healthy attitude toward oneself. *Self and Identity, 2*(2), 85–101. https://doi.org/10.1080/15298860309032

Neff, K. D. (2012). The science of self-compassion. In C. Germer & R. Siegel (Eds.), *Wisdom and compassion in psychotherapy: Deepening mindfulness in clinical practice* (pp. 79–92). The Guilford Press.

References

Argentero, P., & Setti, I. (2011). Engagement and vicarious traumatization in rescue workers. *International Archives of Occupational and Environmental Health, 84*(1), 67–75. https://doi.org/10.1007/s00420-010-0601-8

Association for Play Therapy. (2020). Play therapy best practices. https://cdn.ymaws.com/www.a4pt.org/resource/resmgr/publications/apt_best_practices_-_june_20.pdf

Boellinghaus, I., Jones, F. W., & Hutton, J. (2014). The role of mindfulness and loving-kindness meditation in cultivating self-compassion and other-focused concern in health care professionals. *Mindfulness, 5*(2), 129–138. https://doi.org/10.1007/s12671-012-0158-6

Born, S. L., Heckmann, C., Hillerud, K., Oberg, M., & Baker, C. E. (2022). Self-compassion and play therapists well-being. Manuscript in preparation. South Dakota State University.

Croy, I., Fairhurst, M. T., & McGlone, F. (2022). The role of C-tactile nerve fibers in human social development. *Current Opinion in Behavioral Sciences, 43*, 20–26. https://doi.org/10.1016/j.cobeha.2021.06.010

Dion, L. (2018). *Aggression in play therapy: A neurobiological approach for integrating intensity.* W. W. Norton & Company.

Figley, C. R. (Ed.). (1995). *Compassion fatigue: Coping with secondary traumatic stress disorder in those who treat the traumatized.* Brunner/Mazel.

Figley, C. R. (Ed.). (2002). *Treating compassion fatigue.* Brunner-Routledge.

Foreman, T. (2018). Wellness, exposure to trauma, and vicarious traumatization: A pilot study. *Journal of Mental Health Counseling, 40*(2), 142–155. https://doi.org/10.17744/mehc.40.2.04

Germer, C. (2019, June 20). MSC and diversity, equity and inclusion. Center for Mindful Self-Compassion. https://centerformsc.org/msc-and-diversity-equity-and-inclusion/

Germer, C., & Neff, K. (2019). *Teaching the mindful self-compassion program: A guide for professionals.* The Guilford Press.

Germer, C. K., & Neff, K. D. (2013). Self-compassion in clinical practice. *Journal of Clinical Psychology, 69*(8), 856–867. https://doi.org/10.1002/jclp.22021

Green, A. E., Albanese, B. J., Shapiro, N. M., & Aarons, G. A. (2014). The roles of individual and organizational factors in burnout among community-based mental health service providers. *Psychological Services, 11*(1), 41–49. https://doi.org/10.1037/a0035299

Gilbert, P., Baldwin, M. W., Irons, C., Baccus, J. R., & Palmer, M. (2006). Self-criticism and self-warmth: An imagery study exploring their relation to depression. *Journal of Cognitive Psychotherapy: An International Quarterly, 20*(2), 183–200. https://doi.org/10.1891/jcop.20.2.183

Gottlieb, M., & Shibusawa, T. (2020). The impact of self-compassion on cultural competence: Results from a quantitative study of MSW students. *Journal of Social Work Education, 56*(1), 30–40. https://doi.org/10.1080/10437797.2019.1633976

Harman, R., & Lee, D. (2010). The role of shame and self-critical thinking in the development and maintenance of current threat in post-traumatic stress disorder. *Clinical Psychology and Psychotherapy, 17*(1), 13–24. https://doi.org/10.1002/cpp.636

Hotchkiss, J. T. (2018). Mindful self-care and secondary traumatic stress mediate a relationship between compassion satisfaction and burnout risk among hospice care professionals. *American Journal of Hospice and Palliative Medicine, 35*(8), 1099–1108. https://doi.org/10.1177/1049909118756657

Kelly, A. C., Zuroff, D. C., Foa, C. L., & Gilbert, P. (2010). Who benefits from training in self-compassionate self-regulation? A study of smoking reduction. *Journal of Social and Clinical Psychology, 29*(7), 727–755. https://doi.org/10.1521/jscp.2010.29.7.727

Lawson, G. (2007). Counselor wellness and impairment: A national survey. *Journal of Humanistic Counseling, Education and Development, 46*(1), 20–34. https://doi.org/10.1002/j.2161-1939.2007.tb00023.x

Leary, M. R., Tate, E. B., Adams, C. E., Batts Allen, A., & Hancock, J. (2007). Self-compassion and reactions to unpleasant self-relevant events: The implications of treating oneself kindly. *Journal of Personality and Social Psychology, 92*(5), 887–904. https://doi.org/10.1037/0022-3514.92.5.887

Lenz, A. S., & Smith, R. L. (2010). Integrating wellness concepts within a clinical supervision model. *Clinical Supervisor, 29*(2), 228–245. https://doi.org/10.1080/07325223.2010.518511

Maslach, C., & Jackson, S. E. (1981). The measurement of experienced burnout. *Journal of Organizational Behavior, 2*(2), 99–113. https://doi.org/10.1002/job.4030020205

Meany-Walen, K. K., Cobie-Nuss, A., Eittreim, E., Teeling, S., Wilson, S., & Xander, C. (2018). Play therapists' perceptions of wellness and self-care practices. *International Journal of Play Therapy, 27*(3), 176–186. https://doi.org/10.1037/pla0000067

Morse, G., Salyers, M. P., Rollins, A. L., Monroe-DeVita, M., & Pfahler, C. (2012). Burnout in mental health services: A review of the problem and its remediation. *Administration and Policy in Mental Health, 39*(5), 341–352. https://doi.org/10.1007/s10488-011-0352-1

Neff, K. D. (2003a). The development and validation of a scale to measure self-compassion. *Self and Identity, 2*(3), 223–250.https://doi.org/10.1080/15298860309027

Neff, K. D. (2003b). Self-compassion: An alternative conceptualization of a healthy attitude toward oneself. *Self and Identity, 2*(2), 85–101. https://doi.org/10.1080/15298860309032

Neff, K. D. (2012). The science of self-compassion. In C. Germer & R. Siegel (Eds.), *Wisdom and compassion in psychotherapy: Deepening mindfulness in clinical practice* (pp. 79–92). The Guilford Press.

Neff, K. D., & Beretvas, S. N. (2013). The role of self-compassion in romantic relationships. *Self and Identity, 12*(1), 78–98. https://doi.org/10.1080/15298868.2011.639548

Neff, K. D., Kirkpatrick, K. L., & Rude, S. S. (2007). Self-compassion and adaptive psychological functioning. *Journal of Research in Personality, 41*(1), 139–154. https://doi.org/10.1016/j.jrp.2006.03.004

Neff, K. D., Pisitsungkagarn, K., & Hsieh, Y. (2008). Self-compassion and self-construal in the United States, Thailand, and Taiwan. *Journal of Cross-Cultural Psychology, 39*(3), 267–285. https://doi.org/10.1177/0022022108314544

Neff, K. D., Rude, S. S., & Kirkpatrick, K. L. (2007). An examination of self-compassion in relation to positive psychological functioning and personality traits. *Journal of Research in Personality, 41*(4), 908–916. https://doi.org/10.1016/j.jrp.2006.08.002

Newell, J. M., & MacNeil, G. A. (2010). Professional burnout, vicarious trauma, secondary traumatic stress, and compassion fatigue: A review of theoretical terms, risk factors, and preventive methods for clinicians and researchers. *Best Practices in Mental Health: An International Journal, 6*(2), 57–68.

Magnus, C. M. R., Kowalski, K. C., & McHugh, T.-L. F. (2010). The role of self-compassion in women's self-determined motives to exercise and exercise-related outcomes. *Self and Identity, 9*(4), 363–382. https://doi.org/10.1080/15298860903135073

Patsiopoulos, A. T., & Buchanan, M. J. (2011). The practice of self-compassion in counseling: A narrative inquiry. *Professional Psychology: Research and Practice, 42*(4), 301–307. https://doi.org/10.1037/a0024482

Pearlman, L. A., & Saakvitne, K. W. (1995). *Trauma and the therapist: Countertransference and vicarious traumatization in psychotherapy with incest survivors.* Norton Professional Books.

Richardson, C. M. E., Trusty, W. T., & George, K. A. (2018). Trainee wellness: Self-critical perfectionism, self-compassion, depression, and burnout among doctoral trainees in psychology. *Counselling Psychology Quarterly*, 1–12. https://doi.org/10.1080/09515070.2018.1509839

Rothschild, B. (2006). *Help for the helper: Self-care strategies for managing burnout and stress.* Norton Professional Books.

Sansbury, B. S., Graves, K., & Scott, W. (2015). Managing traumatic stress responses among clinicians: Individual and organizational tools for self-care. *Trauma, 17*(2), 114–122. https://doi.org/10.1177/1460408614551978

Siegel, R. D., & Germer, C. K. (2012). Introduction. In C. K. Germer & R. S. Diegel (Eds.), *Wisdom and compassion in psychotherapy: Deepening mindfulness in clinical practice* (pp. 1–6). The Guilford Press.

Stammers, L. (2017). The neurobiology of touch: Developmental play therapy with a child diagnosed with sensory processing disorder. In J. A. Courtney & R. D. Nolan (Eds.), *Touch in child counseling and play therapy: An ethical and clinical guide* (pp. 35–47). Routledge.

Upton, K. V. (2018). An investigation into compassion fatigue and self-compassion in acute medical care hospital nurses: A mixed methods study. *Journal of Compassionate Health Care, 5*(7). https://doi.org/10.1186/s40639-018-0050-x

Webb, N. B. (2007). *Play therapy with children in crisis: Individual, group, and family treatment* (3rd ed.). The Guilford Press.

Williams, A., Helm, H., & Clemens, E. (2012). The effect of childhood trauma, personal wellness, supervisory working alliance, and organizational factors on vicarious traumatization. *Journal of Mental Health Counseling, 34*(2), 133–153. https://doi.org/10.17744/mehc.34.2.j3l62k872325h583

Wolf, C. P., Thompson, I. A., Thompson, E. S., & Smith-Adcock, S. (2014). Refresh your mind, rejuvenate your body, renew your spirit: A pilot wellness program for counselor education. *Journal of Individual Psychology, 70*(1), 57–75. https://doi.org/10.1353/jip.2014.0001

Yarnell, L. M., & Neff, K. D. (2013). Self-compassion, interpersonal conflict resolutions, and well-being. *Self and Identity, 12*(2), 146–159. https://doi.org/10.1080/15298868.2011.649545

14 Mindfulness-Based Techniques in Play Therapy Supervision

Michelle M. Pliske

Mindfulness-Based Techniques in Play Therapy Supervision

Mindfulness

"Are you there?" Seven-year-old "James" asked this question for the second time while tapping on the play therapist's forehead with his index finger. The therapist, "Jordan," was startled but quickly recovered and redirected the child to continue the play therapy session. The child asked Jordan if it was time to leave when more than 15 minutes were remaining in the session. Upon reviewing this recording in supervision, Jordan acknowledged the exchange and stated, "my mind must have wandered. I remember I was thinking about other things … I'm not sure how he knew, considering I was still tracking his play."

Mindfulness is the non-judgmental awareness cultivated by applying one's attention in a specific way in the present moment (Kabat-Zinn, 2015). Simply put, mindfulness is the art of paying attention. However, attention is multi-faceted. Tracking a child's behavior by phenomenologically naming what is observed is a common play therapy response (Ray, 2011). Jordan's ability to track the child's play behaviors in the session was not in congruence to her presence or attunement while providing that reflection. While presence is a state of openness, attunement is presence within a process of focused attention to self or others (Siegel, 2010). The multitasking nature of the encounter (naming the child's behavior while simultaneously lost in thought) contributed to the moment of rupture between Jordan and her client. Jordan concluded that the child may have felt unimportant or that she didn't care about him, prompting his question on whether he could leave early. Effective interventions with children involve developing a strong working relationship and knowing about the child's life and the events that led to the current state of disequilibrium (Figley, 2002; Newell & MacNeil, 2010). The practice of mindfulness fosters an exercising of one's innate capacity to attend and pay attention, giving rise to awareness (Kabot-Zinn, 2015).

DOI: 10.4324/9781003196075-18

Secondary Traumatic Stress and Compassion Fatigue

Play therapists listen intently and, to some degree, absorb a child's worldview, bearing witness through visual imagery to the emotional pain associated with the child or family's suffering (Gil, 2016). Literature and research document the presence of vicarious traumatization, secondary traumatic stress, and compassion fatigue in helping professions (McCann & Pearlman, 1990; Newell & MacNeil, 2010 Skovholt & Trotter-Mathison, 2016). Play therapy supervisors are essential in reviewing supervisee practices to prevent secondary traumatic stress. This is to assist the supervisee in building sustainable play therapy practices.

Figley (1995) defined secondary traumatic stress as "the natural and conse-quential behaviors and emotions resulting from knowing about a traumatizing event experienced by a client and the stress resulting from helping or wanting to help a traumatized or suffering person" (Figley, 1995, p. 7). Secondary traumatic stress is theorized to have increased prevalence when the nature of the relation-ship results from an empathic encounter (therapist to client) as one bears witness to suffering (Newell, 2017).

Compassion fatigue and vicarious trauma are used interchangeably; however, this author notes that compassion fatigue can occur without exposure to traumatic material. Newell and MacNeil (2010) reported that "the experience of compassion fatigue tends to occur cumulatively over time, whereas vicarious trauma and sec-ondary traumatic stress have a more immediate onset" (p. 61). For play therapists, empathic relationships are crucial, but attunement and the act of caring deeply for a child can result in both secondary traumatization and the cumulative stress of compassion fatigue. Harrison and Westwood (2009) assert training is necessary to effectively apply strategies that support supervisee reduction of long-term compli-cations of secondary traumatic stress and compassion fatigue. Approaching super-vision through mindfulness offers one tool for play therapists to buffer against the cumulative stress which negatively affects client relationships.

Incorporating Mindfulness into Supervision

Presence

Siegel (2007) describes presence as an awareness of the mind, one that mindfulness recreates. Mindful supervisors offer a space where a supervisee can be creative, open to new possibilities, and possess an awareness of what it feels like to be pre-sent without judgment. This mindful practice enables flexibility and receptivity to internal and external feedback (Siegel, 2010). Modeling presence and facilitating mindfulness techniques in supervision allows for awareness of the self in relation to others to emerge. This supervisor practice creates space for grounding and stress reduction during complex clinical case review or crisis support (Kestly, 2016). A supervisor's ability to find mindful presence, in turn, models safety within the room. Many play therapists indicate that creating therapeutic safety and building rapport through presence is their first treatment goal. Understanding how it feels to be present is a parallel process within the supervisory relationship to mirror the therapeutic relationship between play therapists and their child clients.

Understanding Presence Through Polyvagal Theory

Presence depends upon a sense of feeling safe within the room. Porges (2011) coined the term "neuroception of safety" within his conversation on polyvagal theory, meaning the brain continuously monitors the external and internal environment for cues of threat or danger. Porges (2011) identified the body's function to process safety and detect threat. These detection systems operate primarily outside of our conscious awareness through neuroception (Porges, 2011). Neuroception integrates internal and external safety and danger signals and coordinates somatic, affective, and autonomic responses. Porges (2011) largely identifies these primary threats to this system: (a) risk of physical or bodily harm, (b) self-doubts, "shoulds," and unobtainable expectations, (c) incongruence in the environment, and (d) unknown or novel experiences.

   Play therapists' past experiences resonate and shape their neuroception of safety during supervision. Traumatic histories shape perspective; therefore, children will monitor whether a therapist's affect is genuine or authentic. False affect (a bright smile even when a therapist is worried, confused, disoriented) will elevate stress for the child and register as a threat. The same is true in supervision. Supervisees register when there is a threat within the supervisory space. Supervisors who offer reflections through an affect that is incongruent with their physiological state will register as false to their play therapy supervisees. This false state is perceived as a threat, creating a rupture within the supervisory relationship and disrupting the felt sense (neuroception) of safety within the session (Porges, 2011). Mindful supervisors self-monitor their stress levels, striving to "name-to-tame" their emotions to their supervisees. They model through direct teaching what it means to have awareness of presence, subsequently regulating their experience. Supervisors can directly apply mindfulness grounding techniques through modeling during supervision, assuming responsibility for their emotional state, and regulating those emotions to maintain a presence within the room.

Attunement

In a supervisory relationship, attunement is a supervisor's ability to pick up on the nuances of their supervisee's responses, interacting with the supervisee in a way that accurately captures the sense of how they are feeling in the moment (Frawley-O'Dea, 2003). The intention is for a play therapist to feel seen and heard by their supervisor. Supervisors who notice and name the emotions within the space can support a supervisee in understanding the perception of their signals, words, and nonverbal patterns of communication, which have energy and patterned information (Siegel, 2010). Creating a "smart vagus" (Porges, 2011) or ventral state where one is not experiencing threat supports the concept that humans are hardwired for empathic responsiveness within connection: "Mirror neurons make emotions contagious, letting the feelings we witness flow through us, helping us get in synch and follow what is going on with another" (Goleman, 2006, p. 42). Attunement requires presence. For a supervisor to understand their supervisee's experience, they must explore attuned resonances. A supervisor will move their presence into the social sphere as they track their supervisee's internal state for interpersonal attunement through verbal or nonverbal reflections. Supervision becomes an analogous process, and the attunement or "felt sense" a supervisee experiences within the relationship can then be translated into their presence and attunement with child clients.

Mindfulness-based supervision allows for attunement to unfold, and creates a space to respond to supervisees' needs, and a similar process for the families they hold, thereby "holding the holder" (Goodyear-Brown & Stauffer, 2019, p. 42–43). Working within healthcare can quickly shift from being stressful to overwhelming. Supervision that harnesses mindfulness offers a way to rebalance power and control back toward a calm state. Supervisors engaged in mindfulness practices can hold space for supervisees in shifting their stress outwards toward a place of letting go of what is outside their control and focusing on what is within their control.

Resonance

How we feel "felt" within social interaction is a form of resonance that requires vulnerability and humility (Brown, 2010a; Siegel, 2010). Play therapists' resonances are intricately linked to their lived experiences (Fish, 2017; Stauffer, 2019) and bridge the separate worlds of the client and therapist. A play therapist may become activated within a conversation or play sequence. This activation can cue the play therapist to further explore how the therapist's activated resonances interact with the child. Emotions arising, such as joy, sorrow, disgust, anger, may resonate within the play therapist and bring into the room a past experience that needs to be uncovered or unpacked to deepen the analysis of the case or connection with the child. For example, a play therapist unpacked his experience of being bullied in middle school. He described being activated in session (anger and anxiety) while he was with his adolescent client. Unpacking these resonances uncovered the link to his own lived experience of being bullied. The adolescent client brought forth that lived experience through the tone of his voice and profile of his face during conversation in session with his play therapist. The therapist's emotions toward his client, and subsequent "dreading" of scheduled sessions, were resolved following exploration and discovery of the association. Exploring resonances amplifies the personal sensibility within the therapeutic context (Elkaim, 2012). Siegel (2010) states:

> Presence permits us to be open to others, and to ourselves. Attunement is the act of focusing on another person (or ourselves) to bring into our awareness the internal state of the other in interpersonal attunement … resonance is the coupling of these two autonomous entities into a functional whole.
>
> (p. 54)

For play therapists to explore resonances during supervision requires both the presence of safety and the attunement with the supervisor. Exploring how a case resonates with a play therapist requires the therapist to unpack activating stressors. Supervisors who can successfully create safety and build trust within the context of relationship (Bloom, 1994) support that supervisory relationship by providing a foundation for the play therapist to feel activated within a holding space. Content during a session, family system engagement, or organizational and supervisory systems can all create activation and draw upon play therapist resonances.

Supervisors are tasked with the duty to support supervisee personal growth through providing direct, honest, respectful, and constructive feedback (Aasheim, 2012), which may be activating for the play therapist. Giving feedback to play therapists during supervision can be a parallel process (Ekstein & Wallerstein, 1972) for clinical work. Play therapists are tasked with providing direct, honest, respectful, and constructive feedback to parents or allied health professionals during a play therapy case. Mindfully engaging with the self allows for professional growth as a play therapist begins to make known resonances, thus finding balance when they move through conversations that create discomfort. Play therapy supervisors who are authentic, understand vulnerability through presence, and attune to their supervisees can offer co-regulatory support and/or direct teaching of mindfulness and grounding. Mindful supervision assists a play therapist in exploring their resonances, fears, or uncertainties within a trusting relationship.

Trust

Seigel (2010) states, "presence, attunement, and resonance are the way we clinically create the essential condition of trust" (p. 75). Trust will emerge from attunement, and trust within a relationship emerges when one achieves a sense of realness in oneself (Rogers, 1980). When supervisors are congruent, they are genuine and can best aid their supervisees. Deep mutual encounters offer mutual empathy and mutual understanding, providing a quality of humanness (Rogers, 1980; Jordan, 2018). Fundamentally, supervisees who don't trust their supervisor will be more guarded and reluctant to share or expand on their thoughts or explore emotional resonances. This state creates a barrier for quality case analysis and limits the play therapist in professional growth.

Mindfulness-Based Techniques

Employing mindfulness-based techniques in supervision creates a parallel pathway for play therapists to utilize mindfulness in session with their child clients. Certainly, there is room to teach techniques for regulation and mindfulness; however, play therapists can learn a lot more from *what* we do than from hearing *how* we do it. Teaching a direct skill has merit and purpose. Still, teaching by involving the supervisee in mindfulness practice provides a deeper understanding of a way of being, thereby solidifying the embodied state of mindfulness.

Mindful Breathing: The Bee Breath

Play therapists can learn about the power of their breath and integrate *pranayama*. *Prana* is Sanskrit for "breath," translating as "sustaining the body," while *ayama* translates to "extending or drawing out" (Schmaizi, Streeter, & Khalsa, 2016; Dix & McClintic, 2016; Pliske & Balboa, 2019). This technique will support the practice of mindful breathing to calm and regulate the body during moments of perceived stress or environmental threat. *Pranayama* promotes deep relaxation to support mindfulness in the reflection of the self.

When play therapy supervisors perceive stress activation within a supervisee, providing a gentle prompt for breath can aid in bottom-up regulation (Perry, 2006). The Bee Breath uses a humming sound to gently encourage longer exhales (Dix & McClintic, 2016). Play therapists who lengthen their exhale in relation to their inhale can activate the parasympathetic nervous system (a branch of the autonomic nervous system), which decreases heart rate, thereby reducing the "flight or fight" stress response and supporting regulation (Van der Kolk, 2014). We can access our autonomic nervous system and increase regulation within the body through our breath, movement, and touch (Van der Kolk, 2014). The Bee Breath harnesses mindfulness to focus entirely on the breath. The idea is that a simple breathing exercise can reinforce a calm state and always be found within the individual (Dix & McClintic, 2016).

Incorporating the Bee Breath exercise into supervision provided the necessary support for Jordan to regulate. Jordan sat on the sofa staring at the ground. She began by intellectually discussing the merits of her case. She had been working with James for several months. The local forensic team referred him due to physical child abuse. He had been removed from his home by child-protection workers and was placed in kinship foster care with his paternal grandmother. James' father died of an overdose when he was an infant, and his mother was in and out of treatment programs while struggling with addiction. His mother would physically abuse him when intoxicated, always blacked out, and never remembered the abuse. Her confusion added to his confusion as he clearly remembered how he obtained the bruises and the spinal fracture, which landed him in the emergency department and later in an interview with a pediatric forensic team. As Jordan discussed the case, her breathing changed. It began to hitch as she spoke, and her words moved rapidly as she articulated details of James' case.

I asked Jordan to pause and sit with her hands on her knees and close her eyes if she felt comfortable doing so. She did. Reducing the multisensory environment can help one focus more intently as we eliminate distractions. I asked her to inhale through her nose and hum the letter "M" sound, like a bumblebee, upon the exhale. Next, I asked her to focus only on her breath and the sound. The buzzing sound slows the exhale to support the parasympathetic response where the exhale (out) is longer than the inhale (in) (Pliske & Balboa, 2019). Jordan repeated this process three times. I asked her what she noticed in her body. She responded that there was a stronger sense of "being there." When I asked her to expand, she was able to identify having a calm presence and feeling connected to the here and now, no longer lost and overwhelmed by the past.

Body Scan

Body scans are a common technique utilized by EMDR practitioners with clients across the lifespan (Shapiro, 2001). The practice of a body scan is a journey through the body as the supervisee focuses specific attention on the body (Pliske & Balboa, 2019). Supervisors can guide play therapists through a brief body scan starting at the feet, moving through the legs, up into the torso, along the shoulders and arms, into the neck and head. The supervisor is working to open awareness to the body and the impact session content, work-related stress, or other stressors have left imprinted on the body. The goal of a body scan is to increase play therapists' awareness of the stress they hold within their body, which often is compartmentalized in a manner that can become disconnected (Pliske & Balboa, 2019). This disconnect impairs the play therapist's ability to feel emotion and sensation and can give rise to incongruence, threatening the neuroception of safety within a play therapy session. Affect congruence involves body awareness and letting go, tolerating, or accepting emotion and sensation (Wolf & Serpa, 2015). The body scan can be an opportunity to practice *non*-striving or "not asking anything from the body. It is more a receiving of sensations" (Wolf & Serpa, 2015, p. 100). Play therapy supervisors can write their own scripts for a body scan, speaking comfortably and using their own words to guide a play therapist through the body to identify each part and simply notice the sensation(s) within. Connecting with supervisees in this manner is about unconditional positive regard within the relationship (Rogers, 1980), one of acceptance without judgment or a quest to find *why* or *how*, but simply acknowledging what *is*.

The body scan is a technique that ties in beautifully with breathwork. A body scan followed Jordan's reflection on feeling in the "here and now." I asked her to simply notice her body, beginning with her feet and moving upwards. We moved through her legs, torso, arms, neck, and head. Jordan said she had noticed feeling a little lightheaded and confused when she was talking about her case. She stated that she now felt like she had more clarity and didn't feel so alone. Jordan stated she felt "connected" to herself.

STOP (Stop, Take a Step Back, Observe, and Proceed Mindfully)

Engaging mindfulness through the STOP technique is easier said than done. Play therapists may develop an expectation that when implementing this technique, they will find a sense of calm immediately (Wolf & Serpa, 2015). However, the STOP technique is better thought of as a way to become fully present in the moment and observe what is happening, rather than simply reacting to it (Linehan, 2015; Wolf & Serpa, 2015). The goal is to experience the emotion and move through the feeling with acceptance rather than follow an agenda to change the emotional experience.

Play therapist resonances may create reactivity, perpetuating the accumulation of stress contributing to compassion fatigue or burnout. STOP helps a play therapist reorient during activation and notice what they are experiencing. Linehan (2015) details the STOP skill through the following directive, which can be adapted for play therapy practice:

Stop: Play therapists don't need to react impulsively. Rather they can notice and name their emotion while simply being present and remaining in control.

Take a step back: Taking a step back during a play therapy session allows a therapist to have a short break. Play therapists can let go, engage their breath, and not let their emotions drive them to act rashly.

Observe: Simply observing what the play therapist is experiencing internally and externally (stress-response-system scanning for threats) can support a play therapist in recognizing their own resonances during the encounter.

Proceed mindfully: Play therapists can act with awareness, make decisions on how to reflect, or opportunities to re-engage in the play while considering their thoughts and feelings about the situation.

Play therapists utilizing STOP during play therapy sessions can bring those experiences into supervision. Supervision serves as an opportunity to explore the encounter within a secure holding environment. Conversely, play therapy supervisees who become activated while processing difficult case content may benefit from a STOP exercise facilitated by their supervisor. The STOP exercise allows an opportunity for play therapists to pause and then reflect following grounding and regulation. This technique therefore serves as a bottom-up regulatory process to support greater cognitive processing and creative thought during supervisory reflection (Perry, 2006; Pliske & Balboa, 2019).

Jordan reported feeling more connected to her own body, which she interpreted as being in touch with her emotions, regaining a sense of control, while feeling supported to "let it all out." I asked Jordan if we might use a technique to help organize our thinking. Jordan agreed and engaged in the STOP technique to further support the processing of her experience. When reflecting upon her play therapy session, Jordan noticed and named her emotions (confusion, anger, followed by helplessness). When she noticed these emotions, we discussed simply naming them without judgment and taking a step back for regulation. Jordan could reflect the emotion to the child in session and model regulation (movement, stretching, diaphragmatic breath), which also supports the integration of therapeutic powers of play (Fraser, 2014). Jordan's processing yielded activation within her own stress response system. Jordan recalled that James had identified one doll in the dollhouse as the mother. This doll was systematically hitting another doll (child). Jordan's client then moved the child doll under the bed to hide while the mother moved around the dollhouse. The mother eventually went to sleep on the sofa. Jordan's reflection included the observation that during this play, she "checked-out." Jordan states she recalled disconnecting from the scene entirely. Jordan brought this realization into her awareness and discussed strategies for proceeding mindfully to engage coping and regulation during play intensity to keep her grounded in the present moment.

RAIN (Recognize, Acknowledge or Allow, Interest or Investigate, Non-identify)

Play therapists can transform thinking and generate new ideas for solving society's most difficult problems. The work is engaging, never boring, and always changing. This work also asks the clinician to look deeply into their own past, unpack intersecting identities, and critically examine resonances with an expectation of continuous personal growth because working with others fundamentally changes our perspectives. RAIN is a skill or technique that can be difficult to facilitate. It also requires the supervisor to engage in their own work, exploring resonances to best equip them with readiness for holding space for another play therapist. The following, adapted from Wolf & Serpa (2015), serves as an outline for the acronym RAIN:

Recognize: Play therapists are invited to lean into the moment of recognition as that is the moment when awareness emerges (similarly to the "S" in STOP). This becomes an opportunity to realize a play therapy supervisee is in the grip of strong emotion. This allows for truth to emerge when the process is grounded in relational trust.

Acknowledge or Allow: Play therapists are encouraged to allow the therapeutic process to happen, therefore acknowledging that the emotional experience is valid. This involves turning toward and not away from what the play therapist perceives as challenging. Play therapists are habitually asked to engage in work that includes intensity and discomfort. Allowing emotions to emerge and processing those perceptions and experiences during supervision is critical for professional growth.

Interest or Investigate: This process is when a play therapist can become curious about the moment, their emotional world, and lean into their feelings (positive or negative). There is a propensity to numb or avoid emotions society has deemed negative or unpleasant (Brown, 2010a). Having interest is about exploring how a specific emotion manifests in the body during present-day encounters. The play therapist is encouraged to invest time and emotional resources to strengthen their understanding of this process through curiosity and kindness.

Non-identify: Play therapists may notice a physical manifestation of emotion but struggle with the meaning assigned to that emotion. Supervisors who can support play therapists in the journey of experiencing emotion like a storm passing, not taking the process personally, will help increase their supervisee's regulatory capacity and improve self-worth. The subtle, yet important, shift away from "I'm feeling anxious … I'm an anxious person!" toward a thinking process such as, "I'm feeling some anxiety at this moment, and it shall pass," provides an opportunity for play therapists to normalize the human experience and let go of labels that activate the stress response system (shoulds).

Jordan processed her activation and what resonated within her during the play. We wove in the RAIN technique to guide the processing. This was aided by the use of visual art in the form of a sandtray miniature to add an expressive arts component to her processing. Images are powerful tools to elicit emotional content and bring into awareness past experiences. Jordan leaned into the moment in which she felt a strong emotion during that session, prior to "checking-out." Jordan moved through the sandtray miniatures and selected a female tiger with her mouth open and teeth bared. She set the miniature on the table in front of her chair. I asked her to look at her selection, without judgment, and simply allow the emotion she felt to emerge. Jordan's eyes became damp as she investigated the miniature. Jordan said, "It's a like me phenomenon." Jordan had grown up in a household with an alcoholic mother. She remembered feeling afraid as a child, not knowing who would be waiting for her when she got home from school. Jordan described hiding in her room or burying herself in stuffed animals when her mother was struggling. She pointed at the tiger and said, "That's my mother, and I can imagine what James felt in that home. I understand his abuse." Jordan worried aloud if she was a bad therapist and began to shift toward fear of being an imposter. I reminded her we don't need to label ourselves and reflected that some of the most impressive play therapists I have ever had the privilege of working with understood child trauma, not because they read about it in a book, but because they have lived experiences. This is an opportunity for her to lean in, actualize her strengths, and engage in the work with greater knowledge about herself.

Conclusion

Mindfulness is simple in its true form. It increases awareness generating opportunity for action. These practices provide care for the therapist so that they can freely give care in return to their clients. Supervisors who can support the play therapist in directing attention back toward the self in a compassionate and gentle way are offering light and hope during moments that may otherwise feel dark and hopeless. When therapist resonances can be explored within mindful supervision, therapy can progress with the client.

Counteracting the impact of secondary traumatic stress and compassion fatigue is fundamental for play therapist sustainability. Mindful supervision has the potential to become mindful practice and mindful living. Supervisors offer their supervisees a way of being that can fundamentally change the course of treatment for a child and trajectory for a career. Sustainable practices mean continued care for children and families within all our communities.

Jordan often reflected on the encounter during play therapy when James wisely understood the power of presence. She determined this encounter was the start of awakening, a shifting of her practice toward intentional attentive care. She was thankful to James, who had the courage to name what was missing in their relationship. This provided her with an opportunity for deep reflection during supervision. This one encounter changed the course of her practice. Jordan found herself more present and open. Jordan's supervision began to demonstrate a difference in her state of being during sessions. Jordan identified her ability to lean into what was difficult and share what was most vulnerable, knowing she offered a holding space; not in words, but by a way of being, with hands to receive her clients just as they were.

References

Aasheim, L. (2012). *Practical clinical supervision for counselors: An experiential guide.* Springer.

Bloom, S. (1994). The sanctuary model: Developing generic inpatient programs for the treatment of psychological trauma. In M. B. Williams & J. F. Sommer (Eds.), *The handbook of post-traumatic therapy.* Greenwood Press.

Brown, B. (2010a). *The gifts of imperfection: Let go of who you think you're supposed to be and embrace who you are: Your guide to a wholehearted life.* Hazelden Publishing.

Brown, S. (2010b). *Play: How it shapes the brain, opens the imagination, and invigorates the soul.* Penguin Group.

Dix, J., & McClintic, J. (2016). *Imagination yoga inspiring kids to move: Calm curriculum.* [Unpublished manuscript]. Imagination Yoga, LLC.

Ekstein, R., & Wallerstein, R. S. (1972). *The teaching and learning of psychotherapy* (2nd ed.). International University Press.

Elkaïm, M. (2012). Les résonances picturales [Pictorial resonances]. *Cahiers Critiques de Thérapie Familiale et de Pratiques de Réseaux, 48*(1), 149–166. http://doi.org/10.3917/ctf.048.0149

Figley, C. R. (1995). *Compassion fatigue: Coping with secondary traumatic stress disorder in those who treat the traumatized.* Brunner/Mazel.

Figley, C. R. (2002). Compassion fatigue: Psychotherapists' chronic lack of selfcare. *Psychotherapy in Practice, 58*(11), 1433–1411. http://doi.org/10.1002/jclp.10090

Fish, B. (2017). *Art-based supervision: Cultivating therapeutic insight through imagery.* Routledge.

Fraser, T. (2014). Direct teaching. In C. E. Schaefer & A. A. Drewes (Eds.), *The therapeutic powers of play: 20 core agents of change* (2nd ed., pp. 39–50). Wiley.

Frawley-O'Dea, M. G. (2003). Supervision is a relationship too: A contemporary approach to psychoanalytic supervision. *Psychoanalytic Dialogues, 13*(3), 355–366. http://doi.org/10.1080/10481881309348739

Gil, E. (2016). *Posttraumatic play in children: What clinicians need to know.* Guilford Press.

Goleman, D. (2006). *Social intelligence: The new science of human relationships.* Bantam Books.

Goodyear-Brown, P., & Stauffer, S. D. (2019, June). Not taking the trauma home: Holding the holder. *Play Therapy, 14*, 42–46.

Harrison, R. L., & Westwood, M. J. (2009). Preventing vicarious traumatization of mental health therapists: Identifying protective practices. *Psychotherapy: Theory, Research, Practice, Training, 46*(2), 203–219. http://doi.org/ 10.1037/a0016081

Jordan, J. (2018). *Relational cultural therapy* (2nd ed.). American Psychological Association.

Kabat-Zinn, J. (2015). Mindfulness. *Mindfulness, 6,* 1481–1483. http://doi.org/10.1007/s12671-015-0456-x

Kestly, T. A. (2016). Presence and play: Why mindfulness matters. *International Journal of Play Therapy, 25*(1), 14–23. http://doi.org/10.1037/pla0000019

Linehan, M. (2015). *DBT skills training manual* (2nd ed.). Guilford Press.

McCann, I. L., & Pearlman, L. A. (1990). Vicarious traumatization: A contextual model for understanding the effects of trauma on helpers. *Journal of Traumatic Stress, 3,* 131–149. http://doi.org/10.1007/s10615-015-0573-y

Newell, J. M. (2017). *Cultivating professional resilience in direct practice: A guide for human service professionals.* Columbia University Press.

Newell, J. M., & MacNeil, G. A. (2010). Professional burnout, vicarious trauma, secondary traumatic stress, and compassion fatigue: A review of theoretical terms, risk factors, and preventive methods for clinicians and researchers. *Best Practices in Mental Health, 6*(2), 57–68. http://doi.org/10.1080/15555240.2011.540978

Perry, B. D. (2006). The neurosequential model of therapeutics: Applying the principles of neuroscience to clinical work with traumatized and maltreated children. In N. B. Webb (Ed.), *Working with traumatized youth in child welfare* (pp. 27–52). The Guilford Press.

Pliske, M., & Balboa, L. (2019). *Integrating yoga and play therapy: The mind-body approach for healing adverse childhood experiences.* Jessica Kingsley Publishers.

Porges, S. W. (2011). *The polyvagal theory: Neurophysiological foundations of emotions, attachment, communication, and self-regulation.* Norton.

Ray, D. (2011). *Advanced play therapy: Essential conditions, knowledge, and skills for child practice.* Routledge.

Rogers, C. R. (1980). *A way of being.* Mariner Books.

Schmaizi, L., Streeter, C. C., & Khalsa, S. B. S. (2016). Research on the psychophysiology of yoga. In S. B. S. Khalsa, L. Cohen, T. McCall, & S. Telles (Eds.), *The principles and practice of yoga in health care* (pp. 51–68). Handspring Publishing.

Shapiro, F. (2001). *Eye movement desensitization and reprocessing: Basic principles, protocols, and procedures.* Guilford.

Siegel, D. (2007). *The mindful brain: Reflection and attunement in the cultivation of well-being.* Norton.

Siegel, D. (2010). *The mindful therapist: A clinician's guide to mindsight and neural integration.* Norton.

Skovholt, T. M., & Trotter-Mathison, M. (2016). *The resilient practitioner: Burnout and compassion fatigue prevention and self-care strategies for the helping professions* (3rd ed.). Routledge.

Stauffer, S. D. (2019). Ethical use of drawings in play therapy: Considerations for assessment, practice, and supervision. *International Journal of Play Therapy, 28*(4), 183–194. http://doi.org/10.1037/pla0000106

Van der Kolk, B. (2014). *The body keeps the score: Brain, mind, and body in the healing of trauma.* Viking.

Wolf, C., & Serpa, J. G. (2015). *A clinician's guide to teaching mindfulness: The comprehensive session-by-session program for mental health professionals and health care providers.* New Harbinger Publications.

15 Art and Movement in Play Therapy Supervision

Working Through Inevitable Trauma Stuckness

Sarah D. Stauffer and Michelle M. Pliske

Introduction

Sometimes therapists' ideas and feelings about casework are not easily explained in words, especially when their cases are complex, confusing, or triggering. When play therapists feel "stuck," like spinning their wheels in mud without making real movement despite the constant effort made in trauma casework, supervisors can help them explore their resonances more deeply (Cheung & Pau, 2013) and to reflect on the therapeutic relationship (Levine, 2015). Art is moving. Movement sets intentions into motion that are unwitting or unspoken. Play therapist supervisors may use art, such as drawings and imagery (Fish, 2017; Stauffer, 2019) or movement (Devereux, 2015; Federman et al., 2019; Ko, 2014, 2016) to enhance therapists' knowledge of the therapist–child relationship and to increase their understanding of and availability to the child, especially when the child has been affected by traumatic experiences.

Trauma, as a mind–body experience, must be treated at different levels, including the body's role and functions and the client's neurological development and consequences (somatic and relational). Malchiodi (2020) explained, "the mind is defined not only as a function of the brain but as a system that involves the individual in relation to others" (p. 40). Traumatic experiences, particularly those stemming from interpersonal violence, tend to sever the connections between individuals and themselves and between themselves and their communities, and necessitate re-establishing this connection (Herman, 2015). The process begins by establishing safety and proceeds through recognizing and strengthening the mind–body connection affected to integrate traumatic experiences and attain mastery over personal reactions (Herman, 2015; van der Kolk, 2014) on different tiered levels.

The client who has survived a traumatic experience may exhibit somatic symptoms and manifest behavioral and relational consequences, even within the therapist–client relationship. The play therapist, resonating with an aspect of the trauma or the client's reactions to it, must examine their resonances to discover the reverberation felt from their own life experiences (Elkaïm, 2002, 2004) in triadic interaction within the therapeutic relationship. The supervisor acts as a container for the entire therapeutic system and "hold[s] the holder" (Goodyear

DOI: 10.4324/9781003196075-19

Brown & Stauffer, 2019) until the stuckness can be worked through and overcome first in supervision, then in therapy with the client.

Combining logic and creativity is a formula recommended to help supervisees (Koltz, 2008) reap the benefits of the mind–body connection and treat the consequences of the connection that trauma has severed. Therefore, the authors utilize a systemic theory base and relational-cultural theory to highlight several therapeutic powers of play (Schaefer & Drewes, 2014) within the chapter, such as therapeutic relationship, empathy, direct and indirect teaching, self-expression, access to the unconscious, catharsis, creative problem-solving, and resiliency, to support supervisors' interventions and help supervisees overcome difficulties and gain insight into difficult cases. Creating an effective alliance with the supervisee in the context of art and movement supports interactional factors for processing client cases and play therapist resonances. Munns (2008) described that it is wise for therapists to employ activities designed to tap into their deeper and more unconscious feelings to help them "learn something about themselves in a new way" (p. 278).

Using Relational-Cultural and Systemic Theories in Play Therapy Supervision

When the "person of the play therapist emerges [as] a professional … supervision becomes consultation, often initiated by the supervisee to explore the self in relation to play therapy" (Thomas, 2015, p. 4). Jordan (2018) defined relational-cultural theory (RCT) as "the premise that throughout the lifespan human beings grow through and toward connection" (p. 3). Relational-cultural theory applied to supervision expands beyond the exchange between two individuals and provides a lens for a supervisor to understand the exchange between their supervisee and other systems (e.g., client systems, agency, community, larger societal systems) that the supervisee will encounter within their lived experience. The role of a play therapist is often to navigate several different systems simultaneously. The play therapist must attend to the micro encounter with their child client. The therapist also attends to the mezzo encounter. This may include parent consultations, family-system intervention, school advocacy, court advocacy, navigating agency politics/policies/procedures, and understanding neighborhoods and communities in which the child and family live. Play therapists are often tasked with evaluating whether these environments are (un)safe. Play therapists determine whether a family is struggling with poverty or other barriers that may influence treatment. Finally, the play therapist interacts with the larger macro encounters impacting the micro and mezzo systems by influencing policy to initiate social change.

There is an expectation for play therapists to lead the charge in caring for children affected by mental illness. The play therapist is expected to understand the rules, laws, and governance models of health care service delivery, education (private and public sectors), inequity (e.g., marginalization, racism, oppression), and judicial systems for criminal and civil court, for example. These systems all impact the child whom a play therapist serves. The play therapist has to make considerable effort to support growth and healing, and these same systems may neither support nor assist the play therapist in reaching those goals. Play therapists witness unspeakable atrocities and may work within systems not equipped to support their work. The supervising relationship serves to hold space for that supervisee to unpack and counteract the secondary traumatic stress (Figley, 1999) and fatigue experienced within helping professions. Relational-cultural supervision becomes an agent of change to protect and guard against compassion fatigue (Newell, 2017) and burnout (Skovholt & Trotter-Mathison, 2016).

Multiculturalism and Social Justice

Relational-cultural approaches challenge dominant theoretical assumptions to become more inclusive to a spectrum of human experience and identity. Relational-cultural play therapy supervision will employ activities designed to uncover deeper and more unconscious feelings supporting learning about cultural bias, systemic oppression, diversity, and resonances influencing therapists' perspectives, decision-making, or lack of decision-making and "stuckness."

Relationships are embedded within communities and larger cultural systems; therefore, RCT honors multiculturalism as a principle and challenges power and privilege. This, in turn, challenges the supervisor to include the whole of their supervisee's personal and professional experiences within supervision sessions. RCT draws upon the concept of intersectionality, or how intersecting identities interplay within relational theoretical principles to understand human development and power within systems. Relational-cultural play therapy supervision seeks to identify play therapist identities in relationship to the child, family, and community systems.

Concurrently, play therapy supervision also asks the supervisor to utilize expressive arts modalities to understand intersecting identities in relationship to their supervisee. The depth of this examination builds new understandings of the supervisor–supervisee relationship and supports deepening the quality of the supervisory relationship. Just as the presence of a strong therapeutic alliance is necessary for change to occur and predicts better therapeutic outcomes for clients (Stewart & Echterling, 2014), the quality of the supervisory alliance and relationship are essential to improving client care and treatment.

Therapeutic Relationship

Humans have evolved to connect. We seek engagement with each other and need to be in relationships (Stewart & Echterling, 2014). Jordan (2018) asserted, "We need relationships in the same life-sustaining ways that we need air and water. We are simply and essentially interdependent beings" (p. 4). It is a dance of attunement that shifts behavior and expresses the quality of feeling within a shared state of the internal self (Stern, 1985). The concept of shared affect attunement is illustrated in the quality of attachment relationships created by secure connections when one feels understood (Jordan, 2018). Supervisors utilizing movement and the arts provide multiple opportunities for their play therapy supervisees to experience shared affect attunement and opportunity for being seen, heard, and understood.

To illustrate, the second author found herself in deep conversation with a play therapy supervisee regarding their work with a six-year-old girl deeply impacted by trauma. It was suspected that the child had been sexually abused for several years by her paternal uncle. The child told her mother about the "bad touch" that happened during the workday. The child's parents reacted swiftly, and a forensic team interviewed her. The child would not answer any questions during the forensic interview; however, physical evidence supported abuse had occurred by someone, though there were limited possibilities to prosecute without clear disclosure. She was referred to a seasoned play therapist who specialized in trauma.

The play therapist had been working with the child for about 8 months when she reported feeling stuck and worried she was unable to help the child any further. She worried aloud whether the child needed to be referred to another therapist. The therapist wisely asserted that a referral in the middle of trauma treatment felt like a last-resort option. Play therapists understand trauma disrupts attachment and that children seek safety within the playroom (Gil, 2017). Chronic transitions within the therapeutic setting further disrupt trauma reprocessing if children are shuffled from provider to provider (Bloom & Farragher, 2011).

The play therapist engaged in supervision, focusing on the child's specific play behaviors, mannerisms, toy selection, and the repetition of play. Using words to convey a deep understanding, empathy, and analysis of the supervisee's "stuckness" did not advance the treatment. Supervision recreated a parallel process to the play therapy sessions: repetitive and stuck in a tense, focused, analytical cycle. Approaching what felt stuck through a right-brain process, using imagery instead of words, provided an opportunity to zoom out and see possible solutions from a broader perspective.

When using art and movement activities in supervision or therapy, it is important for all participants to remain in a receptive and therapeutic posture. Fish (2017) recommended starting with a supervisory *intention* (p. 67), such as "I am present and open to feedback" or a question, such as "Why do I feel so angry in my client's presence?" The supervisee was prompted to select images from the Dixit game (Roubira & Cardoua, 2016), without overthinking the selection, and she set the supervisory intention to be open and receptive. The images ranged in complexity but offered the ability for the supervisee to project her somatic, felt, lived experience within the playroom onto the images as she processed the case in a new way. The image that caught her attention was one she found herself returning to several times, even though she did not immediately know the meaning behind the image selection. The supervisee finally selected two images and placed them in the center of the table.

The first image depicted a rider on a horse with a rainbow bridge to take that rider from a desolate place to one filled with life and growth. She labeled that image "post-traumatic growth." The second image was of a ribbon being cut, separating one group of people from another. She stated, "My client has been separated from her family in one quick cut. She was suddenly cut off from those she loved. Fighting began between families who once trusted and loved each other." She continued, "This image with the rainbow is where we are and where we want to go, but I can't get there."

The supervisor asked, "What does it feel like in the room?" The supervisee placed two more images on the left side of her first selections. One was of a girl sitting on a highchair playing music as the music sheets floated down around her in a haphazard fashion. The second was of a creature with a large mess littering the floor around them: "It feels like chaos. I feel confused, messy, and disorganized." The play therapist paused and then started to laugh to herself, stating, "You know, I may have just described her attachment style." The therapist described the girl's history, in which the child's mother has struggled with anxiety and has had a difficult time returning to work. This mother often presented as very anxious during family therapy sessions. The child's father, in contrast, has a blunted presentation, seemingly disconnected at times.

The supervisor prompted to expand the therapist's understanding and self-expression further: "What feels missing from the session?" The final two selections were placed on the right side of the supervisee's first two selections. These images represented what the therapist wanted to provide, though she described feeling like she was providing the exact opposite experience to the child. The therapist pointed to the first image of a long road filled with dishes, some covered with a cloche to represent unseen possibilities, and others open for the taking. The final image was of a large eye staring at a tiny animal who appeared frightened, standing on a dinner plate with a fork laying next to it. With emotion evident in her eyes and voice trembling, the therapist described that she may have been so intent on helping the child disclose a name that instead of the open road of possibilities, she was creating a space of intense observation and fear.

The pressure to receive direct disclosure had been building. The district attorney had been calling for the past several weeks to check on the child's progress; parents emailed, left voice messages, and scheduled frequent consultations to inquire about the play therapy process and whether their daughter had "told." The school had been in communication, concerned by some behaviors in the classroom, wondering what they could do to support the therapeutic process in conjunction with a polite, but pressured, inquiry as to how long this all might take. The therapist looked at her images and started to speak but stopped. She started once more and stopped again. She breathed and finally said softly, "I also think I'm feeling pressure because I'm not White. It is almost like the expectations are even greater because I have to prove myself, my worth, to everyone."

Holding an internalized racism with a supervisee's direct experience of systemic institutional racism from the macro level while processing mezzo and micro aspects of this situation highlights a supervisor's challenge. Navigating a multisystem environment to support a play therapist in understanding and clarifying a problem is difficult to do without one or both parties becoming overwhelmed by the enormity of the task. Systemically, the play therapist was simultaneously holding the child's experience (micro); traversing the family, school, and judicial criminal court systems (mezzo); and consciously acknowledging the historical, past, and present microaggressions and overt racism and systemic institutional oppression she experienced (macro).

The supervisor selected an image for the supervisee. This image represented openness to new ideas, with the therapist holding the keys to trauma-processing, providing a platform for supervisor reflection of the therapist's strengths and an unconditional positive regard for the work and process of therapy. The supervisee added her own image to her supervisor's reflections, identifying moments of grit and determination in her life and her hope for the future. The supervisee selected a final image of what she described as teardrops of pain, joy, relief, new beginnings, and hope.

The supervisee reflected on her own lived experiences of being a person of color, growing up in poverty, and learning about child sexual abuse in her own family. The therapist's grandfather had sexually abused her aunt and several of her cousins. She had never experienced molestation herself and described survivor guilt that she was "spared." She reflected upon the process of therapy, and how a therapist can feel rushed or pressured to perform or supply results. This pressure may be felt differently, depending upon identity within society. She identified this in conjunction with her own experience and how she has felt driven to help and protect this child and prove herself to the community. She expressed that the reality of her work was messy and that trauma included a multitude of emotions, both from the child and her own resonances. She responded that her next step was to hold space in a new way, not to scrutinize and analyze to "help and show her worth," but instead to be in the room as herself with all the messy complexities of humanity.

Several weeks later, the therapist reported that "everything had changed" and described the child's play shifting in the room. There were sessions that held positive emotions and appeared to broaden the play with greater exploration and creativity. This reflection was consistent with therapeutic powers of play as key change agents for growth and recovery, offering room for self-expression (Morrison Bennett & Eberts, 2014) and positive emotions (Kottman, 2014). The therapist theorized her transformation of presence during sessions was supported through empathic attunement within the therapeutic relationship. Essentially, she created conditions for interpersonal child-directed play to emerge by contingently and sensitively responding to the child through supportive reflections and authentic warmth (Stewart & Echterling, 2014). The child directly disclosed her sexual abuse experiences to the therapist approximately 2 months later, 10 months into treatment.

Jordan (2018) described an inherent human need of shared affect attunement and secure attachment for survival. Just as Malchiodi (2020) described using expressive arts in therapy to establish "a sense of safety, positive attachment, and prosocial relationships" (p. 52), so too can these concepts be used in play therapy supervision to explore therapists' resonances when trauma cases leave them feeling stuck and helpless in session. Therapists' resonances are inextricably linked to their lived experiences (Fish, 2017; Stauffer, 2019), making play therapists feel vulnerable and inadequate in exploring them, though it is important to do so. Not exploring unresolved trauma resonances may result in an "inability to remain present, a reduction of tracking and facilitative responses, and inability to identify play themes, the inadequate maintenance of the playroom, or a general lack of playfulness and wonder" (Turner, 2019, p. 33).

Supervision is a process undertaken early in a career, but some therapists mistakenly consider themselves "done" with supervision upon obtaining licensure. Jordan (2018) described the common overemphasis on independence, stating, "We are wired to flourish in connection, but our culture pushes us to stand separate and compete… this dilemma and clash generate chronic stress" (p. 4). RCT challenges the notion that we all must find strength in a separate self and individualism. Placing problems that arise during play therapy treatment in individual terms does not consider that play therapists are a part of a community, regardless of the supervisee's developmental phase within their career trajectory.

Trauma work becomes increasingly difficult when done in isolation (Pliske & Balboa, 2019); secure and attuned interpersonal relationships are what repairs and reshapes our perceptions toward growth and healing (Jordan, 2018). Regardless of how knowledgeable one is about theory and practice or seasoned as a practicing play therapist, becoming "stuck" is an inevitable phenomenon when faced with the helplessness and hopelessness of traumatic reactions. Sometimes private practice can translate to an individual and isolating practice experience. Supervisory relationships can support greater vulnerability and exploration of the lived experience, offering mutual empathy and empathic support throughout a career so that a play therapist can continue to engage in self-exploration and find joy in their work.

Exploring Systemic Resonances in Play Therapy Supervision

Systemically, Elkaïm (2002) implored therapists to remain attuned to their own lived experiences and the feelings and reactions that emerge in the therapeutic context. He explained that therapists' resonances emerge because clients "solicit the therapist in a certain manner to provoke a reaction" in the former (Elkaïm, 2002, p. 3, personal translation). In so doing, a systemic triangulation between the client's experiences, the therapist's experiences, and the therapeutic context allows the client "to try to repeat something that has significance for them," and that "reproduces rules from the family system within the therapeutic system" (Elkaïm, 2002, p. 3, personal translation). Children will reproduce their traumatic experiences through play (American Psychiatric Association, 2013; Gil, 2017; van der Kolk, 2014), and these enactments rarely leave the play therapist feeling indifferent. Munns (2008) cautioned play therapists to be particularly attentive to four reactions arising from children's play, notably anger, dependency, sexuality, and competition, to which Stauffer (2019) added previous difficult or traumatic personal or professional experiences that may be triggered.

Through supervision, exploring why and/or how the feelings emerge for the play therapist may help them understand how their own lived experiences function to preserve, maintain, and/or protect different members of the client's family throughout the therapeutic relationship (Elkaïm, 2002). Uncovering these mechanisms and motives raises therapists' awareness, promotes therapists' understanding of children's worldview, and allows for greater latitude in expressing their working hypotheses in session. Resonances provide a veritable vehicle for "use of self" in therapy (e.g., Cheung & Pau, 2013; Kissil et al., 2018) and for acting with a "heightened sensitivity that can prevent harmful behaviors, such as ignoring, minimizing, belittling, or undermining" (Killmer, 2014, p. 3) the client's or supervisee's self-expression.

Putting hands or bodies into movement through creation or human sculpture can enhance the play therapy process through clarifying and (re-)conceptualizing case material, promoting creativity, flexibility, and problem-solving skills (Stauffer, 2019). This allows for new perspectives that can help play therapists break through the stuckness they are experiencing. For example, witnessing a child's violent play in session triggered the first author's previous experiences of physical abuse in such a way that she was initially frozen in responding. Her feelings of fear, utter helplessness, and powerlessness emerged in the moment, cutting access to her ability to track the play and respond empathically to the client.

Through a human sculpture activity, the therapist took a brief moment to concentrate silently on the most difficult moment of the session, then physically positioned herself (spatially in the room and through body posture) to express and illustrate the felt resonances that emerged. She explored the triadic reunion of (1) the child's systematic shooting of all the dolls, hand puppets, and stuffed animals in the playroom (child's experience), in relation to (2) her previous experiences of physically shielding herself against physical attacks (therapist's experience), to better understand (3) the child's communication of power and danger (therapeutic context) to gain insight into her futility in remaining mentally present or in responding to this violence within the therapeutic relationship in session (therapeutic system repetition reproduced from the family system). The awareness raised from sculpting her own responses to the play session in supervision fostered insight.

First, the play therapist set her intention to allow movement in supervision where there had been none in session. Then, she showed the supervision group how she felt in the moment by physically tucking herself into a "cannonball" posture, wherein she crouched to the floor and shielded her head with her hands as she looked down and closed her eyes. There was no movement in the pose, indicative of her inability to move or speak at the moment in session. After a minute of holding this pose, the group offered the following responses: "Seeing what is happening is too difficult to bear," and, "Making yourself small and being silent might allow you to go unnoticed and keep you safe from danger."

After exploring her resonances of past physical violence and the meaning that the group helped her make of her initial posture, she sculpted the ideal posture she would like to adopt with this client during this type of play. She set into motion her intention to welcome and witness his play actively: She stood up straight and tall, leaning slightly forward on one foot, with one hand at her brow and her other hand outstretched, palm up, and moving gently to the left and right from midline to her side. The group offered the following observations: "You can see as far as the eye can see," and, "The world is your oyster, and anything is possible," and "Ahoy, matey, all aboard!" The laughter that ensued changed the tone of the supervisory session from serious and dark to light and playful. The latter statement captured the welcoming gesture intended by the play therapist. She left the supervision session feeling more buoyant, empowered in her ability to witness the violence, all while being attentive to any possible danger ahead and open to the self-expression her client needed to enact through his play.

Coming to awareness of her resonances, aided by sculpting her feelings in the most salient moment of the session, and then sculpting the posture she would ideally like to adopt thereafter, allowed the play therapist to voice her hypotheses when the play repeated in subsequent sessions. She later verbalized to the child, "Sometimes, no matter what you do, you can't control how others treat you," which elicited a silent look from the child; "It must be hard to be at the mercy of powerful others," after which the child looked to the floor and kicked his foot in the air; and, "Having power and control lets you be the one who decides what happens," to which the child responded, "That's right. For once, I get to be the one in control."

Taking personal resonances into account and finding a way to respond empathically to his violent play allowed the therapist to recognize the importance of facilitating the therapeutic powers of play (Shaefer & Drewes, 2014) of therapeutic relationship, empathy, self-expression, access to the unconscious, catharsis, and resiliency to deepen the child's search for self-expression and self-regulation. Having been heard, understood, and joined by the play therapist, the child enacted remnants of the violent play for one or two sessions more before transitioning to using more artful forms of self-expression with natural play materials he chose (e.g., rocks, mineral powders, clay).

Promoting Safety and Understanding Through the Mind–Body Connection

Exploring personal resonances through systemic and relational-cultural lenses allows play therapists to summon their "courage to be imperfect" (Lazarsfeld, as cited in Ansbacher, 1966, p. 152) in the confusion, not-knowing, and complexity that toxic traumatic play evokes. Kissil et al. (2018) reported that participants "accepting their own vulnerabilities and woundedness gave them the freedom to access and use themselves more fully in therapy, and also helped them better see and relate to the humanity and woundedness of their clients" (p. 83). Capitalizing on the mind–body connection can enhance the play therapy relationship, allowing for joining with clients on an experiential level and creating shared understanding (Stauffer, 2019) and changing the dynamics of the relationship to find a new equilibrium (Boszormenyi-Nagy & Krasner, 1986).

Fish (2017) cited the eloquent explanation that Henzell offered about this mind–body connection:

[Embodied images] possess the power to sort, discriminate and combine perceptions from apparently different realms of experience with extraordinary speed and force - just because they avoid lexical structures. The essence of the image, particularly the invited image, is that it directly *presents* rather than indirectly *describes* its concerns.

(Henzell, 1997, p. 75, emphasis in original)

Using art, imagery, and movement in supervision may create a more egalitarian, less authoritative relationship and enhance verbal sharing (Ko, 2014) in individual or group contexts for these very same reasons.

Additional Practices Using Art and Movement in Supervision

Supervision is a relationship about a relationship, typically about other relationships! Play therapy supervision requires the supervisor to maintain the supervisor–play therapist relationship, consisting of setting goals, examining tasks, and creating bonds (Stewart & Echterling, 2014) to support play therapy supervisees in processing the inevitable stuckness of complex cases. To do so, the supervisor must impart knowledge or skills through strategies of instruction, modeling, and guided practice while reinforcing supervisee strengths (Aasheim, 2012). Stewart and Echterling (2008) recommended taking full advantage of the "powerful tools" play therapy may provide the supervision process (p. 283).

Supervisees and supervisors may use art- and movement-based techniques between sessions or during supervision "to clarify case conceptualization and understanding; to illuminate supervisees' thoughts, feelings, and resonances; and to generate hypotheses about the client(s) or relationships within the family or institutional systems that they can later test in session" (Stauffer, 2019, p. 189). These practices may help supervisees through the inevitable stuckness that occurs when trauma treatment becomes difficult to hold as a clinician, allowing them to explore the therapist–client relationship in greater depth and promote movement and transformation in the therapeutic system.

Fish (2017) explained that "the maker of the image is the authority on its meaning" (p. 69), and this applies equally to movement exercises. Likewise, "therapy using authentic movement begins with a lack of movement, in silence, while turning attention inward and focusing on internal listening and relating to the feelings that emerge here and now, without being judgmental" (Federman et al., 2019, p. 16). Therefore, once an intention has been set, the presenter, who will communicate the case and produce either the image or the movement, begins in silence and concentration on that intention and the resonances that emerge in the moment.

Then, as receivers of the message, the supervisor or supervisory group use their play therapy skills, such as tracking, to notice and describe images or movements phenomenologically, creating a bridge between the communicator's and receiver's unconsconcious and allowing the receiver(s) to witness the production so that their resonances emerge. All participants, the communicator and receiver(s), are encouraged to make *no connections* with the case, once presented, nor the "why" they chose to do what they did in creating or in offering observations. The thoughtful communication of those resonances through *suspended discussion* (Fish, 2017, p. 77), wherein meanings are not explained though "wonderings" may be voiced, will allow the presenter to take what they need from the observations offered by the receiver(s).

Applying Drawing and Imagery to (Re-)Conceptualize Cases

Art evokes the creator's personal – and polysemous – meaning-making through the "aesthetic analysis [of] giving the work a title and imagining its message" (Levine, 2015, p. 61). Supervisors and supervisees may glean insight through discussion because "the message coming from aesthetic analysis often is a direct response to the original issue, shedding light upon it in ways that enable us to see what had hitherto been obscured or ignored" (Levine, 2015, p. 61). This type of analysis, which may lend itself to interpretation, should be approached with caution, because it is crucial that the creator "validate interpretations based on their own association, language, and metaphors" (Betts & Groth-Marnat, 2014, p. 275).

Creating or using different types of art or images may evoke supervisee resonances that can be explored in supervision. For example, drawing a picture helps communicate something about the client's or supervisee's presentation in therapy/supervision (e.g., attitude, culture, encouragement level, engagement, social interest). Choosing an image captures resonances/feelings about the therapy/supervision process (e.g., art cards, painting, photo). Sculpting an aspect of therapeutic/supervisory relationship using clay, Play-Doh, or model magic, or making a collage from images/words captures wishes for the client/supervise. Using bricks or LEGO minifigures gives a global impression of the therapy/supervision (Peabody, 2021). And, using any of the above can convey the ideal evolution of the client's/supervisee's or the therapist's/supervisor's posture or attitude, the therapeutic/supervisory process, or the relationship.

Specifically creating *response art*, such as an image, drawing, or other creation with a specific therapeutic aim or supervision intention in mind, offers opportunities to respond to material that arises within the therapeutic process (Fish, 2012, p. 138). It allows supervisees to foster personal introspection, explore countertransference and vicarious trauma, and spur dialogue to process and explore their authentic self. Response art also helps therapists bear difficult material and explore the meaning of their experiences (Fish, 2012, p. 139) when discussed within the confines of a safe supervisory relationship. Elkaïm (2012) emphasized that pictorial resonances, created and explored in supervision, have to be neither esthetically pleasing nor elaborate to serve their purpose in thinking more flexibly about the link established between the therapist and client(s) through the therapist's resonances. According to Elkaïm (2012), the drawing acts as a "springboard to bring the therapist's lived experience into this specific situation" (p. 150, personal translation), which does not act as a substitute for the client's own experiences or as a projection of the therapist's own issues into the therapeutic space (Stauffer, 2019).

For example, one supervisee created response art using watercolors in context to bear witness to complex developmental trauma. The artwork depicted the therapist with long sea-green hair that moved in a wave like pattern, as if the hair were the depths of the sea. She painted a tiny boat adrift, moving through the vast space. She titled the piece "Lost at Sea." She conveyed that the process of therapy felt at times to be moving against the current, not fluid, but awash in new turbulent emotions and barriers altering service delivery. She reported feeling "small" at times, wondering if she was able to make a difference. The process of therapy could yield confusion and hopelessness, yet she was in a position of power tasked by others to be all-knowing and in charge.

This supervisee was able to express more fully through her response art resonances of bearing witness to others' suffering. She described her own lived experiences and re-experiencing some of her own adversity through the eyes of her child clients. Many children's stories echoed her own, and these insights facilitated exploration of countertransference and vicarious trauma.

Directing Movement Activities to Inspire Movement in Therapy

Movement is a foundation for all elements of play. Through movement, one thinks in motion. Through movement, play stimulates the brain, fostering learning, resilience, flexibility, and innovation. Movement provides opportunities to enhance self-efficacy and self-control (e.g., yoga therapy; McLafferty, 2018; Pliske & Balboa, 2019) and to improve balance (e.g., Tai chi; McLafferty, 2018). Totora (2019) commended how clients can improve stress management, quality of life, and pain management; increase vitality and energy; reduce anxiety, depression, and fatigue; build resilience, and accept life's unpredictability through movement. Within a dance movement therapy context, "embodied relational knowing, body memory, and embodied sense-making are highly developed" and may be particularly useful with clients for whom finding words is difficult (Karkou & Meekums, 2017, p. 4).

Using movement in supervision allows therapists to practice attunement dynamics through various body shapes, relational dances, and "rhythmic synchrony" (Devereaux, 2015, p. 88). Attuning to clients' emotions and, from that place of embodied knowing inherent in dance movement therapy, imitating, or reflecting clients' movements to them, or in supervision, as we argue, allows the therapist to nonverbally communicate to the client or for the supervisee to experience for themselves, "I hear you, I understand you, and it's OK" (Deveraux, 2015, p. 88). In supervisory contexts, using movement can guide honest sharing (Ko, 2014) and can help therapists develop kinesthetic empathy through the mind–body connection and body images evoked (Ko, 2016).

In the case example above, wherein the first author's client expressed his desire for power and control through violent play, exploring the play therapist's blockages through human sculpture was essential to creating movement in her conceptualization of the case and in reactivating her empathic responses to the child in subsequent sessions. These movements included only the play therapist. However, it is sometimes helpful for the play therapist to extract themselves from the sculpture to be able to see it in its entirety.

Group sculptures using humans in form and movement have long been used in many supervision contexts, for example, in mapping relationships (Constantine, 1978; Satir, 1972), exploring family dynamics (Baldo & Softas-Nall, 1998), understanding personal history (Platteau, 2016), and exploring therapist resonances. The first author's systemic psychotherapy training regularly included group sculpture for exploring therapists' case resonances. It is helpful to have a group of five to ten or more therapists with whom to process group sculpture to be sure that people and/or systemic dynamics may be adequately represented.

The presenting therapist briefly describes the case, then the sculpting group exits the room, uses 5 to 10 minutes to plan the sculpture, then re-enters the room and uses themselves and other receivers to sculpt their here-and-now resonances. The sculptors may give specific intentions to other group members, asking them to hold a pose physically, look in a certain direction, or move in a particular way. After setting the sculpture into motion for a minute or so, with the presenting therapist watching and taking any desired notes, the members of the sculpture talk about what was difficult for them in the piece, remaining in the here and now of the supervision session, and observers also comment, without connecting what they say to the case.

Then, members may change their position to show what the "ideal" outcome would look like. In the ideal sculpture, the sculpting group gives no notes to members, and each member is free to change position or to move as they feel comfortable. Sculpture often passes in silence, but sometimes a sound may be pertinent to add to the initial resonance movement or the ideal outcome to illustrate or liberate any perceived stuckness. Group members describe how the ideal sculpture felt to them in the moment, observers comment, and the presenting therapist always gets the last word, taking from the experience the therapeutic power of indirect teaching that they needed to gain insight into their case.

Conclusion

Inevitable stuckness in play therapy occurs when holding client-trauma stories becomes difficult for the clinician, who may resonate with aspects of the case that are complex or triggering on micro, mezzo, and/or macro levels. Leaning into these resonances and understanding them from the vantage points of relational-cultural and systemic theories in supervision allows play therapist supervisors to leverage specific therapeutic powers of play and design art and movement activities to augment therapist self-awareness and initiate needed movement in session.

References

Aasheim, L. (2012). *Practical clinical supervision for counselors: An experiential guide.* Springer.

American Psychiatric Association. (2013). Posttraumatic stress disorder. *Diagnostic and statistical manual of mental disorders* (5th ed.). https://doi.org/10.1176/appi.books.9780890425596

Ansbacher, H. L. (Ed.). (1966). Contributors to this issue. *American Journal of Individual Psychology*, *22*(2), 152.

Baldo, T. D., & Softas-Nall, B. C. (1998). Family sculpting in supervision of family therapy. *Family Journal*, *6*(3), 231–234. https://doi.org/10.1177/1066480798063012

Betts, D., & Groth-Marnat, G. (2014). The intersection of art therapy and psychological assessment. In L. Handler & A. D. Thomas (Eds.), *Drawings and assessment in psychotherapy: Research and application* (pp. 268–285). Routledge.

Bloom, S. L., & Farragher, B. (2011). *Destroying sanctuary: The crisis in human service delivery systems*. Oxford University Press.

Boszormenyi-Nagy, I., & Krasner, B. R. (1986). *Between give and take: A clinical guide to contextual therapy*. Mazel.

Cheung, P. K., & Pau, G. Y. K. (2013). Congruence and the therapist's use of self. In M. Baldwin (Ed.), *The use of self in therapy* (3rd ed., pp. 166–185). Routledge.

Constantine, L. L. (1978). Family sculpting and relationship mapping techniques. *Journal of Marriage and Family Therapy*, *4*(2), 13–24.

Devereaux, C. (2015). Moving with the space between us: The dance of attachment security. In C. A. Malchiodi & D. A. Crenshaw (Eds.), *Creative arts and play therapy for attachment problems* (pp. 84–99). Guilford.

Elkaïm, M. (2002, January 10). Thérapie de couple et résonance dans le cadre thérapeutic [Couples therapy and ressonances in therapy]. *Centre de Formation à la Thérapie Familiale*. https://www.systemique.org

Elkaïm, M. (2004). L'expérience personnelle du psychothérapeute: Approche systémique et résonance [The psychotherapist's personal experience: The systemic approach and resonance]. *Psychothérapies*, *24*(3), 145–150. https://doi.org/10.3917/psys.043.0145

Elkaïm, M. (2012). Les résonances picturales [Pictorial resonances]. *Cahiers Critiques de Thérapie Familiale et de Pratiques de Réseaux*, *48*(1), 149–166. https://doi.org/10.3917/ctf.048.0149

Federman, D., Shimoni, S., & Turjeman, N. (2019). "Attentive movement" as a means for treating depression. *Body, Movement and Dance in Psychotherapy*, *14*(1), 14–25. https://doi.org/10.1080/17432979.2019.1586773

Figley, C. R. (1999). Compassion fatigue: Toward a new understanding of the costs of caring. In B. H. Stamm (Ed.), *Secondary traumatic stress: Self-care issues for clinicians, researchers, and educators* (pp. 3–28). Sidran Institute.

Fish, B. J. (2012). Response art: The art of the art therapist. *Art Therapy: Journal of the American Art Therapy Association*, *29*(3), 138–143. https://doi.org/10.1080/07421656.2012.701594

Fish, B. J. (2017). *Art-based supervision: Cultivating therapeutic insight through imagery*. Routledge.

Gil, E. (2017). *Posttraumatic play in children: What clinicians need to know*. Guilford.

Goodyear-Brown, P., & Stauffer, S. D. (2019). Not taking the trauma home: Holding the holder at the organizational level. *Play Therapy*, *14*(2), 42–46.

Henzell, J. (1997). Art, madness and anti-psychiatry. *Art, Psychotherapy, and Psychosis*, 176.

Herman, J. (2015). *Trauma and recovery: The aftermath of violence - From domestic abuse to political terror*. (Original published 1992). Basic Books.

Jordan, J. (2018). *Relational-cultural therapy*. American Psychological Association.

Karkou, V., & Meekums, B. (2017). Dance movement therapy for dementia (review). *Cochrane Database of Systematic Reviews*, *2*, 1–28, (Article no. CD011022). https://doi.org/10.1002/14651858.CD011022.pub2

Killmer, J. M. (2014). Exploring spirituality in systemic supervision. In T. C. Todd & C. L. Storm (Eds.), *The complete systemic supervisor: Context, philosophy, and pragmatics* (2nd ed.). Wiley.

Kissil, K., Carneiro, R., & Aponte, H. J. (2018). Beyond duality: The relationship between the personal and the professional selves of the therapist in the person of the therapist training. *Journal of Family Psychotherapy, 29*(1), 71–86. https://doi.org/10.1080/08975353.2018.1416244

Ko, K. S. (2014). Korean expressive arts therapy students' experiences with movement-based supervision: A phenomenological investigation. *American Journal of Dance Therapy, 31*(2), 141–159. https://doi.org/10.1007/s10465-014-9180-7

Ko, K. S. (2016). Using bodily movement in supervision for expressive arts therapy students: A case study. *Arts in Psychotherapy, 48*, 8–18. https://doi.org/10.1016/j.aip.2015.12.005

Koltz, R. L. (2008). Integrating creativity into supervision using Bernard's discrimination model. *Journal of Creativity in Mental Health, 3*(4), 416–427. https://doi.org/10.1080/15401380802530054

Kottman, T. (2014). Positive emotions. In C. E. Schaefer & A. A. Drewes (Eds.), *The therapeutic powers of play: 20 core agents of change* (2nd ed., pp. 103–120). Wiley.

Levine, E. (2015). *Play and art in child psychotherapy: An expressive art therapy approach.* Jessica Kingsley.

Malchiodi, C. A. (2020). *Trauma and expressive arts therapy: Brain, body, and imagination in the healing process.* Guilford Press.

McLafferty, H. (2018). *Mind-body medicine in clinical practice.* Routledge.

Morrison Bennett, M., & Eberts, S. (2014). Self-expression. In C. Schaefer & A. Drewes (Eds.), *The therapeutic powers of play: 20 core agents of change* (2nd ed., pp. 11–24). Wiley.

Munns, A. (2008). Playful activities for supervisors and trainers. In A. A. Drewes & J. A. Mullen (Eds.), *Supervision can be playful: Techniques for child and play therapist supervisors* (pp. 271–279). Jason Aronson.

Newell, J. M. (2017). *Cultivating professional resilience in direct practice: A guide for human service professionals.* Columbia University Press.

Peabody, M. A. (2021). Building understanding in parent consultation brick by brick. *Play Therapy, 16*(1), 4–7.

Platteau, G. (2016). Métaphores et sculptures du temps en formation [Metaphores and sculptures of time in training]. *Cahiers Critiques de Thérapie Familiale et de Pratiques de Réseaux, 56*(1), 201–220. https://doi.org/10.3917/ctf.056.0201

Pliske, M., & Balboa, L. (2019). *Integrating yoga and play therapy: The mind-body connection for healing adverse childhood experiences.* Jessica Kingsley Publishing.

Roubira, J.-L. (with Cardoua, M.) (2016). *Dixit 7: Revelation [Card game].* Libellud.

Satir, V. M. (1972). *Peoplemaking.* Science and Behavior Books.

Schaefer, C. E., & Drewes, A. A. (Eds.). (2014). *The therapeutic powers of play: 20 core agents of change* (2nd ed.). Wiley.

Skovholt, T. M., & Trotter-Mathison, M. (2016). *The resilient practitioner: Burnout and compassion fatigue prevention and self-care strategies for the helping professions.* Routledge.

Stauffer, S. D. (2019). Ethical use of drawings in play therapy: Considerations for assessment, practice, and supervision. *International Journal of Play Therapy, 28*(4), 183–194. https://doi.org/10.1037/pla0000106

Stern, D. N. (1985). *The interpersonal world of the infant: A view from psychoanalysis and developmental psychology.* Basic Books.

Stewart, A., & Echterling, L. G. (2008). Playful supervision: Sharing exemplary exercises in the supervision of play therapists. In A. A. Drewes & J. A. Mullen (Eds.), *Supervision can be playful: Techniques for child and play therapist supervisors* (pp. 281–307). Jason Aronson.

Stewart, A., & Echterling, L. G. (2014). Therapeutic relationship. In C. Schaefer & A. Drewes (Eds.), *The therapeutic powers of play: 20 Core agents of change* (2nd ed.) (pp. 157–170). Wiley.

Thomas, D. A. (2015). *Intentionality in supervision: Supervising play therapy interns and practitioners.* American Counseling Association. https://www.counseling.org/docs/default-source/vistas/article_387a5c21f16116603abcacff0000bee5e7.pdf?sfvrsn=e44a412c_8

Totora, S. (2019). Children are born to dance! Pediatric medical dance/movement therapy: The view from integrative pediatric oncology. *Children, 6*(1), 14. https://doi.org/10.3390/children6010014

Turner, R. (2019). Play heals us, too! *Play Therapy, 14*(2), 32–35.

van der Kolk, B. A. (2014). *The body keeps the score: Brain, mind, and body in the healing of trauma.* Penguin Books.

16 Virtual Reality and Supervision

Jessica Stone

Introduction

Virtual reality has become accessible to the general consumer through the advent of less-expensive, lightweight, portable units. The expansion of both hardware and software allows virtual reality to be perfectly poised as a powerful addition to the play therapy world, both clinically and within supervision. This powerful platform includes immersive and integrative experiences which can enhance and expand mental health treatment. This chapter will explore the foundation and uses of virtual reality (VR) in play therapy supervision, alongside the contextual history regarding its development and integration.

Beyond the "wow" factor of donning a VR head-mounted display (HMD) unit, important components of therapeutic VR (tVR) include transporting the client, clinician, and/or supervisee to the environment of one's choosing to be interacted with in ways the users see fit. VR utilizes stimuli to create an experience in which all the senses within the user are telling them that the environment and stimuli are real. These experiences create a powerful environment for embodiment, creation, interaction, understanding, and change. Having been found to have profound uses with issues of anxiety, depression, and trauma, VR can assist the supervisee with not only understanding and experiencing how to use the tool within sessions with their clients, but also ways to process their own internal experiences within their work.

Discussed in terms of fundamental play therapy tenets, this chapter discusses the use of VR and Digital Play Therapy™ (Stone, 2020a) within sessions and during supervision to inform the clinician's understanding of the client's needs and experiences. Play therapists who achieve comfort and competence in evaluating and using VR will find a plethora of options for use in case conceptualization, assessment, treatment planning, and interventions. Integrating VR into modern therapeutic practice is an exciting and powerful addition to a play therapist's repertoire and the supervisor's offerings.

DOI: 10.4324/9781003196075-20

History and Literature

Supervision

Throughout this book, the reader has learned about various aspects of general and play therapy specific supervision. This chapter will review a variety of specific components regarding the supervision of mental health treatment providers, along with an incorporation of the play therapy specific mandates delineated by the Association for Play Therapy (APT). The context for the appropriate clinical use of any tool in supervision requires a solid foundation. APT requires that a Registered Play Therapist-Supervisor maintain the following abilities:

a. Demonstrate advanced play therapy skills
b. Facilitate play therapist self-awareness and insight
c. Resolve supervisee reluctance and resistance
d. Utilize a variety of supervisory interventions
e. Facilitate parent consultation and involvement
f. Facilitate play therapist development
g. Build trust and rapport with supervisees
h. Develop professionalism, professional identities, and advocacy skills
i. Incorporate technology in supervision
j. Demonstrate multicultural competency (Association for Play Therapy, 2020, pp. 3–4)

Supervisors have a critical three-part role in the supervisee's progression: (1) assist with cases, (2) provide support, (3) monitor and evaluate progress. The first role is to assist the supervisee with specific cases. This can include ongoing updating and discussion of the case(s) and includes the periodic review of any recorded interactions between the supervisee and client(s). Providing education and support to the supervisee with ongoing case conceptualization allows for the integration of new experiences and material. This material can then be incorporated into the supervisee's learning and the client's care. Education can include didactic, experiential, and independent learning.

The second role is to provide support regarding the experiences, stressors, environments, and more, that the supervisee faces during supervision. There is a desired balance to ensure the supervisor provides support yet does not engage in individual therapy with the supervisee. However, the supervisee's internal state and personal experiences will affect the client's therapeutic experience, the supervisee's clinical process, and the supervisee's educational process. The supervisor's goal is to "assist the supervisee in learning to recognize personal issues and gain insight on how to navigate through compartmentalizing those issues during their work as the counselor" (Mitchell, 2021, p. 180). This supportive role, along with role number one, can also address any transference and/or countertransference concerns.

The third role of the play therapy supervisor is to monitor and evaluate the supervisee's overarching clinical process and abilities to ensure their work meets a high level of care. The supervisor is responsible for the endorsement of the supervisee to move forward toward independence as a clinician. Additionally, the supervisor holds both legal and ethical responsibilities for the supervisee and their work in many circumstances.

Immersive Technologies

Many fields have benefitted from the advancements in immersive technology. These newly popular mediums allow users to interact, create, choose, explore, and play due to their highly motivating, immersive, interactive features. Including VR in play therapy allows education, supervision, and treatment to move beyond imagining, describing, and orchestrating; VR inclusion provides environments and interactions within which one can experience therapeutic engagement of the polyvagal, autonomic, sympathetic, and parasympathetic systems (Spiegel, 2020; Safaryan & Mehta, 2020). Using VR therapeutically, or tXR, is truly a whole-body experience (Stone, 2020b).

Many other professional disciplines have embraced these mediums with great success. The disciplines are quite varied and include many critical aspects of our society. Pediatric medical facilities are now utilizing virtual-reality headsets and tablets during procedures (Burns-Nader, 2019). VR tools are used to assist low-vision patients (Deemer et al., 2019) and provide numerous forms of medical training (Jin et al., 2017). Commercial pilots and the United States military use VR for a variety of simulation training (Presnall, 2019; Ellis, 2018; Szoldra, 2018; Stone, 2017). Virtual reality has also been used as occupational training for those re-entering society after prison (Clarke, 2019; Stone 2020b). These fields have embraced the power of VR in their training process and direct work.

The use of virtual reality in professional training has grown exponentially in the last few years. When researchers compared learning retention between a group instructed with a video and a group that learned from a virtual instructor using VR, the VR group demonstrated a 25% increase in recall accuracy (Bailenson, 2018; Stone 2020b). As found by Bailenson, "People learn better by doing than by watching … those who learn best are simulating motor action in the brain" (2018, p. 39).

In particular, play therapy can benefit from adapting the appropriate use of digital tools for supervision and direct client services. As detailed in the book *Digital Play Therapy* (Stone, 2020a), therapeutic underpinnings and research support the use of digital tools in play therapy. Although mental health professionals have been slower to adopt technology in clinical settings, a variety of programs have been used in general therapeutic sessions (Lamb & Etopio, 2019; Baker, 2019; Stone, 2020a; 2020b; 2019). Further, VR is used with special populations such as veterans (Rizzo & Shilling, 2017) and clients diagnosed with autism spectrum disorder (Grant, 2019; Bellani et al., 2011). Therapeutic use of VR within various mental health therapies, including play therapy, will broaden the scope of treatment and interventions, and expand services to a wider audience.

History of Technology in Mental Health and Play Therapy

Play therapists experienced an explosion of exposure and utilization of technology in play therapy during the COVID-19 period. However, digital tools have been discussed and used in mental health treatment for decades. Starting in the late 1980s, clinicians began exploring and incorporating video games into mental health therapies (Farrell, 1989; Gardner, 1991; Resnick & Sherer, 1995; Clarke & Schoech, 1994). A glimpse into the history of incorporating digital tools into mental health treatment prior to 1989 is provided by Farrell through a review of a list of 150 software programs for use in psychology released by the American Psychological Association. Farrell's review indicated a blossoming interest in incorporating digital tools into mental health treatment. His focus was to discover information about the impact of technology on psychology. At the time, the predominant use of digital tools included clerical and practice management type software and use. Additionally, Farrell queried psychologists regarding their direct clinical use in his research. Test administration assistance, assigning diagnoses, gathering client data, biofeedback, and cognitive retraining were the clinical-use categories included at that time. Farrell found that the top three reasons more than 30% of participating psychologists did not use technology included: lack of time, lack of training or experience, and having a small practice which did not justify the expense of the integration of a computer (Farrell, 1989; Stone, 2020a). Altvater et al. (2017) corroborated these findings in their study of clinician attitudes toward incorporating digital tools into play therapy. Amazingly, mental health professionals' attitudes regarding technology in mental health practices have not changed tremendously in over 30 years (Stone, 2020a).

Ceranoglu (2010) explored the direct use of video games in psychotherapy. His experiences and research yielded four key concepts:

1) "The therapeutic relationship emerged more quickly when video games were used, in contrast with traditional therapy with children" (p. 143)
2) These tools can be used in the evaluation of visuospatial skills and executive functions
3) Digital tools are useful in the evaluation of frustration tolerance
4) Digital tools assist in the evaluation of affective regulation

He continued: "Observing a child's play style and content choice may offer significant clues to intrapsychic conflicts and may provide material needed to elaborate on those conflicts" (p. 143). Stone and Ceranoglu both discuss using digital tools in therapy to assist with building a relationship, evaluating the client's cognitive processing style, and elaborating upon – and clarification of – internal conflicts (Stone, 2020a; Ceranoglu, 2010).

Hull (2016) also discussed the benefits of using technology in the playroom. He posited that the playroom is more inviting when using familiar tools, the initial bonding between the therapist and client is improved, and the "imagination and creativity" offered by digital tools is greatly enhanced (Hull, 2016,

p. 616; Snow et al., 2012; Stone, 2020a). The findings by Ceranoglu, Stone, and Hull emphasize that the available power of the interventions when digital play is incorporated therapeutically is a very impactful modality in play therapy settings.

Virtual Reality (VR)

Virtual reality (VR) utilizes a head mounted display (HMD) unit, or headset, and refers to a collection of fully immersive experiences, including a 360-degree view of video with real-world content, computer-generated content, or a combination of both (Irvine, 2017; Stone, 2020b). VR uses either stand-alone computers along with HMDs or all-in-one units in ways which "eliminate[s] the traditional separation between user and machine, providing more direct and intuitive interaction with information" (Bricken & Byrne, 1993, p. 200). Inside-out or outside-in sensors track body, head, and hand movements to reflect the user's natural movements, which leads to desired levels of immersion and congruency (Stone, 2020a; Maples-Keller et al., 2017).

Historically used in research, academia, and various industry laboratories from the 1960s onward, important technological developments have allowed for mass-consumer access and use. Previously bulky, expensive, and uncomfortable units have been replaced with lighter, smaller, and more immersive HMDs (Virtual Reality Society, n.d.; Brooks, Jr., 1999; Mandal, 2013; Stone, 2020a). Mentored by Mark Bolas, an early VR pioneer, and others, Palmer Luckey ignited this new era of consumer VR with a HMD driven by a personal computer at the age of 19 (Dudley, 2018; Rubin, 2014; Beilinson, 2014).

Utilizing the VR HMD, one is instantly transported to the chosen location or scenario, and multiple senses and bodily systems are engaged. The user is immersed in the content and able to interact with the environment toward a goal of embodiment. VR has the potential for phenomenal expansion in the years to come.

Therapeutic Use of XR (tVR)

To understand the power of VR in play therapy supervision, we must understand some of the underpinnings of therapeutic VR. These underpinnings allow us to conceptualize the supervision of both the use within session by the supervisee with the client, and within supervision itself with the supervisee and supervisor.

As with any therapeutic tool, clinicians at any level and supervisors must attend to the appropriate professional and ethical guidelines provided by licensing, professional, malpractice, and governing entities. Additionally, the Health Insurance Portability and Accountability Act (HIPAA) requirements must be adhered to whenever possible, and if they are not, then appropriate consultation, informed consent, and documentation must be retained. Protection of our clients, supervisees, and ourselves is paramount.

Embodied Cognition

Dr. Jeremy Bailensen, of Stanford University, speaks about the concept of "embodied cognition" in relation to the use of virtual reality in his 2018 book entitled *Experience on Demand*. This concept derives from a movement in the 1990s which posits that "cognitive processes are deeply rooted in the body's interactions with the world" (Wilson, 2002, p. 625). When breaking down the components of the use of therapeutic virtual reality, we must explore the concepts that are presented. Some of these concepts include: cognition, the *self*, other, self-other interaction(s), and self–world interactions. What does it mean to understand the *self*, to interact with others and environments, and to make sense of all of it to formulate ideas, concepts, beliefs, and more?

Cognition

Cognition includes how we gather and use information to function. According to the Oxford-powered Lexico dictionary, cognition is "The mental action or process of acquiring knowledge and understanding through thought, experience, and the senses" (2021a, para. 1). The result of the cognition is "a perception, sensation, notion, or intuition" (Lexico, para. 2). In this exploration of what cognition is and how it forms our beliefs and experiences, particularly relating to virtual reality, we can see that the knowledge we acquire through experience, the senses, and thoughts results in some type of notion, intuition, sensation, or perception. We process and incorporate the input of information into some inclusive understanding.

When using VR, these larger, inclusive understandings culminate from the experiences had within the virtual reality environment. The mind and body are perceiving, sensing, and interacting with the stimulus presented to conceptualize, alter, explore, etc., concepts which are affecting the user. How stimulus and interactions impact cognitions are fundamental components of the therapeutic process. Understanding such processes allows the therapist to employ interventions which effectively address the therapeutic needs.

In a somewhat controversial move, Varela, Thompson, and Rosch (1991) explored the concept of *self* in terms of dissonance between personal experience and cognitive science. At the time, this brought into question many long-held beliefs and conceptualizations. For Varela et al. (1991), the concept of embodiment is described to include the necessary sensory-motor experiences of the physical body, which results in cognition. In other words, we experience things with our body and subsequently translate and incorporate that into cognitions.

The Self

The sense and conceptualization of the *self* are fundamental to the human experience. *Self* is also a very important concept within the use of tVR. What defines the *self* in one's mind and experience creates the structure and boundaries for existence. These created boundaries in turn affect interaction with the world and others. Our interactions then impact cognition. The *self* becomes the barometer for the experience and resulting cognitions and the ensuing actions.

The *self* is defined as "a person's essential being that distinguishes them from others, especially considered as the object of introspection or reflexive action" (Lexico, 2021b, para. 1). Within virtual reality, this concept is essential – when, where, and how does the *self* become distinguishable from the stimulus? How does this distinguishing between *self* and other determine, define, and/or distinguish cognitive processing concepts and components? How fluid or static must one's sense of *self* be to formulate and incorporate cognitions, and is this a constant or is it a process of ebb and flow?

Thagard (2012) proposes that the "*self* is a system consisting of subsystems at four levels – social, individual, neural, and molecular – each of which includes environment, parts, interconnections, and change" (p. 11). This incorporates these concepts into a "subsystem consisting of environmental influences, component parts, interconnections between parts, and regular changes in the properties and relations of the parts" (p. 2). Utilizing Thagard's concept of environment, parts, interconnections, and change, or EPIC, within the subsystems of the *self* (pp. 3–4), we can conceptualize that the interconnections of these components are fundamental to the perception of the concept itself, in this case, of the *self*.

Historically the *self* has been difficult and controversial to define, and there is no agreed-upon definition. However, the definition is cardinal to psychological constructs. The better we understand the fundamental constructs, the more clearly and ethically we can utilize interventions in our work.

Sensorimotor Simulation and Psychological Presence

Returning to the earlier mention of Bailensen and embodied cognition, we can expand the idea of cognition to include the brain and the body. Muscles, organs (including the skin), sensory experiences, and movement also impact and influence cognition and help us understand the world around us (Bailensen, 2018). Through the activation of *sensorimotor simulation*, or the simulated experience of sensory and motor activity, the brain can better apply and conceptualize the associated cognitions. Citing examples of research with dancers, hockey players, and college students learning about bicycles, Bailensen illustrates the concept that "people learn better by doing than by watching" *and* "that those who learn best are simulating motor action in the brain" (2018, p. 39).

In VR, the concept of *psychological presence* includes the experience of actually feeling as though one is in the environment being experienced, even when that environment is virtual. The person is psychologically present in the virtual environment and is engaging with it accordingly. This presence includes one's perceptual and motor systems interacting with the virtual environments in ways that are similar to the physical environment (Bailensen, 2018, p. 19) and therefore translating those into cognitions (Varela et al., 1991). Sensorimotor simulation and psychological presence are key concepts when utilizing virtual reality for a therapeutic purpose. If the mind and body believe they are having the experience, then growth, insight, mastery, and more can be achieved.

The Senses, Experiences, and Cognitions

> When done right, VR experiences – intense, beautiful, violent, touching, erotic, educational, or whatever else you choose them to be – will feel so realistic and immersive they will have the potential, similar to experiences in the real world, to enact profound and lasting changes in us.
>
> (Bailensen, 2018, p. 6)

As discussed above, a central concept to the power of immersive, therapeutic virtual reality is that the body and mind believe that the virtual environment and stimuli are reality. This does not mean that the mind believes that the cartoon bot in Job Simulator (Owlchemy Lab, 2019) is a physically real, breathing, living creature; rather, that the presence and interaction are real. The bot is floating there in front of the person, it is speaking to the person, and there are possible, requested, or expected actions that will follow. The interaction is perceived by the dominant senses as real in that moment. In Supernatural (Within Unlimited, 2020), an exercise program, the dominant senses tell the body and mind that the balls with cones are actually coming toward one's self. The giraffe walking by in NatureTreks (Greener Games, 2019) can be perceived as close or far away and a hand can be outreached to touch it. A haptic response (vibration in the controller) leads the mind to believe contact has been made. A table or chair in any program can be perceived to be real enough to want to place an item on the table or even sit in the chair, only to quickly find that there is no item there to bear the weight of anything.

Through the senses, experiences, and cognitions, the mind and body engage in the VR environment to incorporate the cognitive results – a perception, sensation, notion, or intuition – into the therapeutic process as guided by the clinician (Lexico, 2021a, para. 2). The power of the mind is harnessed by the sensorimotor simulation and psychological presence created within tVR to formulate cognitions which will be interpreted by the client and clinician to advance the treatment plan and case conceptualization, thereby addressing the areas of difficulty for the client.

Supervision Using VR

Applying the concepts discussed above, the supervisor and supervisee are able to embrace and understand the power of utilizing VR tools in play therapy and play therapy supervision. The concepts of the *self* and other, embodiment, sensorimotor stimulation, and psychological presence are all concepts that will present during use and the clinicians (supervisee and supervisor) will need to attend to the impacts of each on the therapeutic or supervisorial processes.

Utilizing VR in supervision includes identifying the supervisee's needs and employing interventions accordingly. As previously discussed in this chapter, supervisors have important roles regarding their supervisees: to assist with cases, provide support, and to monitor and evaluate progress. The supervisor can guide the supervisee through a variety of programs, not only for exposure to the experience, but also to identify and weave together important concepts such as the Therapeutic Powers of Play (Schaefer, 1993; Drewes & Schaefer, 2016) and tVR. Understanding the foundational tenets of play therapy treatment and the core agents of change allows the supervisee and supervisor to appropriately apply them to a variety of mediums.

When utilizing tVR in supervision, the supervisor can choose programs that address the needs of the supervisee. They can plan exercises, pre-populate environments, and choose programs that present experiences that the supervisee needs to understand, work through, and/or process. The immersive qualities of tVR allow the user to integrate within the environment, interact with it, and embody a variety of roles. Utilizing this tool within supervision deepens the supervisee's experience, broadens the understanding of the client's experience, and increases learning integration, recall, and understanding by stimulating motor actions in the brain.

VR can be used in in-person supervision and remotely. It is optimal to have two headsets, but not necessary. With one headset, whether used in-person or remotely, the user of the headset can "cast" the images seen onto a screen for observance, instruction, dialogue, and processing. If each person has a headset, many programs include multiplayer functions to join in the experience together. The supervisor has numerous ways to experience what the supervisee, client, or both utilized, guide the supervisee through therapeutic agents, and process pertinent components for the development of the supervisee.

Supervisory Examples

In line with the three-part role a supervisor has regarding the supervisee's progression, these examples will highlight the use of extended reality with each.

1. Assistance with specific cases:

Debbie is a newly licensed clinician who is working toward her Registered Play Therapist certificate. She has a client who was previously engaged in sessions. However, over the last few weeks the client has withdrawn and does not want to utilize any of the tools or games they have used in the past. Historically, this client has enjoyed drawing, coloring, and creating. A number of possible interventions were discussed during supervision, with a focus on the elements the client has liked in the past. With facilitating communication and enhancing social relationships as the key Therapeutic Powers of Play focal points, interventions which would reintroduce fun and interaction between the therapist and client were the focus (Schaefer & Drewes, 2014). The supervisor suggested trying the VR program Tiltbrush (Google, 2019). Tiltbrush allows for spontaneous art creation utilizing a variety of styles and mediums. Debbie and the supervisor explored the program prior to Debbie using it clinically.

2. Supporting the supervisee with their personal difficulties:

Exploration of any personal difficulties for a supervisee is an important part of the supervision process. The focus should remain on augmenting and supporting the exploration and identification of such difficulties and how they may or may not impact the clinical treatment and experience for clients. In an effort to explore such concerns, the supervisee has a few options. For mindfulness, the supervisee can enter into a program such as NatureTreks (Greener Games, 2019) or TRIPP (TRIPP, Inc, 2019) to relax in a safe environment to verbally or nonverbally get in touch with the issues at hand. For a more active and interactive experience either with the supervisor or independently, the supervisee can create a Virtual Sandtray®© – VR (VSA-VR) (Virtual Sandtray, 2016) to create, communicate, depict, and/or interact with the immersive tray created. The VSA-VR program allows the creator to directly interact with the scene for role-playing or the introduction of additional characters, and more.

3. Ensuring proper growth trajectory over the course of supervision:

Supervisors are tasked with fulfilling the positions of teacher, counselor, and consultant per the discrimination model of supervision (Bernard, 1979; Mitchell, 2021). Over the course of supervision, the supervisor must evaluate the progression and growth of the supervisee to ensure that they can move toward independent practice or the next step within their journey. It is a difficult task at times to provide feedback which reflects the supervisee's shortcomings. In this case, the supervisor might benefit from using meditative or creative programs or Virtual Sandtray (Virtual Sandtray, 2016) as discussed in Scenario 2, or another creative program such as TiltBrush (Google, 2019) to process how the progression in supervision is happening. The supervisee and supervisor can even join in Multibrush (Rendever, 2021) together to create and explore worlds and introduce or create scenarios for case or vignette discussion.

Conclusion

Therapeutic VR includes a number of immersive tools under its umbrella. These devices and programs are becoming more and more accessible to professionals and the general consumer. Perfectly poised to be a powerful addition to the play therapy world, clinicians are beginning to utilize these tools clinically, as well as for educational and supervisorial uses. The immersive, integrative, and embodiment experiences enhance and expand mental health treatment in many ways. This chapter explored the foundations of utilizing tVR numerous ways within supervision and clinical sessions. With proper training, supervision, and experience, VR includes a powerful collection of tools for the play therapy supervisor, supervisee, and general practitioner.

Key Readings and Resources

Bailensen, J. (2018). *Experience on demand: What virtual reality is, how it works, and what it can do.* Norton.

Drewes, A., & Mullen, J. A. (2008). *Supervision can be playful: Techniques for child and play therapist supervisors*. Aronson.

Drewes, A. A., & Schaefer, C. E. (Eds.). (2016). *Play therapy in middle childhood*. Washington, DC: American Psychological Association.

Fazio-Griffith, L., & Marino, R. (2020). *Techniques and interventions for play therapy and clinical supervision*. IGI Global.

Korea Times. (2020). Bringing the dead back to life: South Korean VR documentary 'Meeting You' [Video]. https://www.youtube.com/watch?v=7RF44KdzyAc

Irvine, K. (2017). XR: VR, AR, MR – What's the difference? https://www.viget.com/articles/xr-vr-ar-mr-whats-the-difference/

NatureTreks. (2021). https://naturetreksvr.com/ and https://www.youtube.com/watch?v=EyH9F1mYPEs

Sculpt, V. R. (2021). https://www.sculptrvr.com/

Slater, M. (2012). The sense of embodiment in virtual reality. *Presence, 21*(4), 373–387.

Stone, J. (2020a). *Digital play therapy: A clinician's guide to comfort and competence*. Routledge.

Stone, J. (2020b). Extended reality therapy: The use of virtual, augmented, and mixed reality in mental health treatment. In R. Kowert & T. Quandt (Eds.), *Video game debate 2: Revisiting the physical, social, and psychological effects of video games* (pp. 95–106). Routledge.

TiltBrush (2021). https://www.tiltbrush.com/

TRIPP. (2021). https://www.tripp.com/ and https://yhoo.it/3i8GJvK

Virtual Sandtray. (2021). https://www.virtualsandtray.org/ and https://www.youtube.com/channel/Ucd0lQCtuoy6P4Moy7px01Rw/feed

References

Altvater, R. A., Singer, R. R., & Gil, E. (2017). Part 1: Modern trends in the playroom – preferences and interactions with tradition and innovation. *International Journal of Play Therapy, 26*(4), 239–249.

Association for Play Therapy. (2020). Credentialling standards for registered play therapist-supervisor™. https://cdn.ymaws.com/www.a4pt.org/resource/resmgr/credentials/2020_credentials/rpt-s_standards.pdf

Baker, L. (2019). Therapy in the digital age. In J. Stone (Ed.), *Integrating technology into modern therapies* (pp. 37–47). Routledge.

Bailensen, J. (2018). *Experience on demand: What virtual reality is, how it works, and what it can do*. Norton.

Beilinson, J. (2014, May 28). Palmer Luckey and the virtual reality resurrection. https://www.popularmechanics.com/technology/gadgets/a12956/palmer-luckey-and-the-virtual-reality-resurrection-16834760/

Bellani, M., Fornasari, L., Chittaro, L., & Brambilla, P. (2011). Virtual reality in autism: State of the art. *Epidemiology and Psychiatric Sciences, 20*(3), 235–238.

Bernard, J. M. (1979). Supervisor training: A discrimination model. *Counselor Education and Supervision, 19*(1), 60–68.

Bricken, M., & Byrne, C. M. (1993). Summer students in virtual reality: A pilot study on educational applications of virtual reality technology. In A. Wexelblat (Ed.), *Virtual reality applications and explorations* (pp. 199–218). Academic Press Professional.

Brooks Jr., F. P. (1999, November/December). *What's real about virtual reality? Computer graphics and applications special report*. http://www.cs.unc.edu/%7Ebrooks/WhatsReal.pdf

Burns-Nader, S. (2019). Technological tools for supporting pediatric patients through procedures. In J. Stone (Ed.), *Integrating technology into modern therapies* (pp. 181–193). Routledge.

Ceranoglu, T. A. (2010). Video games in psychotherapy. *American Psychological Association, 14*(2), 141–146.

Clarke, B., & Schoech, D. (1994). A computer-assisted game for adolescents: Initial development and comments. *Computers in Human Services, 11*(1–2), 121–140.

Clarke, M. (2019, July). Some prisons are using virtual reality for reentry and other programs. https://www.prisonlegalnews.org/news/2019/jul/2/some-prisons-are-using-virtual-reality-reentry-and-other-programs/

Deemer, A., Swenor, B., Fujiwara, K., Deermeik, J., Ross, N., Natale, D., Bradley, C., Werblin, F., & Massof, R. (2019). Preliminary evaluation of two digital image processing strategies for head-mounted magnification for low vision patients. *Translational Vision Science and Technology, 8*(1), 1–8.

Dudley, D. (2018, December). Virtual reality used to combat isolation and improve health. *AARP Magazine.* https://www.aarp.org/home-family/personal-technology/info-2018/vr-explained.html

Ellis, C. (2018, September). Are VR simulators in the future of pilot training? https://www.aircharterservice.com/about-us/news-features/blog/are-vr-flight-simulators-the-future-of-pilot-training

Farrell, A. D. (1989). Impact of computers on professional practice: A survey of current practices and attitudes. *Professional Psychology: Research and Practices, 20*(3), 172–178.

Gardner, J. E. (1991). Can the Mario Bros. help? Nintendo games as an adjunct in psychotherapy with children. *Psychotherapy: Theory, Research, Practice, and Training, 28*(4), 667–670.

Google. (2019). *Tiltbrush.* https://www.tiltbrush.com/

Grant, R. J. (2019). Utilizing technological interventions with children and adolescents with autism spectrum disorder (ASD). In J. Stone (Ed.), *Integrating technology into modern therapies: A clinician's guide to developments and interventions* (pp. 124–136). Routledge.

Greener Games. (2019). *Nature Treks VR.* [virtual reality program]. https://www.greenergames.net/

Hull, K. (2016). Technology in the playroom. In K. J. O'Connor, C. E. Schaefer, & L. D. Braverman (Eds.), *Handbook of play therapy* (2nd ed., pp. 6613–6627). Wiley.

Irvine, K. (2017). XR: VR, AR, MR – What's the difference? https://www.viget.com/articles/xr-vr-ar-mr-whats-the-difference/

Jin, W., Birckhead, B., Perez, B., & Hoffe, S. (2017). Augmented and virtual reality: Exploring a future role in radiation oncology education and training. *Applied Radiation Oncology,* 13–20. https://www.researchgate.net/publication/327228829

Lamb, R., & Etopio, E. (2019). VR has it. In J. Stone (Ed.), *Integrating technology into modern therapies* (pp. 80–93). Routledge.

Lexico. (2021a). *Cognition.* https://www.lexico.com/en/definition/cognition

Lexico. (2021b). *Self.* https://www.lexico.com/en/definition/self

Mandal, S. (2013). Brief introduction of virtual reality & its challenges. *International Journal of Scientific and Engineering Research, 4*(4), 304–309. https://www.ijser.org/researchpaper/Brief-Introduction-of-Virtual-Reality-its-Challenges.pdf

Maples-Keller, J. L., Bunnell, B. E., Kim, S. J., & Rothbaum, B. O. (2017). The use of virtual reality technology in the treatment of anxiety and other psychiatric disorders. *Harvard Review of Psychiatry, 25*(3), 103–113.

Mitchell, A. E. (2021). Gestalt play therapy supervision. In L. Fazio-Griffith & R. Marino (Eds.), *Techniques and interventions for play therapy and clinical supervision* (pp. 173–187). IGI Global.

Owlchemy Labs. (2019). Job simulator: Time to job. [virtual reality program]. https://jobsimulatorgame.com/

Presnall, B. (2019). International military cooperation with medical VR training. https://www.researchgate.net/publication/334733435_International_military_cooperation_with_medical_VR_training_International_military_cooperation_with_medical_VR_training

Rendever. (2021). Multibrush. https://vrdynamite.com/product/multibrush/

Resnick, H., & Sherer, M. (1995). Computer games in the human services – A review. *Computers in Human Services, 11*(1–2), 17–29.

Rizzo, A., & Shilling, R. (2017). Clinical virtual reality tools to advance the prevention, assessment, and treatment of PTSD. *European Journal of Psychotraumatology, 8*(5), 1–21.

Rubin, P. (2014). The inside story of oculus Rift and how virtual reality became reality. https://www.wired.com/2014/05/oculus-rift-4/

Safaryan, K., & Mehta, M. R. (2020). Enhanced theta rhythmicity and emergence of eta oscillation in virtual reality. *Researchgate.* https://www.biorxiv.org/content/10.1101/2020.06.29.178186v1

Schaefer, C. E. (1993). What is play and why is it therapeutic? In C. Schaefer (Ed.), *The therapeutic powers of play* (pp. 1–15). Jason Aaronson.

Schaefer, C. E., & Drewes, A. (Eds.). (2014). *The therapeutic powers of play: 20 core agents of change* (2nd ed.). Wiley.

Snow, M. S., Winburn, A., Crumrine, L., & Jackson, E. (2012). The iPad playroom a therapeutic technique. http://www.mlppubsonline.com/display_article.php?id=1141251

Spiegel, B. (2020). *VRx: How virtual therapeutics will revolutionize medicine.* Basic Books.

Stone, A. (2017, July). How virtual reality is changing military training. https://insights.samsung.com/2017/07/13/how-virtual-reality-is-changing-military-training/

Stone, J. (2019). Digital games. In J. Stone & C. Schaefer (Eds.), *Game play* (3rd ed.). Wiley.

Stone, J. (2020a). *Digital play therapy: A clinician's guide to comfort and competence.* Routledge.

Stone, J. (2020b). Extended reality therapy: The use of virtual, augmented, and mixed reality in mental health treatment. In R. Kowert & T. Quandt (Eds.), *Video game debate 2: Revisiting the physical, social, and psychological effects of video games* (pp. 95–106). Routledge.

Szoldra, P. (2018, October). The airforce used vr to train pilots in half the time at a fraction of the cost. https://taskandpurpose.com/air-force-vr-pilot-training

Thagard, P. (2012). The self as a system of multilevel interacting mechanisms. http://cogsci.uwaterloo.ca/Articles/Thagard.self.phil-psych.2012.pdf

TRIPP, Inc. (2019). TRIPP [virtual reality program]. https://www.tiltbrush.com/

Varela, F. J., Thompson, E., & Rosch, E. (1991). *The embodied mind: Cognitive science and the human experience.* MIT Press.

Virtual Reality Society. (n.d.). The history of virtual reality. https://www.vrs.org.uk/virtual-reality/history.html

Virtual Sandtray (2016). *Virtual reality* [virtual reality program]. https://www.virtualsandtray.org/virtual-reality/

Wilson, M. (2002). Six views of embodied cognition. *Psychonomic Bulletin and Review, 9*(4), 625–636.

Within unlimited. (2020). *Supernatural.* https://www.getsupernatural.com/

Index

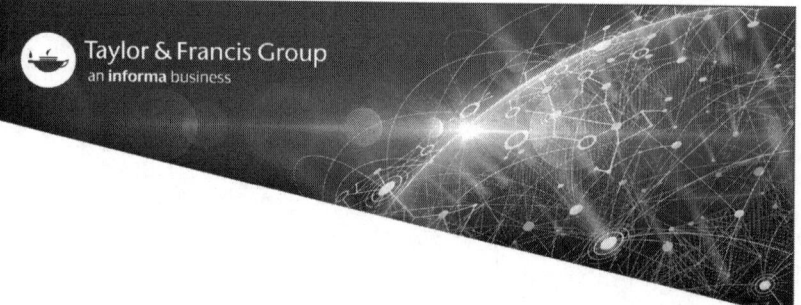
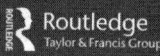
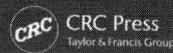